Melloni's Illustrated REVIEW OF HUMAN ANATOMY

Melloni's Illustrated

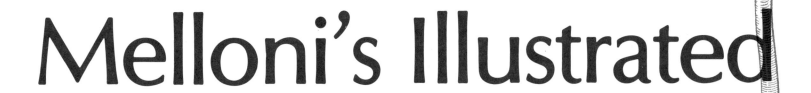

By Structures: Arteries
Bones
Muscles
Nerves
Veins

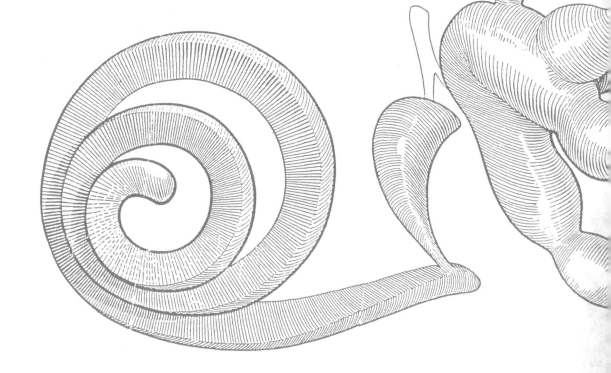

REVIEW OF HUMAN ANATOMY

June L. Melloni, Ph.D.
Ida Dox
H. Paul Melloni
B. John Melloni, Ph.D.

Illustrated by the authors

J.B. Lippincott Company Philadelphia
London   Mexico City   New York
St. Louis   São Paulo   Sydney

Acquisitions Editor: Lisa A. Biello
Developmental Editor: Delois Patterson
Design Coordinator: Michelle Gerdes
Cover Designer: Stephen Cymerman
Production Manager: Carol A. Florence
Production Editor: Rosanne Hallowell
Production Coordinator: Barney Fernandes
Compositor: McFarland Graphics
Text Printer/Binder: Kingsport Press
Cover Printer: The Lehigh Press, Inc.

1   3   5   6   4   2

LIBRARY OF CONGRESS
Library of Congress Cataloging-in-Publication Data
Melloni's illustrated review of human anatomy : by structures—arteries,
bones, muscles, nerves, veins / June L. Melloni . . . [et al.] ; illustrated
by the authors.
     p. cm.
   Includes index.
   ISBN 0-397-50956-1
   1. Anatomy, Human—Atlases.   2. Anatomy, Human—Outlines, syllabi,
etc.   I. Melloni, June L.   II. Title: Illustrated review of human anatomy.
QM25.M45 1988
611'.0022'2—dc19   88-722
                                                        CIP

PREFACE

Students of the health sciences recognize the importance of learning human anatomy and devote considerable time and effort to mastering the discipline. With the information explosion in medicine, and subsequent changes in curricula, the time allotted to the study of anatomy has been compressed. This compression of time requires restructuring the way in which anatomic information is presented so that retrieval of pertinent data can be achieved more rapidly than through present methods. *Melloni's Illustrated Review of Human Anatomy* attempts to meet this need.

The format of the book includes a careful balance of text and illustrations. These two components, textual and pictorial, are placed on opposing pages—the text on the left page, the illustrations on the right. Information is grouped into five sections devoted to *arteries, bones, muscles, nerves,* and *veins.*

The special attention given to the pictorial component of the book reflects a conviction that illustrations are not only essential to comprehension but they serve as building blocks toward long-term memory. Accordingly, illustrations were methodically planned to bring the text alive and were rendered with painstaking care for the more than 1,000 entries in the text. Every anatomic structure described in the text of the book is illustrated. The illustrations are coordinated with the text by means of color and a large bold letter for easy identification. Many of the illustrations are one of a kind.

In most textbooks, illustrations of veins take a back seat to those of arteries, probably because of the many variations associated with veins. In this review book, veins received equal attention because of their tremendous importance. Whenever possible, variations are included in addition to the most common configuration.

At first glance, it may appear that the same structures are portrayed repetitiously throughout the book. Closer scrutiny will show that, although some structures were indeed depicted several times to provide orientation for the principal entries, efforts were made to modify them in a way that would enhance the instructional value of the book. Different perspectives, different emphases, and variations in form are used to enable the reader to gain complete orientation and thus solidify comprehension.

The textual component of the book has two distinctive features. First, it is composed of an alphabetized list of anatomic terms (entries) with relevant information arranged in tabular form. This method of organization was chosen for rapid access and to permit information about each entry to be in one place.

Second, since regional terminology changes more frequently than the Latin, entries were alphabetized in the Latin nomenclature (Nomina Anatomica) to keep the book current as long as possible. If the reader is not familiar with the Latin terms, an index of equivalent English terms is provided at the back of the book. However, many of the Latin terms are sufficiently similar to their English counterparts to allow the reader to go directly to the alphabetized entries in any of the five sections.

The combination of concise description and single-concept illustration is expected to achieve the aim of the book as it was conceptualized by the senior author, June L. Melloni, while taking gross anatomy at Georgetown University School of Medicine. It is a book written from the student's perspective, one that she and other students were looking for but were unable to find. The book's unique format makes it suitable as a ready reference for finding significant information quickly—an important factor for students preparing for examinations. Because of the large number of illustrations, this book could also be used by health practitioners when instructing patients. It could, additionally, prove useful as a reference for students and practitioners in the many allied health fields.

The authors have a combined experience of nearly 100 years of writing and illustrating complex information in basic, clinical, and investigative sciences. June Melloni, in addition to her expertise in anatomy, specializes in evaluation and instructional design. She conducts studies in the field of medical education to determine the instructional value of different media from the learners' perspective. She also develops instructional materials in the health sciences that address the needs of the learner. Two authors, Ida Dox and B. John Melloni, started sketching anatomic structures and writing about them in the early 1950s while taking gross anatomy at the Johns Hopkins University School of Medicine. B. John Melloni, as Professional Lecturer in Anatomy, had the opportunity to dissect numerous cadavers, which provided a wealth of material for this book.

Along with sharing the responsibility of writing and illustrating this book, each author had a specific task. One important task was deciding the placement of labels. H. Paul Melloni had the responsibility of integrating the labels with the illustrations so that they not only inform the mind but, in addition, direct the eyes.

Excellent contributions to the illustrative section were provided by Peter J. Melloni and Roy G. Melloni, who made many of the complex registered color overlays. For their talents and interest, the authors are grateful. Throughout the course of this work, the authors have enjoyed a cordial relationship with the publisher, the J.B. Lippincott Company, who has supported the project with encouraging enthusiasm.

Readers' comments and suggestions for enhancing the usefulness of this book will be appreciated. They should be directed to June L. Melloni, Ph.D., 9308 Renshaw Drive, Bethesda, Maryland 20817.

June L. Melloni, Ph.D.
Ida Dox
H. Paul Melloni
B. John Melloni, Ph.D.

CONTENTS

ARTERIES

	ARTERY	ORIGIN	BRANCHES	DISTRIBUTION
A	**a. alveolaris inferior** *alveolar a., inferior* *dental a., inferior*	maxillary artery	dental, peridental, mental, mylohoid	mandible, chin, lower lip, gums, roots of teeth to pulp
B	**aa. alveolares superiores anteriores** *alveolar a.'s, anterior superior* *dental a.'s, anterior superior*	infraorbital artery	dental, peridental	incisor and cuspid teeth of upper jaw, mucous membrane of maxillary sinus
C	**a. alveolaris superior posterior** *alveolar a., posterior superior* *dental a., posterior superior*	maxillary artery	dental, peridental	molar and bicuspid teeth of upper jaw, maxillary sinus, gums
D	**a. angularis** *angular a.*	terminal branch of facial artery	none	lacrimal sac, orbicularis oculi muscle
E	**aorta** *aorta*			see specific branches below
	aorta abdominalis *abdominal aorta*	continuation of thoracic aorta of the aortic hiatus of the diaphragm	celiac trunk, superior mesenteric, inferior mesenteric, inferior phrenic, renal, middle suprarenal, testicular (in male), ovarian (in female), middle sacral, lumbar, common iliac	
	aorta ascendens *ascending aorta*	left ventricle	right coronary, left coronary	
	aorta thoracica *thoracic aorta*	continuation of arch of aorta at fourth thoracic vertebra	pericardial, bronchial, esophageal, mediastinal, superior phrenic, posterior intercostal, subcostal	
	arcus aortae *arch of aorta*	continuation of ascending aorta directly in back of the manubrium of sternum	brachiocephalic trunk, left common carotid, left subclavian	
F	**a. appendicularis** *appendicular artery*	ileocolic artery	none	vermiform appendix
G	**a. arcuata pedis** *arcuate a. of foot* *metatarsal a.*	dorsal artery of foot	second, third, and fourth metatarsal arteries	foot, sides of toes
H	**aa. arcuatae renis** *arcuate a.'s of the kidney*	interlobar arteries	interlobular arteries	parenchyma of kidney

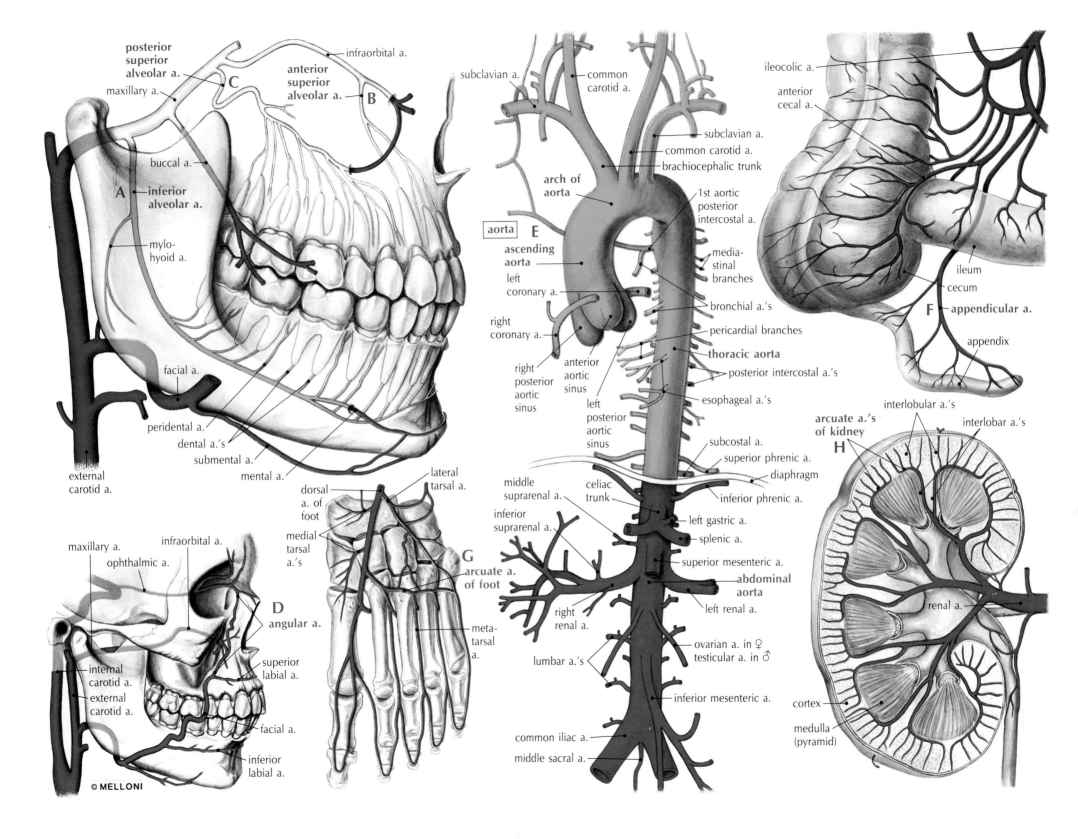

posterior superior alveolar a.

maxillary a.

infraorbital a.

anterior superior alveolar a.

buccal a.

A inferior alveolar a.

mylo-hyoid a.

facial a.

peridental a.

dental a.'s

submental a.

mental a.

external carotid a.

B

C

maxillary a.

infraorbital a.

ophthalmic a.

D angular a.

internal carotid a.

external carotid a.

superior labial a.

facial a.

inferior labial a.

© MELLONI

lateral tarsal a.

dorsal a. of foot

medial tarsal a.'s

G arcuate a. of foot

meta-tarsal a.

subclavian a.

common carotid a.

subclavian a.

common carotid a.

brachiocephalic trunk

arch of aorta

1st aortic posterior intercostal a.

aorta E

ascending aorta

left coronary a.

right coronary a.

right posterior aortic sinus

anterior aortic sinus

left posterior aortic sinus

media-stinal branches

bronchial a.'s

pericardial branches

thoracic aorta

posterior intercostal a.'s

esophageal a.'s

subcostal a.

superior phrenic a.

diaphragm

inferior phrenic a.

middle suprarenal a.

celiac trunk

inferior suprarenal a.

left gastric a.

splenic a.

superior mesenteric a.

abdominal aorta

right renal a.

left renal a.

ovarian a. in ♀ testicular a. in ♂

lumbar a.'s

inferior mesenteric a.

common iliac a.

middle sacral a.

ileocolic a.

anterior cecal a.

ileum

cecum

F appendicular a.

appendix

interlobular a.'s

interlobar a.'s

arcuate a.'s of kidney

H

renal a.

cortex

medulla (pyramid)

	ARTERY	ORIGIN	BRANCHES	DISTRIBUTION
A	**arcus palmaris superficialis** *palmar arch, superficial*	ulnar artery	common palmar digital arteries	fingers and matrix of fingernails
B	**arcus plantaris** *plantar arch*	lateral plantar artery	three perforating arteries, four plantar metatarsal arteries, numerous branches to the muscles, skin, and fasciae in the sole	sole of foot
C	**a. auricularis posterior** *auricular a., posterior*	external carotid artery	stylomastoid, auricular, occipital, parotid	middle ear, mastoid air cells, auricle, parotid gland, digastric, stylohyoid, and sternocleidomastoid muscles
D	**a. auricularis profunda** *auricular a., deep*	maxillary artery	temporomandibular	tympanic membrane, external acoustic meatus, temporomandibular joint
E	**a. axillaris** *axillary artery*	continuation of subclavian artery in axilla beginning at outer border of first rib	highest thoracic, thoracoacromial, lateral thoracic, subscapular, posterior humeral circumflex, anterior humeral circumflex	pectoralis major and minor, deltoid, serratus anterior, subscapularis, long head of biceps, teres major and minor muscles; acromion, sternoclavicular joint, mammary gland (in female), shoulder joint, head of humerus
F	**a. basilaris** *basilar a.*	from union of right and left vertebral arteries	anterior inferior cerebellar, labyrinthine, pontine, superior cerebellar, posterior cerebral	pons, internal ear, cerebellum, pineal body, superior medullary velum, tela choroidea of the third ventricle, temporal and occipital lobes
G	**a. brachialis** *brachial a.*	continuation of axillary artery at lower border of teres major muscle	deep brachial, nutrient of humerus, superior ulnar collateral, inferior ulnar collateral, muscular, radial, ulnar	shoulder, arm, forearm, hand, elbow joint.
H	**aa. bronchiales** *bronchial a.'s*	thoracic aorta and third posterior intercostal artery	none	walls of bronchi and bronchioles, bronchial lymph nodes, esophagus
I	**a. buccalis** *buccal a.* *buccinator a.*	maxillary artery	none	buccinator muscle, cheek, and gums
J	**a. bulbi penis** *a. of bulb of penis*	internal pudendal artery	none	bulb of penis, corpus spongiosum, bulbourethral gland
K	**a. bulbi vestibuli [vaginae]** *a. of bulb of vestibule [of vagina]*	internal pudendal artery	none	bulb of vestibule, greater vestibular glands

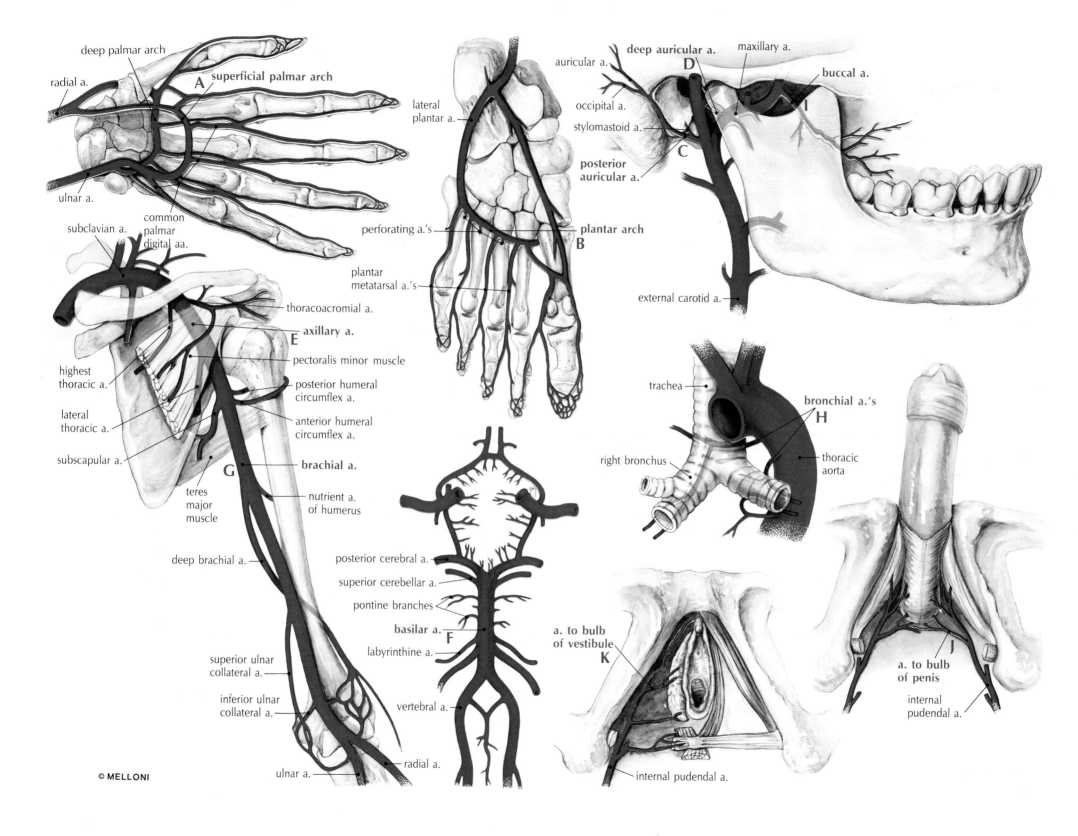

deep palmar arch

radial a.

A **superficial palmar arch**

ulnar a.

common palmar digital aa.

subclavian a.

thoracoacromial a.

E **axillary a.**

pectoralis minor muscle

posterior humeral circumflex a.

anterior humeral circumflex a.

highest thoracic a.

lateral thoracic a.

subscapular a.

teres major muscle

G

brachial a.

nutrient a. of humerus

deep brachial a.

superior ulnar collateral a.

inferior ulnar collateral a.

radial a.

ulnar a.

© MELLONI

lateral plantar a.

perforating a.'s

plantar metatarsal a.'s

plantar arch

B

posterior auricular a.

auricular a.

occipital a.

stylomastoid a.

posterior auricular a.

deep auricular a.

D

maxillary a.

buccal a.

I

C

external carotid a.

posterior cerebral a.

superior cerebellar a.

pontine branches

basilar a. **F**

labyrinthine a.

vertebral a.

trachea

bronchial a.'s

H

right bronchus

thoracic aorta

a. to bulb of vestibule

K

internal pudendal a.

a. to bulb of penis

internal pudendal a.

J

	ARTERY	ORIGIN	BRANCHES	DISTRIBUTION
A	**a. canalis pterygoidei** *a. of pterygoid canal* *Vidian a.*	maxillary artery, internal carotid artery, or greater palatine artery	pharyngeal	upper pharynx, auditory tube, and tympanic cavity
B	**a. carotis communis** *carotid a., common*	right side: brachiocephalic trunk left side: highest part of aortic arch	external carotid, internal carotid	head
C	**a. carotis externa** *carotid a., external*	common carotid artery	superior thyroid, ascending pharyngeal, lingual, facial, occipital, posterior auricular, superficial temporal, maxillary	skull, face, and neck
D	**a. carotis interna** *carotid a., internal*	common carotid artery	cervical part: carotid sinus petrous part: caroticotympanic, artery of the pterygoid canal cavernous part: cavernous, inferior hypophyseal, meningeal cerebral part: ophthalmic, anterior choroidal, anterior cerebral, posterior communicating, middle cerebral, superior hypophyseal	middle ear, brain, hypophysis, choroid plexus, orbit
E	**a. centralis retinae,** *central a. of retina*	ophthalmic artery	superior, inferior	retina
F	**a. cerebelli inferior anterior** *cerebellar a., anterior inferior*	basilar artery	labyrinthine, posterior spinal	anterior part of inferior surface of cerebellum
G	**a. cerebelli inferior posterior** *cerebellar a., posterior inferior*	vertebral artery	medial, lateral	posterior part of inferior surface of cerebellum, medulla oblongata, choroid plexus of fourth ventricle
H	**a. cerebelli superior** *cerebellar a., superior*	basilar artery near its termination	none	superior surface of cerebellum, pons, pineal body, superior medullary velum, choroid plexus of third ventricle
I	**a. cerebri anterior** *cerebral a., anterior*	internal carotid artery	precommunicating (central) part: anterior communicating, central branches postcommunicating (cortical) part: medial frontobasal, callosomarginal, paracentral, precuneal, pericallosal	corpus callosum, caudate nucleus, internal capsule, corpus striatum frontal lobe, parietal lobe, corpus callosum

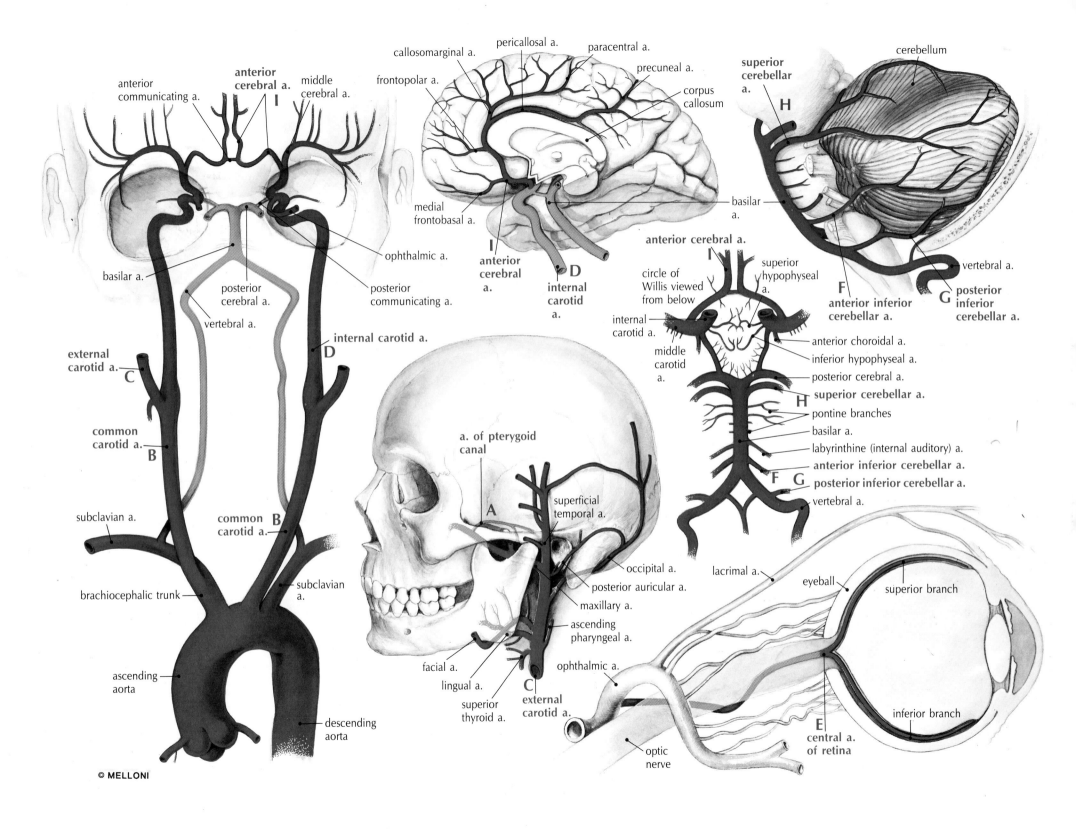

anterior communicating a.

anterior cerebral a.

middle cerebral a.

I

callosomarginal a.

pericallosal a.

paracentral a.

frontopolar a.

precuneal a.

corpus callosum

cerebellum

superior cerebellar a.

H

basilar a.

medial frontobasal a.

I

anterior cerebral a.

D

internal carotid a.

basilar a.

ophthalmic a.

F

G

vertebral a.

anterior inferior cerebellar a.

posterior inferior cerebellar a.

basilar a.

posterior cerebral a.

vertebral a.

posterior communicating a.

anterior cerebral a.

superior hypophyseal a.

I

circle of Willis viewed from below

internal carotid a.

middle carotid a.

anterior choroidal a.

inferior hypophyseal a.

posterior cerebral a.

superior cerebellar a.

H

pontine branches

basilar a.

labyrinthine (internal auditory) a.

anterior inferior cerebellar a.

F G

posterior inferior cerebellar a.

vertebral a.

internal carotid a.

D

external carotid a.

C

common carotid a.

B

subclavian a.

common carotid a.

B

brachiocephalic trunk

subclavian a.

ascending aorta

descending aorta

a. of pterygoid canal

A

superficial temporal a.

occipital a.

posterior auricular a.

maxillary a.

ascending pharyngeal a.

ophthalmic a.

facial a.

lingual a.

superior thyroid a.

external carotid a.

C

lacrimal a.

eyeball

superior branch

inferior branch

E

central a. of retina

optic nerve

© MELLONI

	ARTERY	ORIGIN	BRANCHES	DISTRIBUTION
A	**a. cerebri media** *cerebral a., middle*	internal carotid artery	sphenoidal (central) part: medial striate, lateral striate	lentiform nucleus, internal capsule, caudate nucleus, corpus striatum
			insular (cortical) part: insular, lateral frontobasal, anterior temporal, medial temporal, posterior temporal	insula, inferior frontal gyrus and lateral part of the orbital surface of the frontal lobe, motor and auditory areas
			terminal (cortical) part: central sulcus, precentral sulcus, postcentral sulcus, anterior parietal, posterior parietal, angular gyrus	precentral, middle, inferior frontal, and postcentral gyri; lateral surface of parietal and temporal lobes
B	**a. cerebri posterior** *cerebral a., posterior*	basilar artery	precommunicating (central) part: posteromedial central	thalamus (anterior part), lateral wall of third ventricle, globus pallidus
			postcommunicating (choroidal) part: posterolateral central, thalamus, posteromedial choroidal, postero-lateral choroidal, peduncular	lateral geniculate body, choroidal plexus of third and lateral ventricles, cerebral peduncle, thalamus (posterior part), colliculi, pineal body, medial geniculate body
			terminal (cortical) part: lateral occipital, medial occipital	uncus, parahippocampal, medial and lateral occipito-temporal gyri, occipital lobe (posterior part), cuneus, precuneus, visual area of cerebral cortex
C	**a. cervicalis ascendens** *cervical a., ascending*	inferior thyroid artery	spinal	muscles of neck, vertebral canal, bodies of vertebrae
D	**a. cervicalis produnda** *cervical a., deep*	costocervical trunk	spinal	spinal cord, posterior deep neck muscles
E	**a. cervicalis superficialis** *cervical a., superficial*	thyrocervical trunk and occasionally transverse cervical artery	ascending, descending	trapezius and adjacent muscles
F	**a. choroidea anterior** *choroid a., anterior*	internal carotid artery or middle cerebral artery	optic tract, lateral geniculate body, choroid plexus, internal capsule, caudate nucleus, amygdaloid body, hypothalamus	choroid plexus of inferior horn of lateral ventricle
G	**a. choroidea posterior** *choroid a., posterior*	posterior cerebral artery	medial, lateral	choroid plexus of ateral ventricle and third ventricle
H	**aa. ciliares anteriores** *ciliary a.'s, anterior*	muscular branches of ophthalmic artery	none	conjunctiva, iris

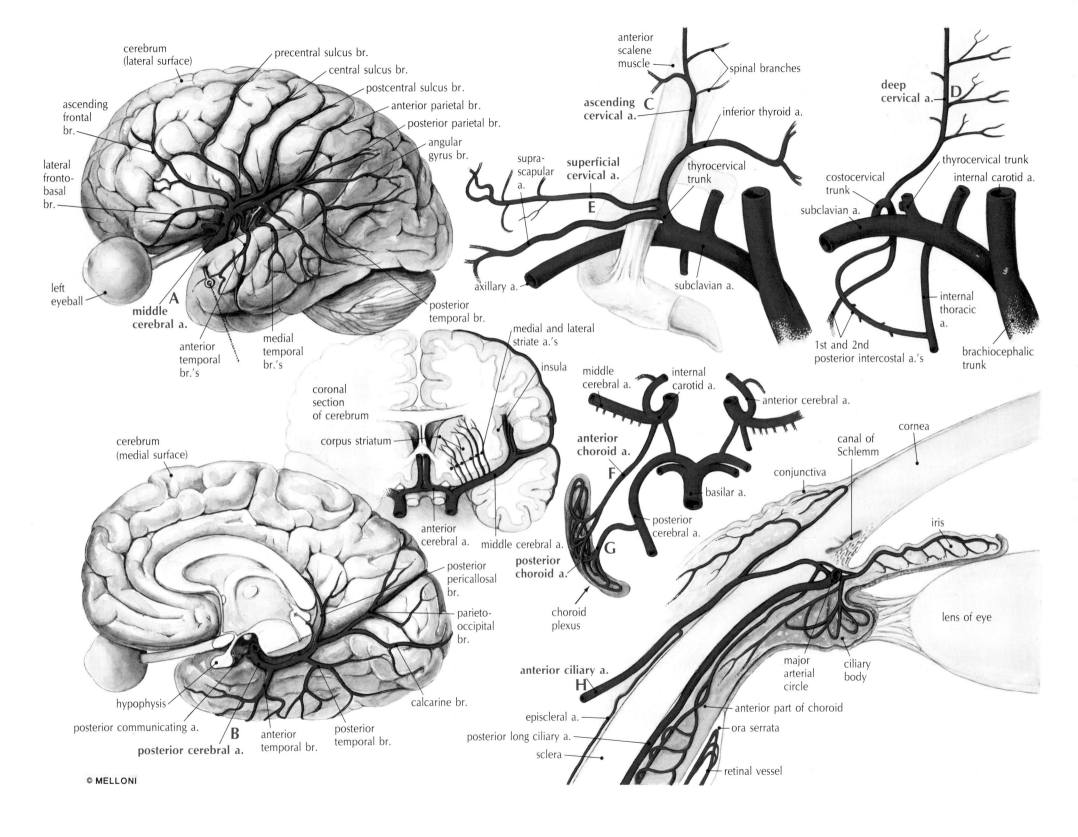

cerebrum (lateral surface)

precentral sulcus br.

central sulcus br.

postcentral sulcus br.

anterior parietal br.

posterior parietal br.

angular gyrus br.

ascending frontal br.

lateral fronto-basal br.

left eyeball

middle cerebral a.

A

anterior temporal br.'s

medial temporal br.'s

posterior temporal br.

anterior scalene muscle

spinal branches

ascending cervical a.

C

inferior thyroid a.

supra-scapular a.

superficial cervical a.

E

thyrocervical trunk

axillary a.

subclavian a.

deep cervical a.

D

thyrocervical trunk

costocervical trunk

internal carotid a.

subclavian a.

internal thoracic a.

1st and 2nd posterior intercostal a.'s

brachiocephalic trunk

coronal section of cerebrum

corpus striatum

medial and lateral striate a.'s

insula

anterior cerebral a.

middle cerebral a.

middle cerebral a.

internal carotid a.

anterior cerebral a.

anterior choroid a.

F

basilar a.

posterior cerebral a.

posterior choroid a.

G

choroid plexus

cornea

canal of Schlemm

conjunctiva

iris

cerebrum (medial surface)

posterior pericallosal br.

parieto-occipital br.

lens of eye

hypophysis

posterior communicating a.

B

posterior cerebral a.

anterior temporal br.

posterior temporal br.

calcarine br.

anterior ciliary a.

H

episcleral a.

posterior long ciliary a.

sclera

major arterial circle

ciliary body

anterior part of choroid

ora serrata

retinal vessel

© MELLONI

	ARTERY	ORIGIN	BRANCHES	DISTRIBUTION
A	**aa. ciliares posteriores breves** *ciliary a.'s, short posterior*	ophthalmic artery	none	choroid layer and ciliary processes of eye
B	**aa. ciliares posteriores longae** *ciliary a.'s, long posterior*	ophthalmic artery	none	iris, ciliary body of eye
C	**a. circumflexa femoris lateralis** *circumflex a., lateral femoral*	deep femoral artery	ascending, descending, transverse	head and neck of femur; thigh muscles
D	**a. circumflexa femoris medialis** *circumflex a., medial femoral*	deep femoral artery	deep, ascending, transverse, acetabular	hip joint, adductor muscles of thigh
E	**a. circumflexa humeri anterior** *circumflex a., anterior humeral*	axillary artery	ascending, descending	head of humerus and shoulder joint; deltoid, biceps, and coracobrachialis muscles; tendons of long head of biceps and pectoralis major muscles
F	**a. circumflexa humeri posterior** *circumflex a., posterior humeral*	axillary artery	descending, nutrient, articular, acromial, muscular	shoulder joint; deltoid, teres major, teres minor, and triceps muscles
G	**a. circumflexa ilium profunda** *circumflex iliac a., deep*	external iliac artery	ascending	internal oblique, transversus abdominis, iliacus, psoas, and sartorius muscles
H	**a. circumflexa ilium superficialis** *circumflex iliac a., superficial*	femoral artery	none	superficial inguinal lymph nodes, skin of groin
I	**a. circumflexa scapulae** *circumflex a., scapular*	subscapular artery	none	subscapularis, teres major, teres minor, long head of triceps, and deltoid muscles
J	**a. colica dextra** *colic a., right*	superior mesenteric artery or ileocolic artery	none	ascending colon

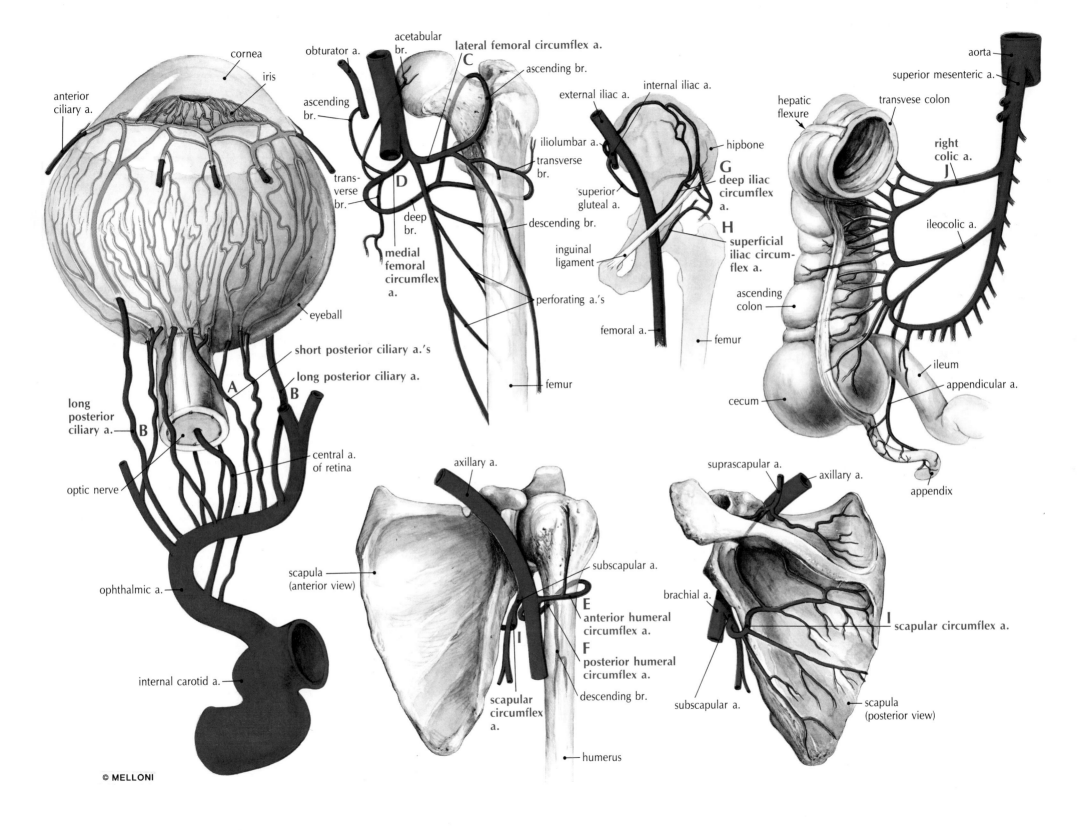

anterior ciliary a.

cornea

iris

obturator a.

acetabular br.

lateral femoral circumflex a.

ascending br.

aorta

superior mesenteric a.

ascending br.

C

ascending br.

external iliac a.

internal iliac a.

hepatic flexure

transvese colon

right colic a.

J

trans-verse br.

D

iliolumbar a.

transverse br.

hipbone

G

deep iliac circumflex a.

eyeball

deep br.

superior gluteal a.

descending br.

H

superficial iliac circum-flex a.

ascending colon

ileocolic a.

short posterior ciliary a.'s

inguinal ligament

medial femoral circumflex a.

long posterior ciliary a.

perforating a.'s

femoral a.

femur

ileum

appendicular a.

A

B

long posterior ciliary a.

B

femur

cecum

central a. of retina

optic nerve

appendix

axillary a.

suprascapular a.

axillary a.

scapula (anterior view)

subscapular a.

brachial a.

I

scapular circumflex a.

ophthalmic a.

E

anterior humeral circumflex a.

F

posterior humeral circumflex a.

I

internal carotid a.

scapular circumflex a.

descending br.

subscapular a.

scapula (posterior view)

humerus

© MELLONI

	ARTERY	ORIGIN	BRANCHES	DISTRIBUTION
A	**a. colica media** *colic a., middle*	superior mesenteric artery just caudal to the pancreas	right, left	transverse colon
B	**a. colica sinistra** *colic a., left*	inferior mesenteric artery	ascending, descending	descending colon, left half of transverse colon
C	**a. collateralis media** *collateral a., middle*	deep brachial artery	anastomotic	elbow joint; triceps and anconeus muscles
D	**a. collateralis radialis** *collateral a., radial*	continuation of deep brachial artery	anastomotic	brachioradialis and brachialis muscles, elbow joint
E	**a. collateralis ulnaris inferior** *collateral a., inferior ulnar*	brachial artery about 5 cm above elbow	anastomotic	elbow joint, arm muscles at back of elbow
F	**a. collateralis ulnaris superior** *collateral a., superior ulnar*	brachial artery and occasionally deep brachial artery	anastomotic	triceps muscle, elbow joint
G	**a. communicans anterior** *communicating a., anterior*	anterior cerebral artery	anteromedial	joins the right and left anterior cerebral arteries
H	**a. communicans posterior** *communicating a., posterior*	internal carotid artery	hypophyseal	joins the internal carotid artery with the posterior cerebral artery
I	**aa. conjunctivales anteriores** *conjunctival a.'s, anterior*	anterior ciliary arteries	none	conjunctiva
J	**aa. conjunctivales posteriores** *conjunctival a.'s, posterior*	peripheral tarsal arch	none	conjunctiva
K	**a. coronaria dextra** *coronary a., right*	aorta at right anterior aortic sinus	posterior interventricular (posterior descending), marginal, sinoatrial nodal, atrioventricular nodal	right atrium, right and left ventricles, sinoatrial node, atrioventricular node, interventricular septum

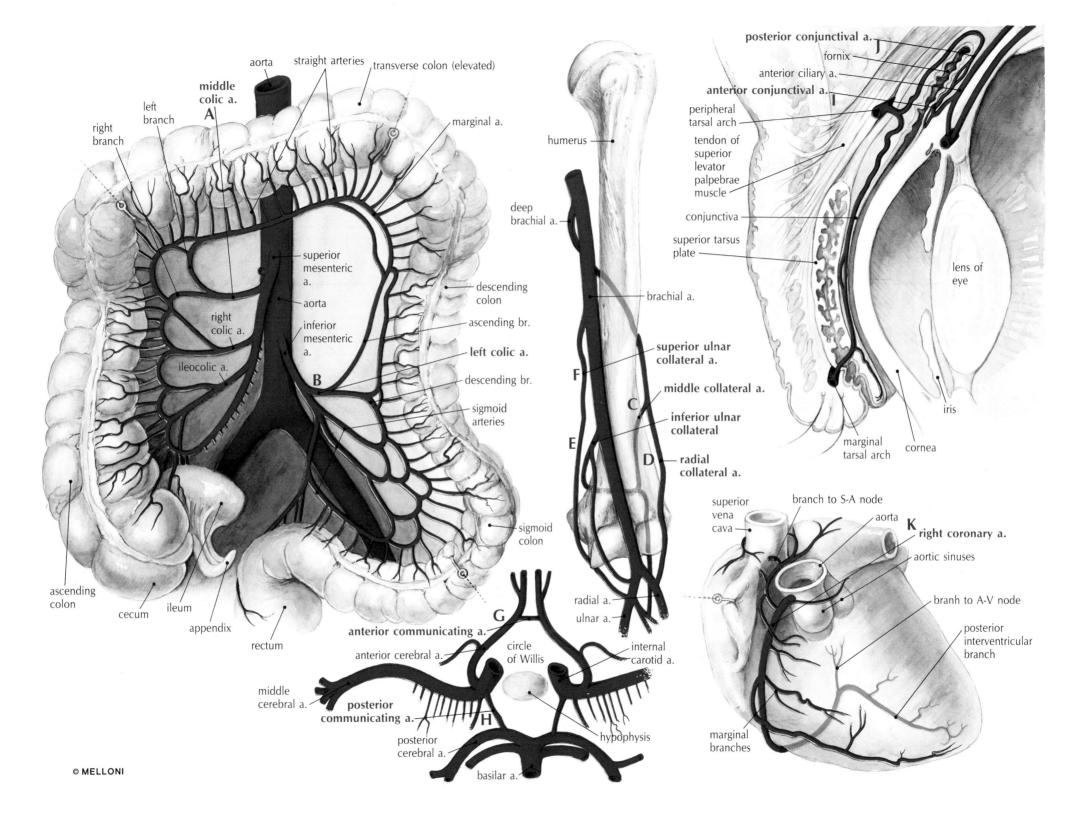

aorta
straight arteries
transverse colon (elevated)

middle colic a.

left branch

A

right branch

marginal a.

superior mesenteric a.

right colic a.

aorta

inferior mesenteric a.

left colic a.

ileocolic a.

B

descending colon

ascending br.

descending br.

sigmoid arteries

sigmoid colon

ascending colon

cecum

ileum

appendix

rectum

middle cerebral a.

anterior cerebral a.

anterior communicating a.

circle of Willis

internal carotid a.

posterior communicating a.

G

H

posterior cerebral a.

hypophysis

basilar a.

humerus

deep brachial a.

brachial a.

superior ulnar collateral a.

F

middle collateral a.

C

inferior ulnar collateral

E

D

radial collateral a.

radial a.

ulnar a.

posterior conjunctival a.

fornix

J

anterior ciliary a.

anterior conjunctival a.

I

peripheral tarsal arch

tendon of superior levator palpebrae muscle

conjunctiva

superior tarsus plate

lens of eye

marginal tarsal arch

cornea

iris

superior vena cava

branch to S-A node

aorta

K **right coronary a.**

aortic sinuses

branh to A-V node

posterior interventricular branch

marginal branches

© MELLONI

	ARTERY	ORIGIN	BRANCHES	DISTRIBUTION
A	**a. coronaria sinistra** *coronary a., left*	aorta at left aortic sinus behind the pulmonary trunk	anterior interventricular (anterior descending), circumflex, occasionally sinoatrial nodal	left atrium, left and right ventricles, sinoatrial node, interventricular septum
B	**a. cremasterica** *cremasteric a.*	inferior epigastric artery	none	coverings of spermatic cord including cremaster muscle
C	**a. cystica** *cystic a.*	right branch of proper hepatic artery	superficial, deep	gallbladder
D	**aa. digitales palmares communes** *digital a.'s, common palmar*	superficial palmar arch	proper palmar, digital	fingers, matrix of fingernails
E	**aa. digitales palmares propriae** *digital a.'s, proper palmar* *collateral digital a.'s*	common palmar digital arteries	dorsal	middle and distal phalanges, matrix of fingernails
F	**aa. digitales plantares communes** *digital a.'s, common plantar*	plantar metatarsal arteries	proper plantar, digital	toes
G	**aa. digitales plantares propriae** *digital a.'s, proper plantar*	common plantar digital arteries	none	toes
H	**a. dorsalis clitoridis** *dorsal a. of clitoris*	internal pudendal artery	none	dorsum, glans, and prepuce of clitoris
I	**a. dorsalis nasi** *dorsal nasal a.* *dorsal a. of the nose*	ophthalmic artery	none	skin of nose
J	**a. dorsalis pedis** *dorsal a. of foot*	continuation of anterior tibial artery at ankle joint	lateral tarsal, medial tarsal, arcuate, first dorsal metatarsal, deep plantar	foot

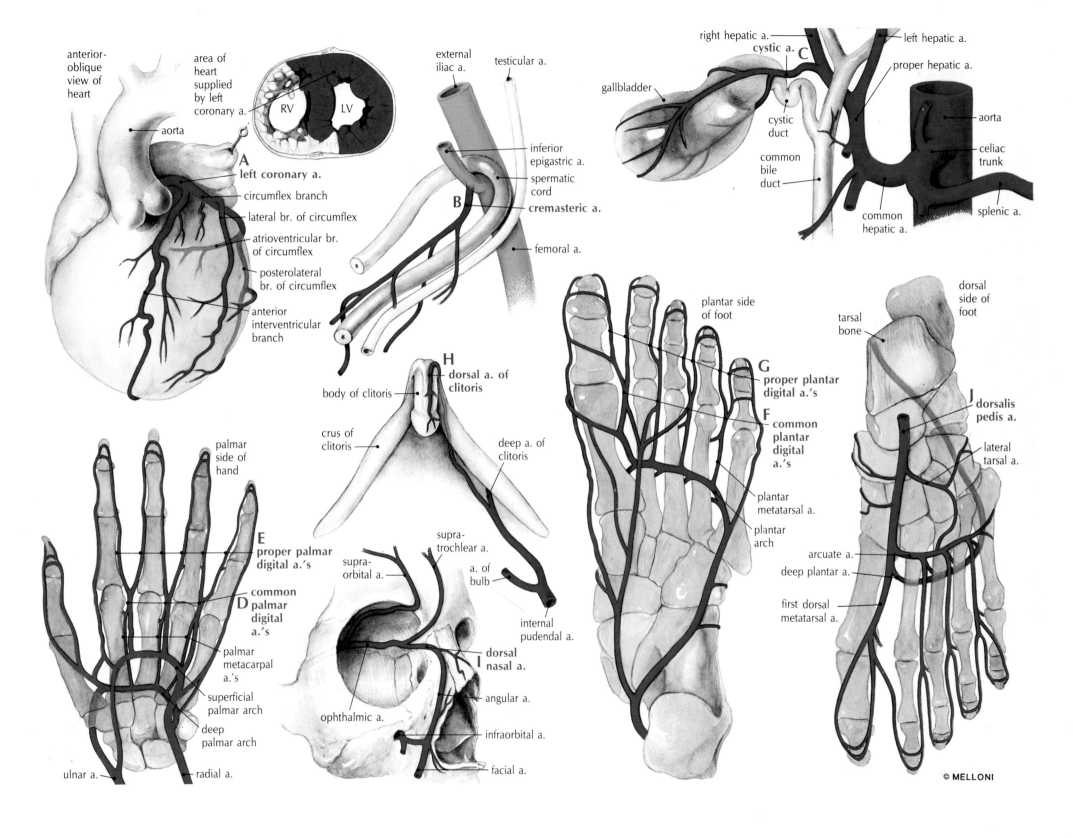

anterior-oblique view of heart

area of heart supplied by left coronary a.

RV   LV

aorta

A **left coronary a.**

circumflex branch

lateral br. of circumflex

atrioventricular br. of circumflex

posterolateral br. of circumflex

anterior interventricular branch

external iliac a.

testicular a.

inferior epigastric a.

spermatic cord

cremasteric a.

B

femoral a.

right hepatic a.

left hepatic a.

cystic a. **C**

proper hepatic a.

gallbladder

cystic duct

aorta

celiac trunk

common bile duct

common hepatic a.

splenic a.

H

dorsal a. of clitoris

body of clitoris

crus of clitoris

deep a. of clitoris

plantar side of foot

tarsal bone

dorsal side of foot

G proper plantar digital a.'s

J **dorsalis pedis a.**

lateral tarsal a.

F common plantar digital a.'s

palmar side of hand

plantar metatarsal a.

plantar arch

E **proper palmar digital a.'s**

D **common palmar digital a.'s**

supra-trochlear a.

supra-orbital a.

a. of bulb

internal pudendal a.

I **dorsal nasal a.**

palmar metacarpal a.'s

superficial palmar arch

deep palmar arch

ophthalmic a.

angular a.

arcuate a.

deep plantar a.

first dorsal metatarsal a.

infraorbital a.

ulnar a.

radial a.

facial a.

© MELLONI

	ARTERY	ORIGIN	BRANCHES	DISTRIBUTION
A	**a. dorsalis penis** *dorsal a. of penis*	internal pudendal artery	none	glans, prepuce, and skin of penis; fibrous sheath of corpus cavernosum
B	**a. ductus deferentis** *a. of ductus deferens*	superior vesical artery or umbilical artery	ureteric	ureter, ductus deferens, seminal vesicle, testis
C	**a. epigastrica inferior** *epigastric a., inferior* *deep epigastric a.*	external iliac immediately above inguinal ligament	cremasteric, pubic, artery of round ligament of uterus, muscular, cutaneous	rectus abdominis and cremaster muscles; skin
D	**a. epigastrica superficialis** *epigastric a., superficial*	femoral artery about 1 cm below inguinal ligament	none	lower part of abdominal wall, superficial inguinal lymph nodes, skin
E	**a. epigastrica superior** *epigastric a., superior*	internal thoracic artery	none	rectus abdominis and diaphragm muscles, skin of the abdomen
F	**a. episcleralis** *episcleral a.*	anterior ciliary artery	none	sclera, limbus, conjunctiva, iris, ciliary body
G	**a. ethmoidalis anterior** *ethmoidal a., anterior*	ophthalmic artery	meningeal, nasal	anterior and middle ethmoidal air cells, frontal sinus, nasal cavity, dura mater
H	**a. ethmoidalis posterior** *ethmoidal a., posterior*	ophthalmic artery	meningeal, nasal	posterior ethmoidal air cells, nasal cavity, dura mater
I	**a. facialis** *facial a.* *maxillary a., external*	external carotid artery	cervical part: ascending palatine, tonsillar, glandular, submental facial part: inferior labial, superior labial, lateral nasal, angular	tonsil, soft palate, submandibular gland muscles of expression

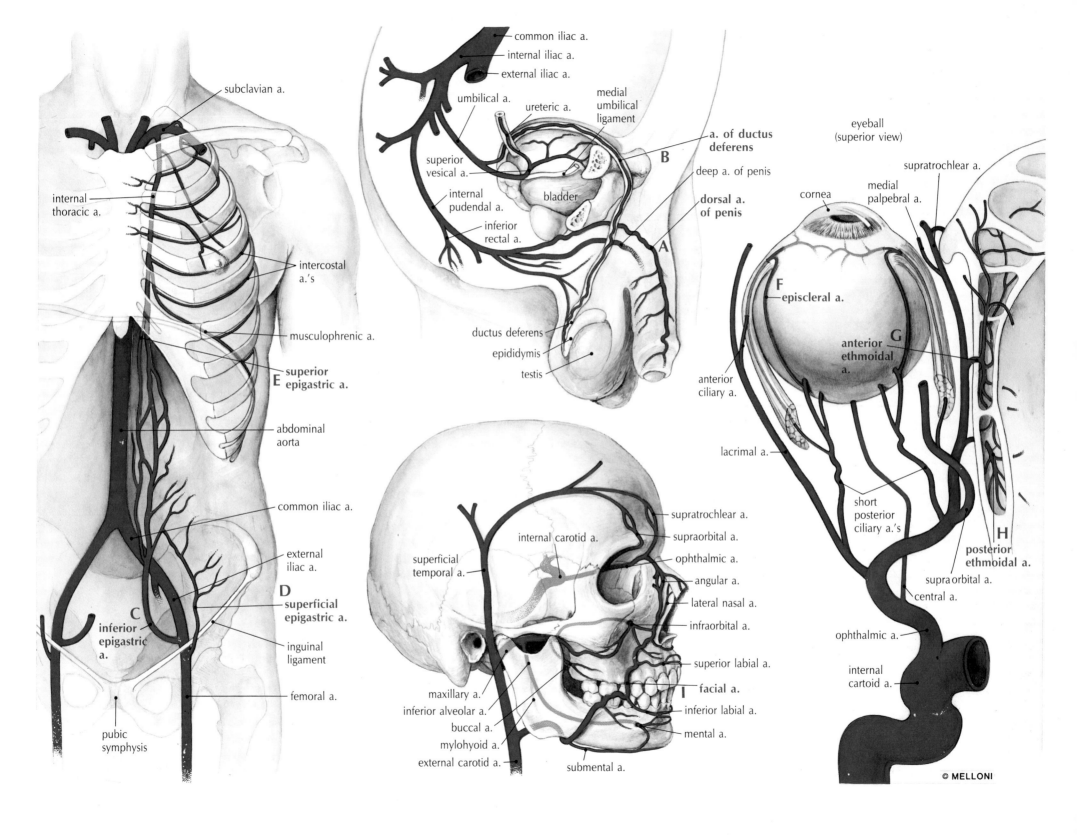

subclavian a.

internal
thoracic a.

intercostal
a.'s

musculophrenic a.

E **superior
epigastric a.**

abdominal
aorta

common iliac a.

external
iliac a.

D
**superficial
epigastric a.**

C
**inferior
epigastric
a.**

inguinal
ligament

femoral a.

pubic
symphysis

common iliac a.

internal iliac a.

external iliac a.

umbilical a.

ureteric a.

medial
umbilical
ligament

superior
vesical a.

bladder

**a. of ductus
deferens**

B

deep a. of penis

internal
pudendal a.

inferior
rectal a.

A

**dorsal a.
of penis**

ductus deferens

epididymis

testis

anterior
ciliary a.

eyeball
(superior view)

supratrochlear a.

medial
palpebral a.

cornea

F
episcleral a.

**anterior
ethmoidal
a.**

G

lacrimal a.

short
posterior
ciliary a.'s

**posterior
ethmoidal a.**

H

supraorbital a.

central a.

ophthalmic a.

internal
cartoid a.

supratrochlear a.

supraorbital a.

internal carotid a.

ophthalmic a.

angular a.

lateral nasal a.

infraorbital a.

superior labial a.

superficial
temporal a.

maxillary a.

inferior alveolar a.

buccal a.

mylohyoid a.

external carotid a.

submental a.

I **facial a.**

inferior labial a.

mental a.

© MELLONI

ARTERY	ORIGIN	BRANCHES	DISTRIBUTION
A **a. femoralis** *femoral a.*	continuation of external iliac artery immediately below the level of the inguinal ligament	superficial epigastric, superficial circumflex iliac, external pudendal, deep femoral, descending genicular	lower abdominal wall, external genitalia, muscles of thigh, superficial inguinal lymph nodes
B **aa. gastricae breves** *gastric a.'s, short* *vasa brevia*	splenic artery and occasionally left gastroepiploic (omental)	none	fundus of stomach
C **a. gastrica dextra** *gastric a., right*	proper hepatic artery and occasionally common hepatic or gastroduodenal artery	none	pyloric end of stomach along lesser curvature
D **a. gastrica sinistra** *gastric a., left*	celiac trunk	esophageal, pyloric, cardiac (stomach)	lesser curvature of stomach, esophagus
E **a. gastroduodenalis** *gastroduodenal a.*	common hepatic artery	right gastroepiploic (omental), superior pancreaticoduodenal, retroduodenal, pyloric, pancreatic, retroduodenal, supraduodenal (occasionally)	duodenum, stomach, pancreas, greater omentum
F **a. gastroepiploica dextra** *gastroepiploic a., right* *gastro-omental a., right*	gastroduodenal artery	epiploic (omental), gastric	stomach, greater omentum, duodenum
G **a. gastroepiploica sinistra** *gastroepiploic a., left* *gastro-omental a., left*	splenic artery	epiploic (omental), gastric	stomach, greater omentum
H **a. genus descendens** *genicular a., descending* *descending a. of the knee*	femoral artery	saphenous, articular, muscular	knee joint and neighboring muscles
I **a. genus inferior lateralis** *genicular a., lateral inferior* *lateral inferior artery of the knee*	popliteal artery	none	knee joint
J **a. genus inferior medialis** *genicular a., medial inferior* *medial inferior artery of the knee*	popliteal artery	none	knee joint, proximal end of tibia, popliteus muscle
K **a. genus media** *genicular a., middle* *middle artery of the knee*	popliteal artery	none	cruciate ligaments and synovial membrane of knee joint

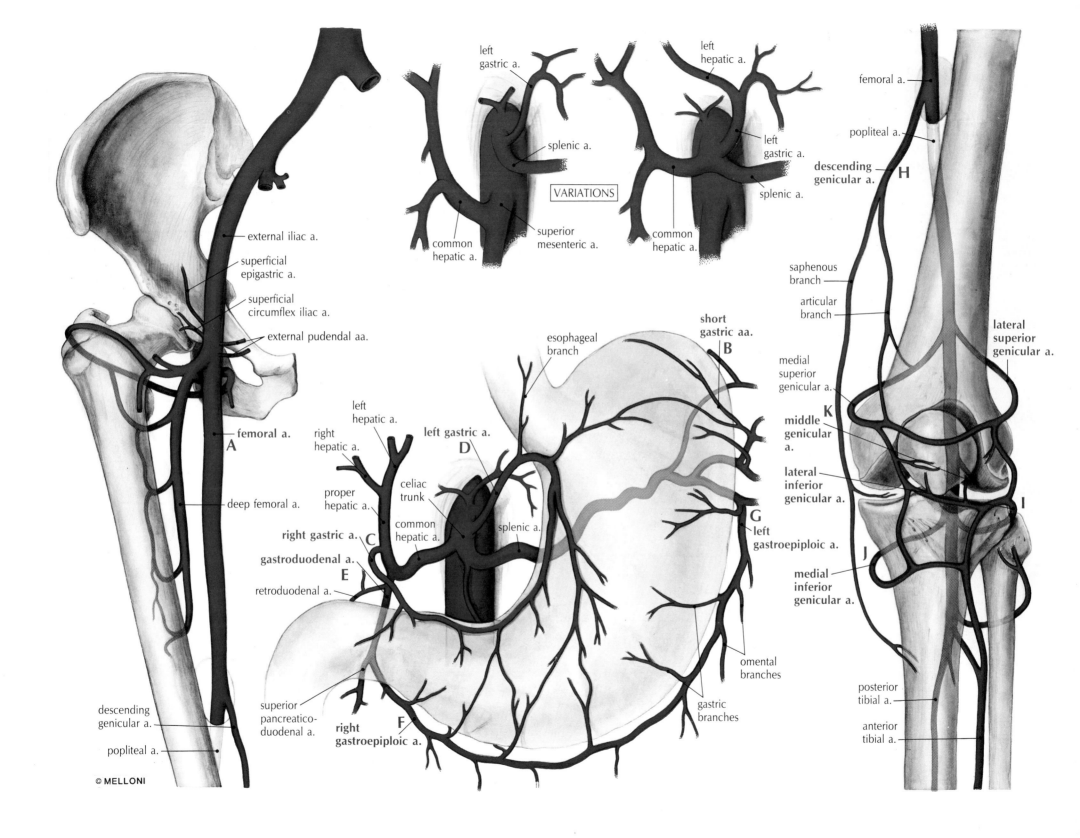

external iliac a.

superficial epigastric a.

superficial circumflex iliac a.

external pudendal aa.

femoral a.

A

deep femoral a.

descending genicular a.

popliteal a.

© MELLONI

left gastric a.

splenic a.

VARIATIONS

common hepatic a.

superior mesenteric a.

left hepatic a.

left gastric a.

splenic a.

common hepatic a.

esophageal branch

short gastric aa.

B

left hepatic a.

right hepatic a.

left gastric a.

D

celiac trunk

proper hepatic a.

right gastric a. **C**

common hepatic a.

splenic a.

gastroduodenal a.

E

retroduodenal a.

G left gastroepiploic a.

omental branches

gastric branches

superior pancreatico- duodenal a.

right **F** gastroepiploic a.

femoral a.

popliteal a.

descending genicular a. **H**

saphenous branch

articular branch

lateral superior genicular a.

medial superior genicular a.

K

middle genicular a.

lateral inferior genicular a.

lateral superior genicular a.

I

J

medial inferior genicular a.

posterior tibial a.

anterior tibial a.

	ARTERY	ORIGIN	BRANCHES	DISTRIBUTION
A	**a. genus superior lateralis** *genicular a., lateral superior* *lateral superior artery of the knee*	popliteal artery	none	lower part of femur, knee joint, patella, and neighboring muscles
B	**a. genus superior medialis** *genicular a., medial superior* *medial superior artery of the knee*	popliteal artery	none	femur, knee joint, patella, and neighboring muscles
C	**a. glutea inferior** *gluteal a., inferior*	internal iliac artery	muscular, coccygeal, sciatic, vesical, articular, anastomotic	muscles of buttock and back of thigh
D	**a. glutea superior** *gluteal a., superior*	internal iliac artery	superficial, deep, muscular, nutrient, articular	muscles of buttock, ilium
E	**a. hepatica communis** *hepatic a., common*	celiac trunk	gastroduodenal, proper hepatic, occasionally right gastric	stomach, pancreas, duodenum, liver, gallbladder
F	**a. hepatica dextra** *hepatic a., right*	proper hepatic artery	cystic, caudate lobar, anterior (left) segmental, posterior (right) segmental	liver, gallbladder
G	**a. hepatica propria** *hepatic a., proper*	common hepatic artery	right hepatic, left hepatic, right gastric	liver, gallbladder, pyloric end of stomach
H	**a. hepatica sinistra** *hepatic a., left*	proper hepatic artery	caudate lobar, medial segmental, lateral segmental	liver
I	**a. hyaloidea** *(disappears before birth)* *hyaloid a.*	central artery of retina	none	lens of eye
J	**a. hypophysialis inferior** *hypophyseal a., inferior*	internal carotid artery (cavernous part)	none	hypophysis
K	**a. hypophysialis superior** *hypophyseal a., superior*	internal carotid artery (cerebral part), posterior cerebral artery or anterior cerebral artery	none	hypophysis

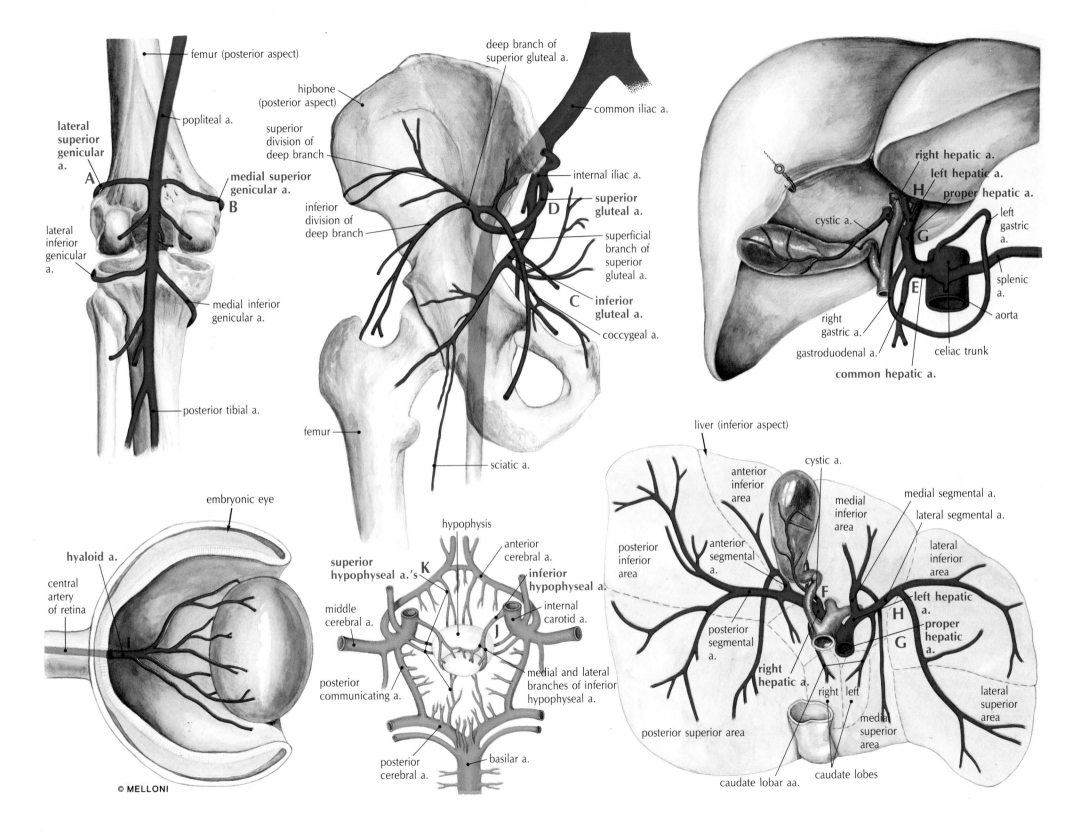

femur (posterior aspect)

popliteal a.

lateral superior genicular a.

A

medial superior genicular a.

B

lateral inferior genicular a.

medial inferior genicular a.

posterior tibial a.

deep branch of superior gluteal a.

hipbone (posterior aspect)

common iliac a.

superior division of deep branch

internal iliac a.

inferior division of deep branch

D

superior gluteal a.

superficial branch of superior gluteal a.

C **inferior gluteal a.**

coccygeal a.

femur

sciatic a.

right hepatic a.

left hepatic a.

proper hepatic a.

cystic a.

H

G

left gastric a.

splenic a.

right gastric a.

E

aorta

gastroduodenal a.

celiac trunk

common hepatic a.

embryonic eye

hyaloid a.

central artery of retina

I

hypophysis

anterior cerebral a.

superior hypophyseal a.'s

K

inferior hypophyseal a.

middle cerebral a.

internal carotid a.

J

posterior communicating a.

medial and lateral branches of inferior hypophyseal a.

posterior cerebral a.

basilar a.

liver (inferior aspect)

cystic a.

anterior inferior area

medial inferior area

medial segmental a.

lateral segmental a.

posterior inferior area

anterior segmental a.

lateral inferior area

posterior segmental a.

F

left hepatic a.

H

proper hepatic a.

G

right hepatic a.

right | left

lateral superior area

posterior superior area

medial superior area

caudate lobes

caudate lobar aa.

© MELLONI

	ARTERY	ORIGIN	BRANCHES	DISTRIBUTION
A	**aa. ileales** *ileal a.'s*	superior mesenteric artery	none	ileum
B	**a. ileocolica** *ileocolic a.*	superior mesenteric artery and occasionally right colic artery	colic (ascending), anterior cecal, posterior cecal, appendicular, ileal	cecum, appendix, ascending colon, ileum
C	**a. iliaca communis** *iliac a., common*	abdominal aorta about the level of L4	internal iliac, external iliac	pelvis, gluteal region, perineum, lower limb, lower abdominal wall
D	**a. iliaca externa** *iliac a., external*	common iliac artery	inferior epigastric, deep circumflex iliac	abdominal wall, external genitalia, cremaster muscle, lower limb
E	**a. iliaca interna** *iliac a., internal* *hypogastric a.*	continuation of common iliac artery	anterior trunk: inferior vesical, middle rectal, uterine, obturator, internal pudendal, inferior gluteal, vaginal, umbilical posterior trunk: iliolumbar, lateral sacral, superior gluteal	wall and viscera of pelvis, external genitalia, buttock, medial side of thigh
F	**a. iliolumbalis** *iliolumbar a.*	internal iliac artery (posterior trunk)	iliac, lumbar, spinal	greater psoas and quadratus lumborum muscles, gluteal and abdominal walls, ilium, cauda equina
G	**a. infraobitalis** *infraorbital a.*	maxillary artery	anterior superior alveolar, orbital, middle superior alveolar	maxilla, maxillary sinus and teeth, cheek, side of nose, lower eyelid, lacrimal sac, rectus inferior and obliquus inferior muscles
H	**aa. intercostales anteriores** *intercostal a.'s, anterior*	internal thoracic artery	muscular, cutaneous	upper six intercostal spaces, pectoralis major and minor muscles, skin of breast
I	**aa. intercostales posteriores I et II** *intercostal a.'s I and II, posterior*	highest intercostal artery	dorsal	upper thoracic wall
J	**aa. intercostales posteriores III-XI** *intercostal a.'s III-XI, posterior*	thoracic aorta	dorsal, collateral, lateral cutaneous	nine lower intercostal spaces; anterior serratus, pectoralis major and minor muscles; mammary gland

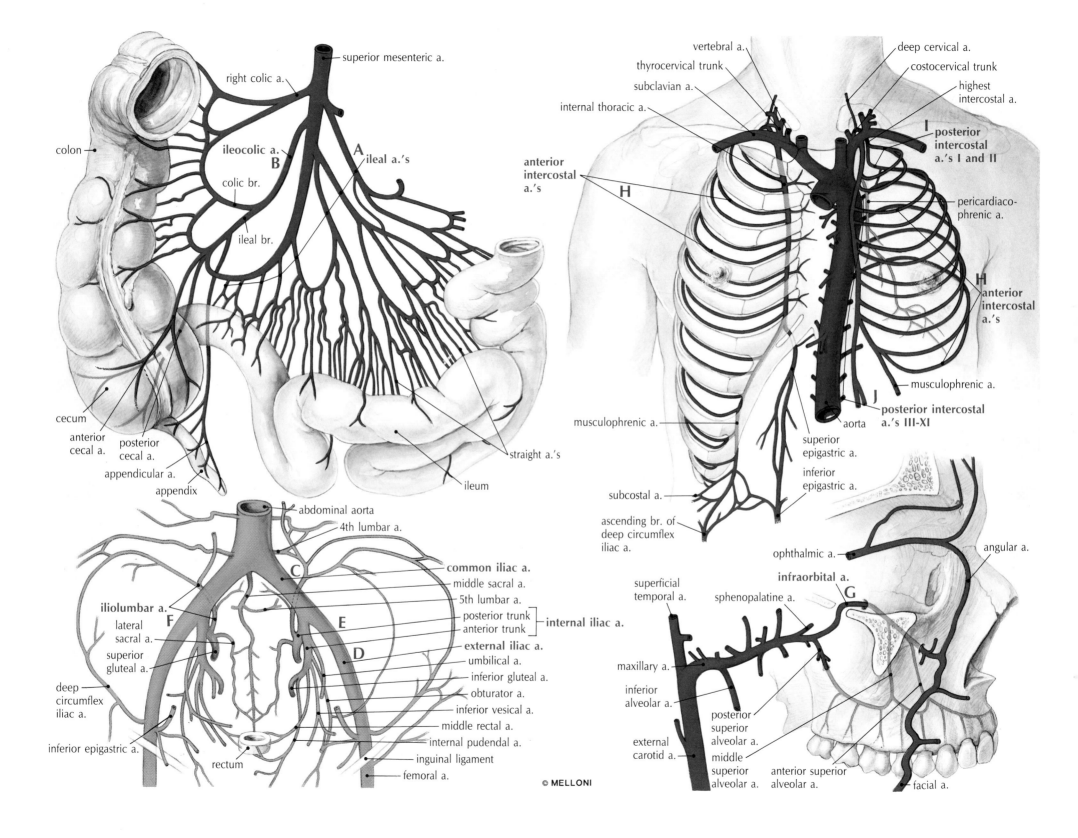

superior mesenteric a.

right colic a.

ileocolic a.

B

colic br.

ileal br.

colon

A

ileal a.'s

cecum

anterior cecal a.

posterior cecal a.

appendicular a.

appendix

straight a.'s

ileum

abdominal aorta

4th lumbar a.

common iliac a.

middle sacral a.

5th lumbar a.

posterior trunk

anterior trunk

internal iliac a.

external iliac a.

umbilical a.

inferior gluteal a.

obturator a.

inferior vesical a.

middle rectal a.

internal pudendal a.

inguinal ligament

femoral a.

C

E

D

iliolumbar a.

F

lateral sacral a.

superior gluteal a.

deep circumflex iliac a.

inferior epigastric a.

rectum

© MELLONI

vertebral a.

thyrocervical trunk

subclavian a.

internal thoracic a.

deep cervical a.

costocervical trunk

highest intercostal a.

I posterior intercostal a.'s I and II

anterior intercostal a.'s

H

pericardiacophrenic a.

H anterior intercostal a.'s

musculophrenic a.

musculophrenic a.

aorta

J posterior intercostal a.'s III-XI

superior epigastric a.

inferior epigastric a.

subcostal a.

ascending br. of deep circumflex iliac a.

ophthalmic a.

infraorbital a.

G

angular a.

superficial temporal a.

sphenopalatine a.

maxillary a.

inferior alveolar a.

external carotid a.

posterior superior alveolar a.

middle superior alveolar a.

anterior superior alveolar a.

facial a.

	ARTERY	ORIGIN	BRANCHES	DISTRIBUTION
A	**a. intercostalis suprema** *intercostal a., highest* *intercostal a., superior*	costocervical trunk	first and second posterior intercostal	first and second intercostal spaces
B	**aa. interlobares renis** *interlobar a.'s of kidney*	branches of segmental arteries of kidney (lobar arteries)	arcuate	between pyramids of kidney
C	**aa. interlobulares hepatis** *interlobular a.'s of liver*	right and left branches of the proper hepatic artery	none	between lobules of liver
D	**aa. interlobulares renis** *interlobular a.'s of kidney*	arcuate arteries of kidney	afferent	glomeruli of kidney
E	**a. interossea anterior** *interosseous a., anterior* *volar interosseous a.*	common interosseous artery	median, nutrient	deep muscles of front of forearm, radius, ulna
F	**a. interossea communis** *interosseous a., common*	ulnar artery	anterior and posterior interosseous	deep muscles in back of forearm, radius, ulna
G	**a. interossea posterior** *interosseous a., posterior* *dorsal interosseous a.*	common interosseous artery	recurrent interosseous	deep muscles of back of forearm
H	**a. interossea recurrens** *interosseous a., recurrent*	posterior interosseous artery	none	elbow joint
I	**aa. jejunales** *jejunal a.'s*	superior mesenteric artery	none	jejunum
J	**a. labialis inferior** *labial a., inferior*	facial artery	none	labial glands, muscles and mucous membrane of lower lip
K	**a. labialis superior** *labial a., superior*	facial artery	septal, alar	nasal septum and ala of nose, upper lip

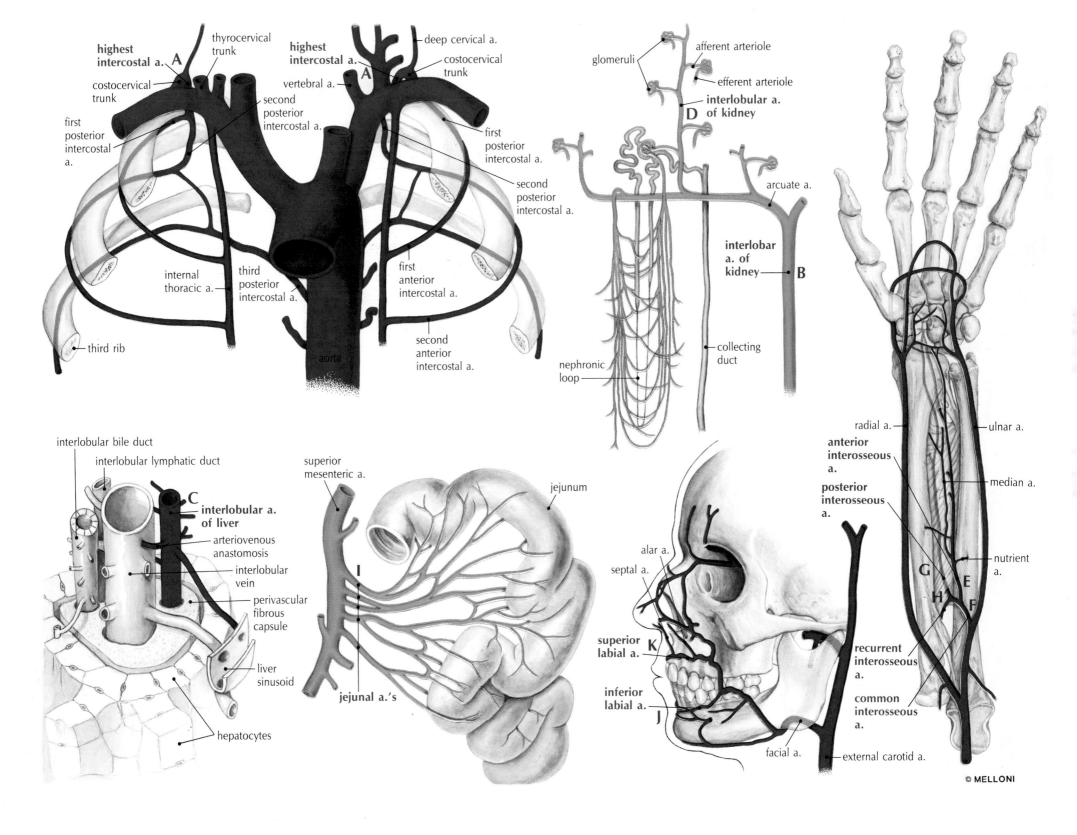

highest intercostal a. **A**
thyrocervical trunk
costocervical trunk
deep cervical a.
highest intercostal a. **A**
costocervical trunk
first posterior intercostal a.
vertebral a.
second posterior intercostal a.
first posterior intercostal a.
second posterior intercostal a.
internal thoracic a.
third posterior intercostal a.
first anterior intercostal a.
second anterior intercostal a.
third rib
aorta

glomeruli
afferent arteriole
efferent arteriole
interlobular a. of kidney **D**
arcuate a.
interlobar a. of kidney **B**
collecting duct
nephronic loop

interlobular bile duct
interlobular lymphatic duct
C
interlobular a. of liver
arteriovenous anastomosis
interlobular vein
perivascular fibrous capsule
liver sinusoid
hepatocytes

superior mesenteric a.
jejunum
I
jejunal a.'s

alar a.
septal a.
superior labial a. **K**
inferior labial a. **J**
facial a.
external carotid a.

radial a.
ulnar a.
anterior interosseous a.
median a.
posterior interosseous a.
nutrient a.
G
H
E
F
recurrent interosseous a.
common interosseous a.

© MELLONI

	ARTERY	ORIGIN	BRANCHES	DISTRIBUTION
A	**a. labyrinthi** *labyrinthine a.* *internal auditory a.*	basilar artery or anterior inferior cerebellar artery	vestibular, cochlear	internal ear
B	**a. lacrimalis** *lacrimal a.*	ophthalmic artery	lateral palpebral, zygomatic, recurrent meningeal, muscular	lacrimal gland, upper and lower eyelids, conjunctiva, eye muscles
C	**a. laryngea inferior** *laryngeal a., inferior*	inferior thyroid artery	none	larynx
D	**a. laryngea superior** *laryngeal a., superior*	superior thyroid artery and occasionally external carotid artery	none	larynx
E	**a. lingualis** *lingual a.*	external carotid artery	suprahyoid, sublingual, dorsal lingual, deep lingual	tongue, sublingual gland, tonsil, gums, epiglottis
F	**a. lingualis, rami dorsales** *lingual a.'s, dorsal*	lingual artery	none	posterior part of tongue, palatoglossal arch, soft palate, tonsil, epiglottis
G	**aa. lumbales** *lumbar a.'s*	abdominal aorta	dorsal, spinal	lumbar vertebrae, back muscles, spinal cord
H	**a. lumbalis ima** *lumbar a., lowest* *lumbar a., 5th*	median sacral artery	none	sacrum
I	**a. malleolaris anterior lateralis** *malleolar a., anterior lateral*	anterior tibial artery	none	lateral side of ankle
J	**a. malleolaris anterior medialis** *malleolar a., anterior medial*	anterior tibial artery	none	medial side of ankle
K	**a. masseterica** *masseteric a.*	maxillary artery	none	masseter muscle

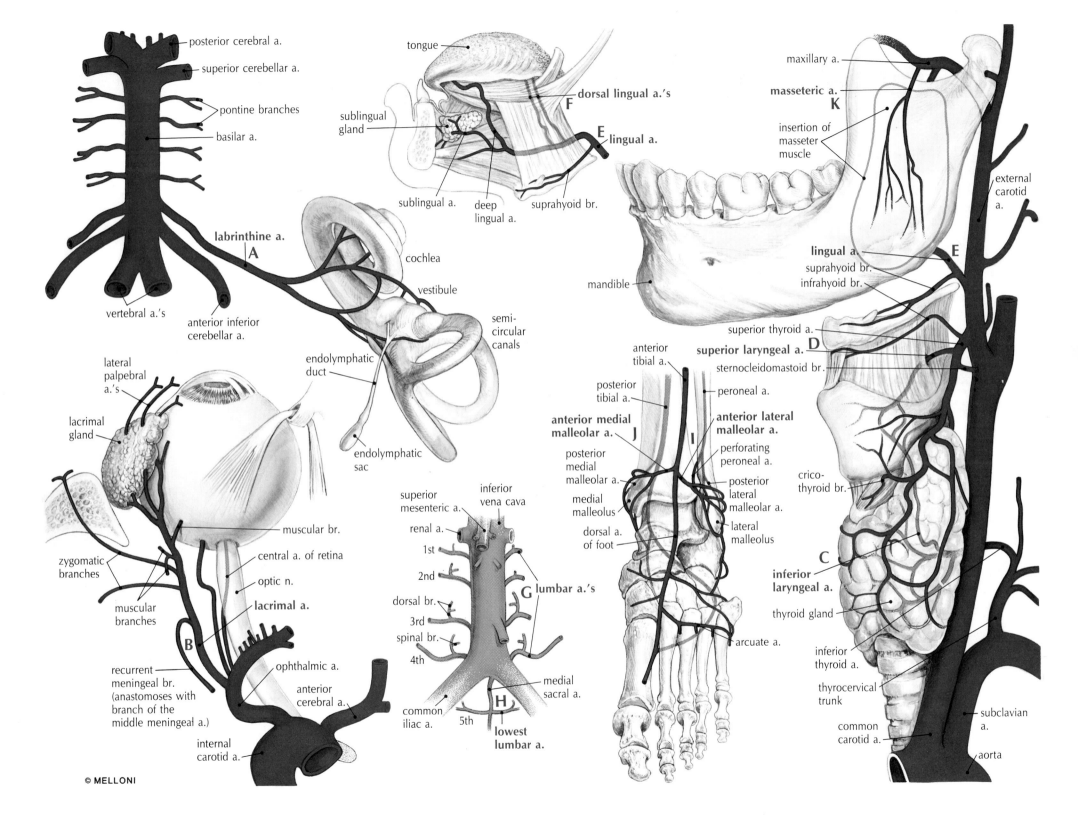

posterior cerebral a.

superior cerebellar a.

pontine branches

basilar a.

labrinthine a.

A

vertebral a.'s

anterior inferior
cerebellar a.

lateral
palpebral
a.'s

lacrimal
gland

zygomatic
branches

muscular
branches

recurrent
meningeal br.
(anastomoses with
branch of the
middle meningeal a.)

internal
carotid a.

muscular br.

central a. of retina

optic n.

lacrimal a.

B

ophthalmic a.

anterior
cerebral a.

cochlea

vestibule

semi-
circular
canals

endolymphatic
duct

endolymphatic
sac

tongue

dorsal lingual a.'s

F

sublingual
gland

E **lingual a.**

sublingual a.

deep
lingual a.

suprahyoid br.

superior
mesenteric a.

inferior
vena cava

renal a.

1st

2nd

dorsal br.

3rd

spinal br.

4th

G lumbar a.'s

medial
sacral a.

common
iliac a.

5th

H

**lowest
lumbar a.**

anterior
tibial a.

posterior
tibial a.

**anterior medial
malleolar a.**

J

posterior
medial
malleolar a.

medial
malleolus

dorsal a.
of foot

peroneal a.

**anterior lateral
malleolar a.**

I

perforating
peroneal a.

posterior
lateral
malleolar a.

lateral
malleolus

arcuate a.

maxillary a.

masseteric a.

K

insertion of
masseter
muscle

external
carotid
a.

lingual a.

E

suprahyoid br.

infrahyoid br.

mandible

superior thyroid a.

superior laryngeal a.

D

sternocleidomastoid br.

crico-
thyroid br.

C

**inferior
laryngeal a.**

thyroid gland

inferior
thyroid a.

thyrocervical
trunk

common
carotid a.

subclavian
a.

aorta

© MELLONI

	ARTERY	ORIGIN	BRANCHES	DISTRIBUTION
A	**a. maxillaris** *maxillary a.* *internal maxillary a.*	external carotid artery	mandibular part: deep auricular, anterior tympanic, inferior alveolar, middle meningeal, accessory meningeal	ear, temporomandibular joint, cranial dura mater, pterygoid muscles, mandible, mandibular teeth
			pterygoid part: deep anterior temporal, deep posterior temporal, pterygoid, masseteric, buccal	temporalis, pterygoid, masseter, and buccinator muscles
			pterygopalatine part: posterior superior alveolar, infraorbital, descending palatine, artery of the pterygoid canal, pharyngeal, sphenopalatine	gums, soft palate, sinuses, auditory tube, roof of nose, maxilla, maxillary teeth
B	**a. mediana** *median a.*	anterior interosseous artery	none	median nerve, palm
C	**aa. medullares** *medullary a.'s* *bulbar a.'s*	vertebral artery and its branches	none	medulla oblongata
D	**a. meningea anterior** *meningeal a., anterior*	anterior ethmoidal artery	none	dura mater
E	**a. meningea media** *meningeal a., middle*	maxillary artery	frontal, parietal, petrosal, superior tympanic, ganglionic, anastomotic, temporal	cranium, dura mater, tensor tympani muscle, trigeminal ganglion, tympanic cavity
F	**aa. meningei posteriores** *meningeal a.'s, posterior*	ascending pharyngeal artery	none	dura mater and bones of posterior cranial fossa
G	**a. mesenterica inferior** *mesenteric a., inferior*	abdominal aorta at level of L3 or L4	left colic, sigmoid, superior rectal	transverse, descending, and sigmoid colon; rectum
H	**a. mesenterica superior** *mesenteric a., superior*	abdominal aorta one cm below celiac trunk	inferior pancreaticoduodenal, jejunal, ileal, ileocolic, right colic, middle colic	small intestine, cecum, ascending colon, and part of the transverse colon
I	**aa. metacarpales dorsales** *metacarpal a.'s dorsal*	dorsal carpal branch or radial artery	dorsal digital	dorsal sides of fingers

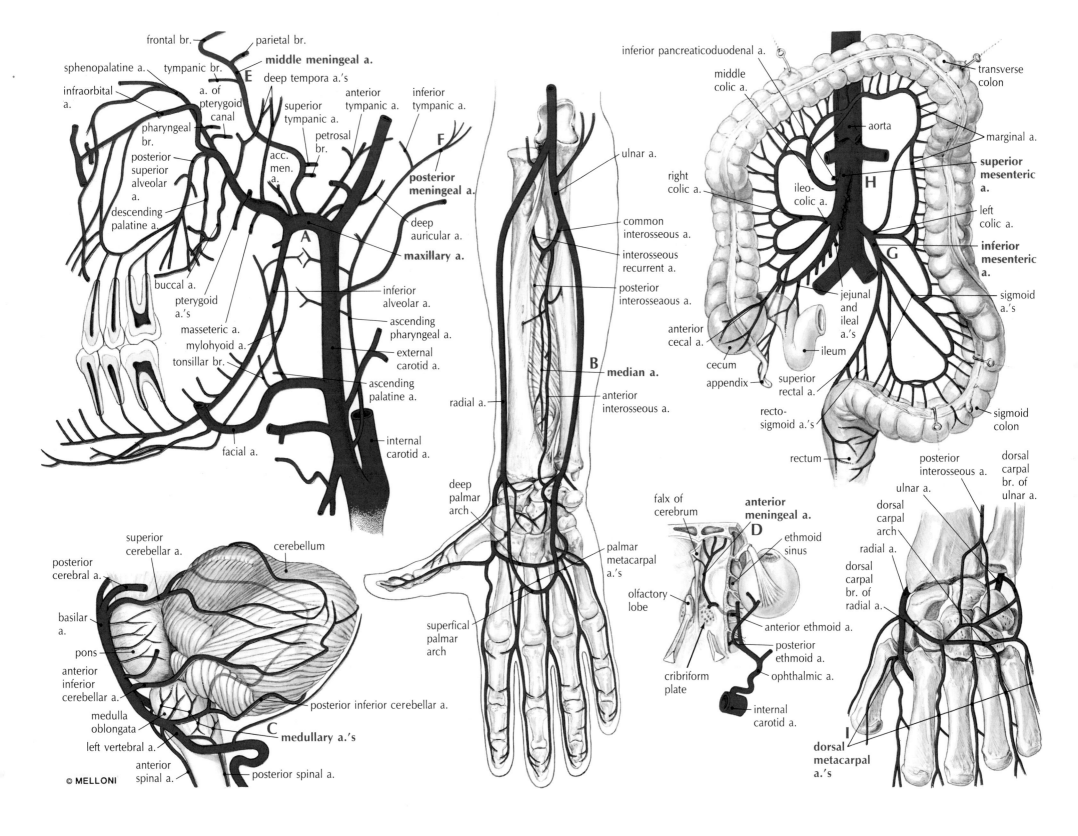

frontal br.
parietal br.
tympanic br.
middle meningeal a.
sphenopalatine a.
E
deep tempora a.'s
infraorbital a.
a. of pterygoid canal
anterior tympanic a.
inferior tympanic a.
superior tympanic a.
pharyngeal br.
petrosal br.
acc. men. a.
F
posterior meningeal a.
posterior superior alveolar a.
deep auricular a.
maxillary a.
descending palatine a.
A
inferior alveolar a.
buccal a.
ascending pharyngeal a.
pterygoid a.'s
masseteric a.
external carotid a.
mylohyoid a.
tonsillar br.
ascending palatine a.
facial a.
internal carotid a.

ulnar a.
common interosseous a.
interosseous recurrent a.
posterior interosseaous a.
radial a.
B median a.
anterior interosseous a.
deep palmar arch
palmar metacarpal a.'s
superfical palmar arch

inferior pancreaticoduodenal a.
middle colic a.
transverse colon
aorta
marginal a.
right colic a.
ileo-colic a.
H
superior mesenteric a.
left colic a.
inferior mesenteric a.
jejunal and ileal a.'s
G
sigmoid a.'s
anterior cecal a.
cecum
ileum
appendix
superior rectal a.
recto-sigmoid a.'s
sigmoid colon
rectum

superior cerebellar a.
cerebellum
posterior cerebral a.
basilar a.
pons
anterior inferior cerebellar a.
posterior inferior cerebellar a.
medulla oblongata
C medullary a.'s
left vertebral a.
anterior spinal a.
posterior spinal a.

© MELLONI

falx of cerebrum
anterior meningeal a.
D
ethmoid sinus
olfactory lobe
anterior ethmoid a.
posterior ethmoid a.
cribriform plate
ophthalmic a.
internal carotid a.

posterior interosseous a.
dorsal carpal br. of ulnar a.
ulnar a.
dorsal carpal arch
radial a.
dorsal carpal br. of radial a.
I
dorsal metacarpal a.'s

	ARTERY	ORIGIN	BRANCHES	DISTRIBUTION
A	**aa. metacarpales palmares** *metacarpal a.'s, palmar* *metacarpal a.'s, volar* *palmar interosseous a.'s*	deep palmar arch	none	metacarpal bones
B	**a. metatarsalis dorsalis I** *metatarsal a., first dorsal*	dorsal artery of foot	none	medial side of great toe and adjoining sides of great and second toes
C	**aa. metatarsales plantares** *metatarsal a.'s, plantar*	plantar arch	plantar digital, perforating	toes
D	**a. musculophrenica** *musculophrenic a.*	internal thoracic artery	anterior intercostal	diaphragm; seventh, eighth, and ninth intercostal spaces; abdominal muscles
E	**a. mylohyoideus** *mylohyoid a.*	inferior alveolar artery	none	mylohyoid muscle
F	**a. nasalis lateral** *nasal a., lateral*	facial artery or superior labial artery	none	ala and dorsum of nose
G	**aa. nasales posteriores laterales** *nasal a.'s, posterior lateral*	sphenopalatine artery	none	frontal, ethmoidal, maxillary, and sphenoid sinuses
H	**aa. nasales posteriores septales** *septal a.'s of the nose, posterior*	sphenopalatine artery	none	nasal septum
I	**a. nutricia fibulae** *nutrient a. of fibula*	peroneal artery	none	fibula
J	**aa. nutriciae humeri** *nutrient a.'s of humerus*	brachial artery or deep brachial artery	none	humerus
K	**a. nutricia tibiae** *nutrient a. of tibia*	posterior tibial artery	none	tibia

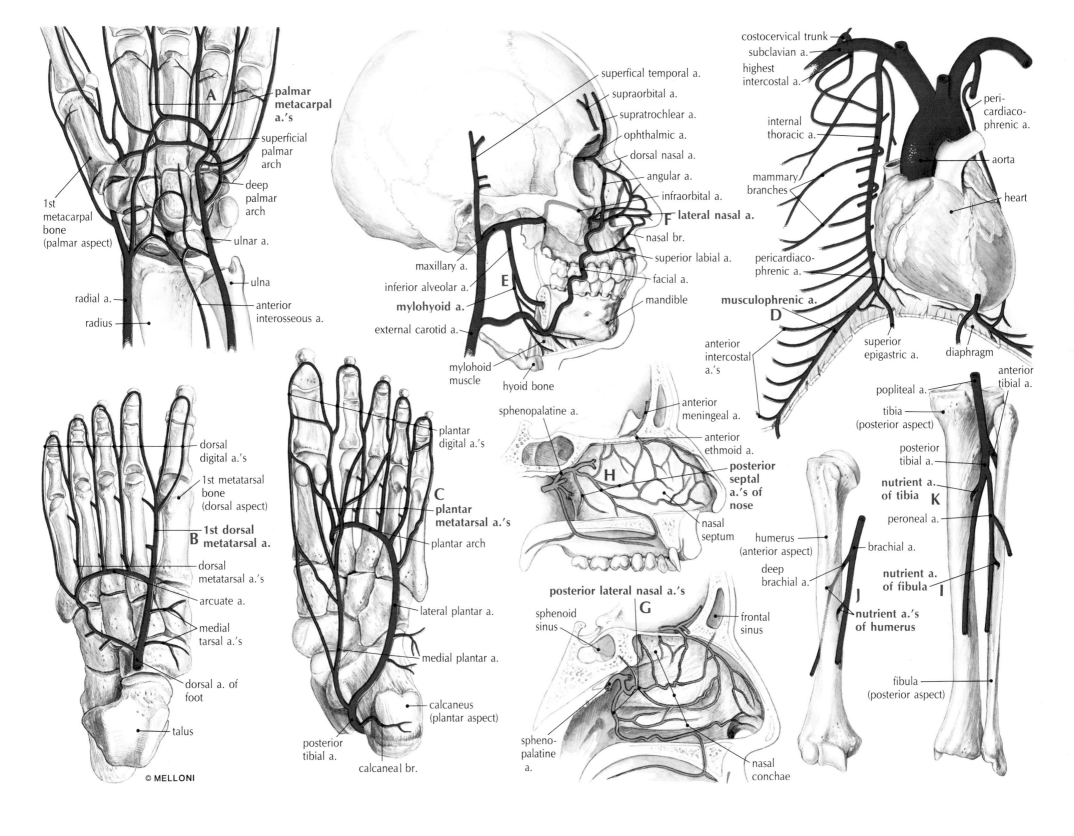

palmar metacarpal a.'s

A

superficial palmar arch

deep palmar arch

1st metacarpal bone (palmar aspect)

ulnar a.

ulna

radial a.

radius

anterior interosseous a.

dorsal digital a.'s

1st metatarsal bone (dorsal aspect)

B **1st dorsal metatarsal a.**

dorsal metatarsal a.'s

arcuate a.

medial tarsal a.'s

dorsal a. of foot

talus

© MELLONI

plantar digital a.'s

C **plantar metatarsal a.'s**

plantar arch

lateral plantar a.

medial plantar a.

calcaneus (plantar aspect)

posterior tibial a.

calcaneal br.

superfical temporal a.

supraorbital a.

supratrochlear a.

ophthalmic a.

dorsal nasal a.

angular a.

infraorbital a.

F **lateral nasal a.**

nasal br.

superior labial a.

facial a.

mandible

maxillary a.

inferior alveolar a.

E

mylohyoid a.

external carotid a.

mylohoid muscle

hyoid bone

sphenopalatine a.

anterior meningeal a.

anterior ethmoid a.

posterior septal a.'s of nose

H

nasal septum

posterior lateral nasal a.'s

sphenoid sinus

G

frontal sinus

spheno-palatine a.

nasal conchae

costocervical trunk

subclavian a.

highest intercostal a.

internal thoracic a.

peri-cardiaco-phrenic a.

aorta

mammary branches

heart

pericardiaco-phrenic a.

musculophrenic a.

D

anterior intercostal a.'s

superior epigastric a.

diaphragm

popliteal a.

anterior tibial a.

tibia (posterior aspect)

posterior tibial a.

nutrient a. of tibia

K

peroneal a.

nutrient a. of fibula

I

humerus (anterior aspect)

brachial a.

deep brachial a.

J

nutrient a.'s of humerus

fibula (posterior aspect)

	ARTERY	ORIGIN	BRANCHES	DISTRIBUTION
A	**a. obturatoria** *obturator a.*	internal iliac artery	pubic, acetabular iliac, vesical, anterior branch, posterior branch	pelvic muscles, hip joint, bladder, iliac fossa
B	**a. occipitalis** *occipital a.*	external carotid artery	sternocleidomastoid, auricular, meningeal, descending, mastoid, occipital	dura mater, mastoid air cells, muscles of neck, scalp
C	**a. ophthalmica** *ophthalmic a.*	internal carotid artery	orbital part: lacrimal, supraorbital, posterior ethmoidal, anterior ethmoidal, medial palpebral, supratrochlear, dorsal nasal	orbit and surrounding parts
			ocular part: central artery of the retina, short posterior ciliary, long posterior ciliary, anterior ciliary	muscles and bulb of eye
D	**a. ovarica** *ovarian a.* *gonadal a.*	abdominal aorta at level of L2	ureteric, capsular, tubal	ovary, ureter, uterus, skin of labium majus
E	**a. palatina ascendens** *palatine a., ascending*	facial artery	none	soft palate, auditory tube, tonsils
F	**a. palatina descendens** *palatine a., descending*	maxillary artery	greater and lesser palatine	soft palate, hard palate, palatine glands, tonsil, gums
G	**a. palatina major** *palatine a., major* *palatine a., greater*	descending palatine artery	none	hard palate, palatine glands, gums
H	**aa. palatinae minores** *palatine a.'s, minor* *palatine a.'s, lesser*	descending palatine artery	none	soft palate, tonsil
I	**aa. palpebrales laterales** *palpebral a.'s, lateral*	lacrimal artery	none	upper and lower eyelids, conjunctiva
J	**aa. palpebrales mediales** *palpebral a.'s, medial*	ophthalmic artery	superior, inferior	upper and lower eyelids, nasolacrimal duct
K	**a. pancreatica dorsalis** *pancreatic a., dorsal* *pancreatic a., superior*	splenic artery	right (anastomotic), left (inferior pancreatic)	pancreas

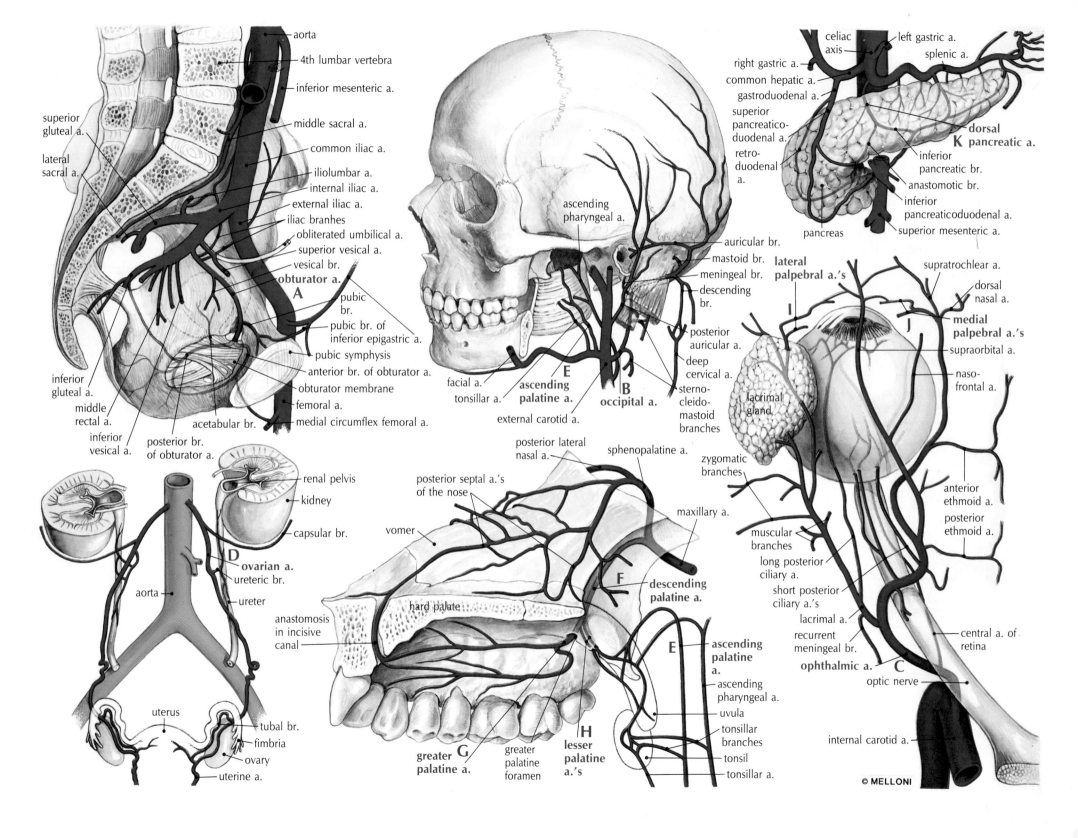

aorta
4th lumbar vertebra
inferior mesenteric a.
middle sacral a.
common iliac a.
iliolumbar a.
internal iliac a.
external iliac a.
iliac branhes
obliterated umbilical a.
superior vesical a.
vesical br.
obturator a.
pubic br.
pubic br. of inferior epigastric a.
pubic symphysis
anterior br. of obturator a.
obturator membrane
femoral a.
medial circumflex femoral a.

superior gluteal a.
lateral sacral a.
inferior gluteal a.
middle rectal a.
inferior vesical a.
posterior br. of obturator a.
acetabular br.
A

renal pelvis
kidney
capsular br.
D ovarian a.
ureteric br.
ureter
aorta
anastomosis in incisive canal
uterus
tubal br.
fimbria
ovary
uterine a.

celiac axis
left gastric a.
splenic a.
right gastric a.
common hepatic a.
gastroduodenal a.
superior pancreatico-duodenal a.
retro-duodenal
dorsal K pancreatic a.
inferior pancreatic br.
anastomotic br.
inferior pancreaticoduodenal a.
superior mesenteric a.
pancreas

ascending pharyngeal a.
auricular br.
mastoid br.
meningeal br.
descending br.
posterior auricular a.
deep cervical a.
sterno-cleido-mastoid branches
facial a.
E
ascending palatine a.
tonsillar a.
B occipital a.
external carotid a.

lateral palpebral a.'s
supratrochlear a.
dorsal nasal a.
medial palpebral a.'s
supraorbital a.
naso-frontal a.
I
J
lacrimal gland
zygomatic branches
anterior ethmoid a.
posterior ethmoid a.
muscular branches
long posterior ciliary a.
short posterior ciliary a.'s
lacrimal a.
recurrent meningeal br.
ophthalmic a.
C
central a. of retina
optic nerve
internal carotid a.

posterior lateral nasal a.
sphenopalatine a.
posterior septal a.'s of the nose
vomer
maxillary a.
F
descending palatine a.
hard palate
E
ascending palatine a.
ascending pharyngeal a.
uvula
tonsillar branches
tonsil
tonsillar a.
greater G palatine a.
greater palatine foramen
H lesser palatine a.'s

© MELLONI

	ARTERY	ORIGIN	BRANCHES	DISTRIBUTION
A	**a. pancreatica magna** *pancreatic a., great*	splenic artery	none	pancreas
B	**a. pancreatica inferior** *pancreatica a., inferior* *pancreatic a., transverse*	dorsal pancreatic artery	none	pancreas
C	**a. pancreaticoduodenalis inferior** *pancreaticoduodenal a., inferior*	superior mesenteric artery	anterior, posterior	head of pancreas, duodenum
D	**aa. pancreaticoduodenales superiores** *pancreaticoduodenal a.'s, superior*	gastroduodenal artery	pancreatic, duodenal, anastomotic	head of pancreas, duodenum
E	**aa. perforantes** *(usually three in number)* *perforating a.'s*	deep femoral artery	nutrient, muscular, cutaneous	back of thigh, buttock, femur
F	**a. pericardiacophrenica** *pericardiacophrenic a.*	internal thoracic artery	none	diaphragm, pleura, pericardium
G	**a. perinealis** *perineal a.*	internal pudendal artery	posterior scrotal/labial, transverse	perineum, external genitalia
H	**a. peronea** *peroneal a.* *fibular a.*	posterior tibial artery	nutrient (fibula), perforating, communicating, lateral malleolar, calcaneal	tibialis posterior, soleus, and flexor hallucis longus muscles; lateral and back side of ankle and heel
I	**a. pharyngea ascendens** *pharyngeal a., ascending*	external carotid artery	pharyngeal, inferior tympanic, posterior meningeal, tonsillar	pharynx, soft palate, meninges, muscles of back of head
J	**a. phrenica inferior** *phrenic a., inferior*	abdominal aorta or celiac trunk	superior suprarenal, anterior, lateral, recurrent	diaphragm, adrenal gland
K	**aa. phrenica superiores** *phrenic a.'s, superior*	thoracic aorta	none	diaphragm
L	**a. plantaris lateralis** *plantar a., lateral*	posterior tibial artery	muscular, continues to form plantar arch	muscles and skin of foot and toes, lateral side of sole

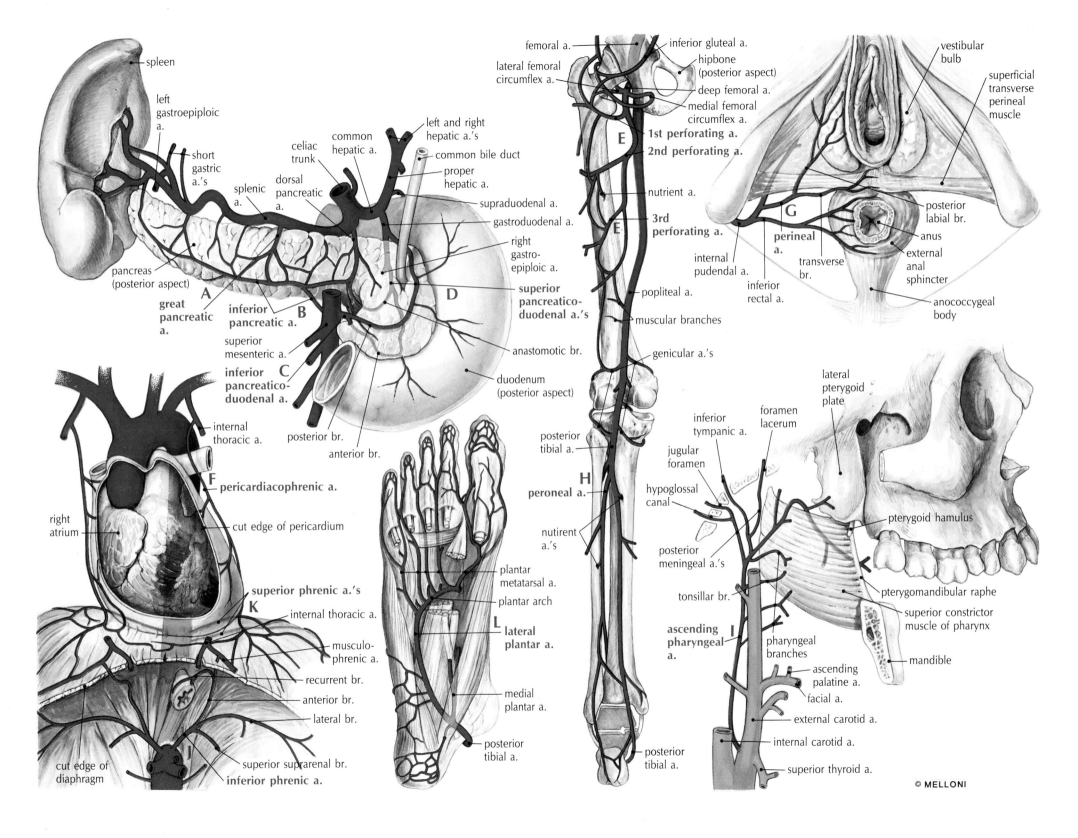

spleen

left
gastroepiploic
a.

short
gastric
a.'s

splenic
a.

dorsal
pancreatic
a.

celiac
trunk

common
hepatic a.

left and right
hepatic a.'s

common bile duct

proper
hepatic a.

supraduodenal a.

gastroduodenal a.

right
gastro-
epiploic
a.

**superior
pancreatico-
duodenal a.'s**

pancreas
(posterior aspect)

**great
pancreatic
a.**

A

**inferior
pancreatic a.**

B

C

superior
mesenteric a.

**inferior
pancreatico-
duodenal a.**

posterior br.

anterior br.

D

anastomotic br.

duodenum
(posterior aspect)

internal
thoracic a.

F

pericardiacophrenic a.

right
atrium

cut edge of pericardium

superior phrenic a.'s

K

internal thoracic a.

musculo-
phrenic a.

recurrent br.

anterior br.

lateral br.

cut edge of
diaphragm

superior suprarenal br.

inferior phrenic a.

femoral a.

lateral femoral
circumflex a.

inferior gluteal a.

hipbone
(posterior aspect)

deep femoral a.

medial femoral
circumflex a.

E

1st perforating a.

2nd perforating a.

nutrient a.

E

**3rd
perforating a.**

internal
pudendal a.

popliteal a.

muscular branches

genicular a.'s

posterior
tibial a.

H

peroneal a.

nutrient
a.'s

posterior
tibial a.

plantar
metatarsal a.

plantar arch

L

**lateral
plantar a.**

medial
plantar a.

posterior
tibial a.

vestibular
bulb

superficial
transverse
perineal
muscle

G

posterior
labial br.

anus

external
anal
sphincter

**perineal
a.**

transverse
br.

inferior
rectal a.

anococcygeal
body

lateral
pterygoid
plate

inferior
tympanic a.

foramen
lacerum

jugular
foramen

hypoglossal
canal

posterior
meningeal a.'s

tonsillar br.

**ascending
pharyngeal
a.**

I

pharyngeal
branches

ascending
palatine a.

facial a.

external carotid a.

internal carotid a.

superior thyroid a.

pterygoid hamulus

pterygomandibular raphe

superior constrictor
muscle of pharynx

mandible

© MELLONI

	ARTERY	ORIGIN	BRANCHES	DISTRIBUTION
A	**a. plantaris medialis** *plantar a., medial*	posterior tibial artery	deep, superficial	muscles and skin of foot and toes, medial side of sole
B	**a. poplitea** *popliteal a.*	continuation of femoral artery at the adductor hiatus	cutaneous, sural, medial superior genicular, lateral superior genicular, middle genicular, medial inferior genicular, lateral inferior genicular; it divides at the distal border of the popliteal muscle and continues as anterior and posterior tibial arteries	muscles of thigh and calf around region of knee, knee joint, and skin
C	**a. princeps pollicis** *principal a. of thumb*	radial artery	radial artery of index finger, nutrient	first metacarpal and skin of thumb
D	**a. profunda brachii** *deep brachial artery* *deep a. of arm*	brachial artery	nutrient, deltoid, radial collateral, middle collateral	humerus, elbow joint, muscles of arm
E	**a. profunda clitoridis** *deep a. of clitoris*	internal pudendal artery	none	corpus cavernosum of clitoris
F	**a. profunda femoris** *deep femoral artery* *deep artery of the thigh*	femoral artery	medial femoral circumflex, lateral femoral circumflex, perforating	adductor, extensor, and flexor muscles of thigh; hip joint; gluteal muscles; head and neck of femur
G	**a. profunda linguae** *deep lingual a.* *deep a. of tongue* *ranine a.*	lingual artery	none	tongue
H	**a. profunda penis** *deep a. of penis*	internal pudendal artery	none	corpus cavernosum of penis
I	**a. pudenda externa** *pudendal a., external*	femoral artery	anterior scrotal (male), anterior labial (female), inguinal	skin of lower abdomen, skin of scrotum and penis (in male), labium majus (in female)
J	**a. pudenda interna** *pudendal a., internal*	internal iliac artery	inferior rectal, perineal, artery of the bulb of penis or vestibule, posterior labial/scrotal, urethral, deep artery of the penis or clitoris, dorsal artery of the penis or clitoris	external genitalia, muscles of perineum, anus
K	**a. pulmonalis dextra** *pulmonary a., right*	pulmonary trunk	branches are named according to the segment which they supply (e.g., apical, posterior descending, posterior ascending)	right lung

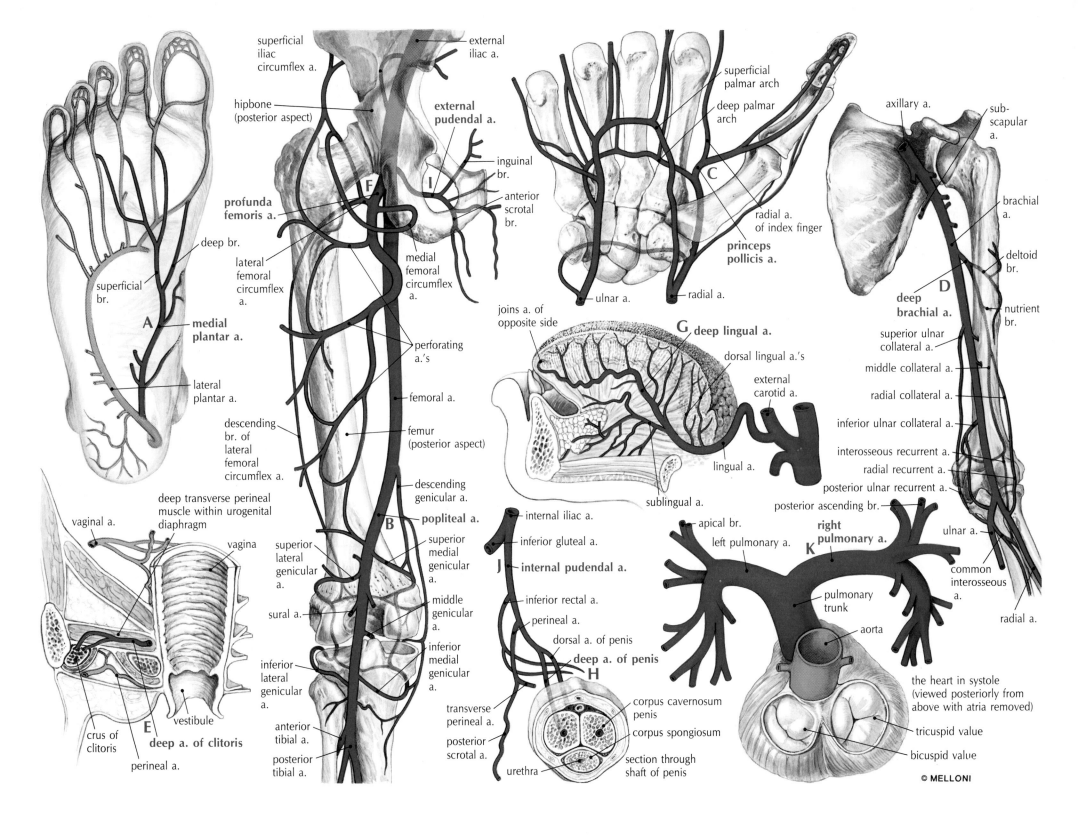

superficial
iliac
circumflex a.

external
iliac a.

hipbone
(posterior aspect)

**external
pudendal a.**

inguinal
br.

F

I

anterior
scrotal
br.

medial
femoral
circumflex
a.

**profunda
femoris a.**

lateral
femoral
circumflex
a.

perforating
a.'s

femoral a.

femur
(posterior aspect)

descending
br. of
lateral
femoral
circumflex a.

descending
genicular a.

popliteal a.

B

superior
lateral
genicular
a.

superior
medial
genicular
a.

sural a.

middle
genicular
a.

inferior
lateral
genicular
a.

inferior
medial
genicular
a.

anterior
tibial a.

posterior
tibial a.

deep br.

superficial
br.

A

**medial
plantar a.**

lateral
plantar a.

vaginal a.

deep transverse perineal
muscle within urogenital
diaphragm

vagina

superficial
palmar arch

deep palmar
arch

C

radial a.
of index finger

**princeps
pollicis a.**

ulnar a.

radial a.

axillary a.

sub-
scapular
a.

brachial
a.

deltoid
br.

D

nutrient
br.

**deep
brachial a.**

superior ulnar
collateral a.

middle collateral a.

radial collateral a.

inferior ulnar collateral a.

interosseous recurrent a.

radial recurrent a.

posterior ulnar recurrent a.

ulnar a.

common
interosseous
a.

radial a.

joins a. of
opposite side

G **deep lingual a.**

dorsal lingual a.'s

external
carotid a.

lingual a.

sublingual a.

crus of
clitoris

E

vestibule

perineal a.

deep a. of clitoris

internal iliac a.

inferior gluteal a.

internal pudendal a.

J

inferior rectal a.

perineal a.

dorsal a. of penis

deep a. of penis

H

transverse
perineal a.

posterior
scrotal a.

urethra

corpus cavernosum
penis

corpus spongiosum

section through
shaft of penis

apical br.

left pulmonary a.

**right
pulmonary a.**

K

pulmonary
trunk

aorta

the heart in systole
(viewed posteriorly from
above with atria removed)

tricuspid value

bicuspid value

© MELLONI

	ARTERY	ORIGIN	BRANCHES	DISTRIBUTION
A	**a. pulmonalis sinistra** *pulmonary a., left*	pulmonary trunk	branches are named according to the segment which they supply (e.g., apical, anterior descending, posterior, anterior ascending)	left lung
B	**a. radialis** *radial a.*	brachial artery	forearm group: muscular, recurrent radial wrist group: palmar carpal, superficial palmar, dorsal carpal hand group: first dorsal metacarpal, princeps pollicis, radialis indicis	muscles of forearm intercarpal articulations and bones of wrist, distal part of radius and ulna medial side of index finger, skin and muscles of thumb
C	**a. radialis indicis** *radial a. of index finger*	radial artery or princeps pollicis	none	lateral side of index finger
D	**a. rectalis inferior** *rectal a., inferior,* *inferior hemorrhoidal a.*	internal pudendal artery	none	rectum, muscles and skin of anal region
E	**a. rectalis media** *rectal a., middle* *middle hemorrhoidal a.*	internal iliac artery	vaginal in females	rectal musculature, seminal vesicles and prostate gland (in male)
F	**a. rectalis superior** *rectal a., superior* *superior hemorrhoidal a.*	continuation of inferior mesenteric artery	none	rectal musculature
G	**a. recurrens radialis** *recurrent a., radial*	radial artery just below elbow	none	supinator, brachioradialis, and brachialis muscles; elbow joint
H	**a. recurrens tibialis anterior** *recurrent a., anterior tibial*	anterior tibial artery	none	tibialis anterior muscle, front and sides of the knee joint
I	**a. recurrens tibialis posterior** *recurrent a., posterior tibial*	anterior tibial artery	none	tibiofibular joint, knee joint

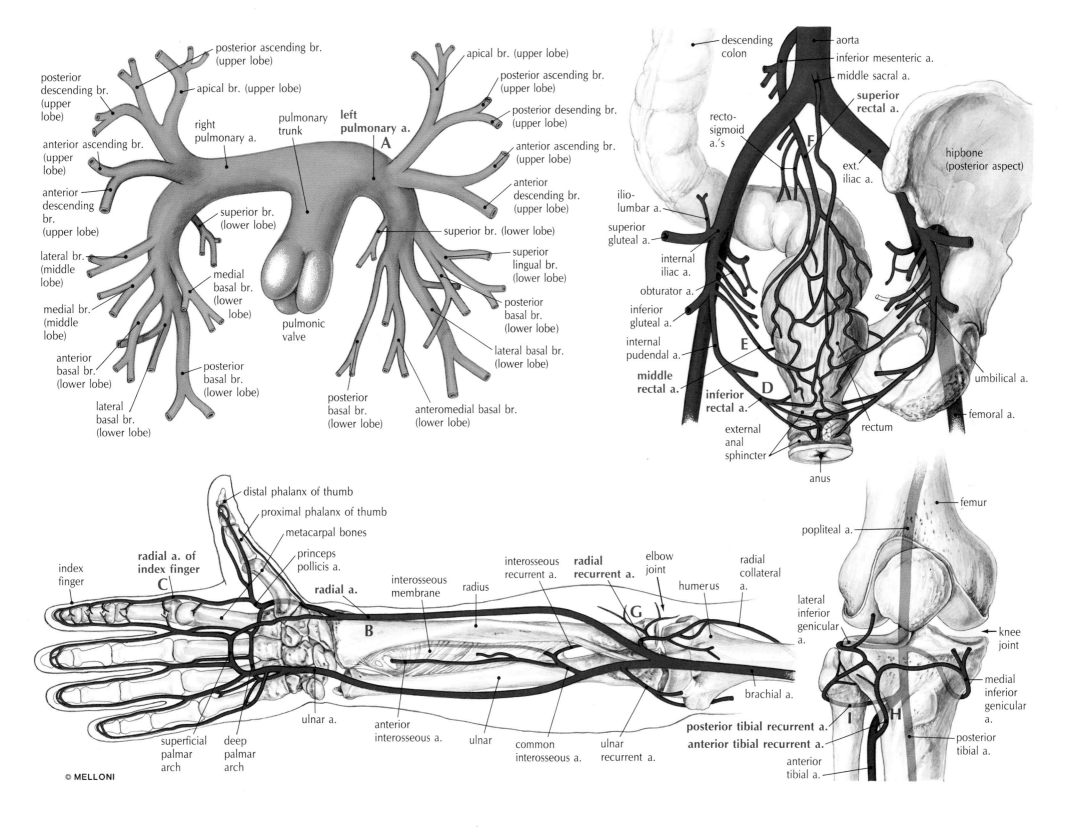

posterior ascending br. (upper lobe)

apical br. (upper lobe)

posterior descending br. (upper lobe)

apical br. (upper lobe)

posterior ascending br. (upper lobe)

right pulmonary a.

pulmonary trunk

left pulmonary a.

posterior desending br. (upper lobe)

anterior ascending br. (upper lobe)

anterior ascending br. (upper lobe)

anterior descending br. (upper lobe)

A

anterior descending br. (upper lobe)

superior br. (lower lobe)

superior br. (lower lobe)

lateral br. (middle lobe)

medial basal br. (lower lobe)

superior lingual br. (lower lobe)

medial br. (middle lobe)

pulmonic valve

posterior basal br. (lower lobe)

anterior basal br. (lower lobe)

posterior basal br. (lower lobe)

lateral basal br. (lower lobe)

lateral basal br. (lower lobe)

posterior basal br. (lower lobe)

anteromedial basal br. (lower lobe)

descending colon

aorta

inferior mesenteric a.

middle sacral a.

recto-sigmoid a.'s

superior rectal a.

F

ext. iliac a.

hipbone (posterior aspect)

ilio-lumbar a.

superior gluteal a.

internal iliac a.

obturator a.

inferior gluteal a.

internal pudendal a.

middle rectal a.

E

D

inferior rectal a.

umbilical a.

femoral a.

rectum

external anal sphincter

anus

distal phalanx of thumb

proximal phalanx of thumb

metacarpal bones

princeps pollicis a.

radial a. of index finger

C

radial a.

interosseous membrane

radius

interosseous recurrent a.

radial recurrent a.

elbow joint

radial collateral a.

humerus

index finger

B

G

femur

popliteal a.

lateral inferior genicular a.

knee joint

medial inferior genicular a.

ulnar a.

superficial palmar arch

deep palmar arch

anterior interosseous a.

ulnar

common interosseous a.

ulnar recurrent a.

brachial a.

posterior tibial recurrent a.

anterior tibial recurrent a.

I

H

anterior tibial a.

posterior tibial a.

© MELLONI

	ARTERY	ORIGIN	BRANCHES	DISTRIBUTION
A	**a. recurrens ulnaris** *recurrent a., ulnar*	ulnar artery	anterior, posterior	brachialis and pronator teres muscles
B	**a. renalis** *renal a.*	abdominal aorta about the level of L1	inferior suprarenal, ureteral, anterior branch, posterior branch	kidney, adrenal gland, ureter
C	**aa. retroduodenales** *retroduodenal a.'s* *posterior pancreaticoduodenal a.'s*	gastroduodenal artery	none	duodenum, head of pancreas, bile duct
D	**aa. sacrales laterales** *sacral a.'s, lateral*	internal iliac	spinal	sacrum, sacral canal
E	**a. sacralis media** *sacral a., middle*	aorta at bifurcation	small lumbar (a. lumbalis ima)	sacrum, rectum
F	**a. scapularis dorsalis** *scapular a., dorsal*	subclavian artery or transverse cervical artery	muscular	levator scapulae, trapezius, rhomboids, and latissimus dorsi muscles
G	**aa. sigmoideae** *sigmoid a.'s*	inferior mesenteric artery	none	sigmoid colon, lower part of descending colon
H	**a. sphenopalatina** *sphenopalatine a.* *nasopalatine a.*	maxillary artery	posterior lateral nasal, posterior septal	frontal, ethmoidal, maxillary, and sphenoidal sinuses, nasopharynx
I	**a. spinalis anterior** *spinal a., anterior*	vertebral artery near termination	central	spinal cord
J	**a. spinalis posterior** *spinal a., posterior*	posterior inferior cerebellar artery or vertebral artery	dorsal, ventral	spinal cord
K	**a. splenica** *splenic a.* *lienal a.*	celiac trunk	pancreatic, splenic, short gastric, left gastroepiploic (omental)	spleen, pancreas, stomach, greater omentum
L	**a. sternocleidomastoidea** *sternocleidomastoid a.*	occipital artery, superior thyroid artery, and occasionally external carotid artery	none	sternocleidomastoid muscle

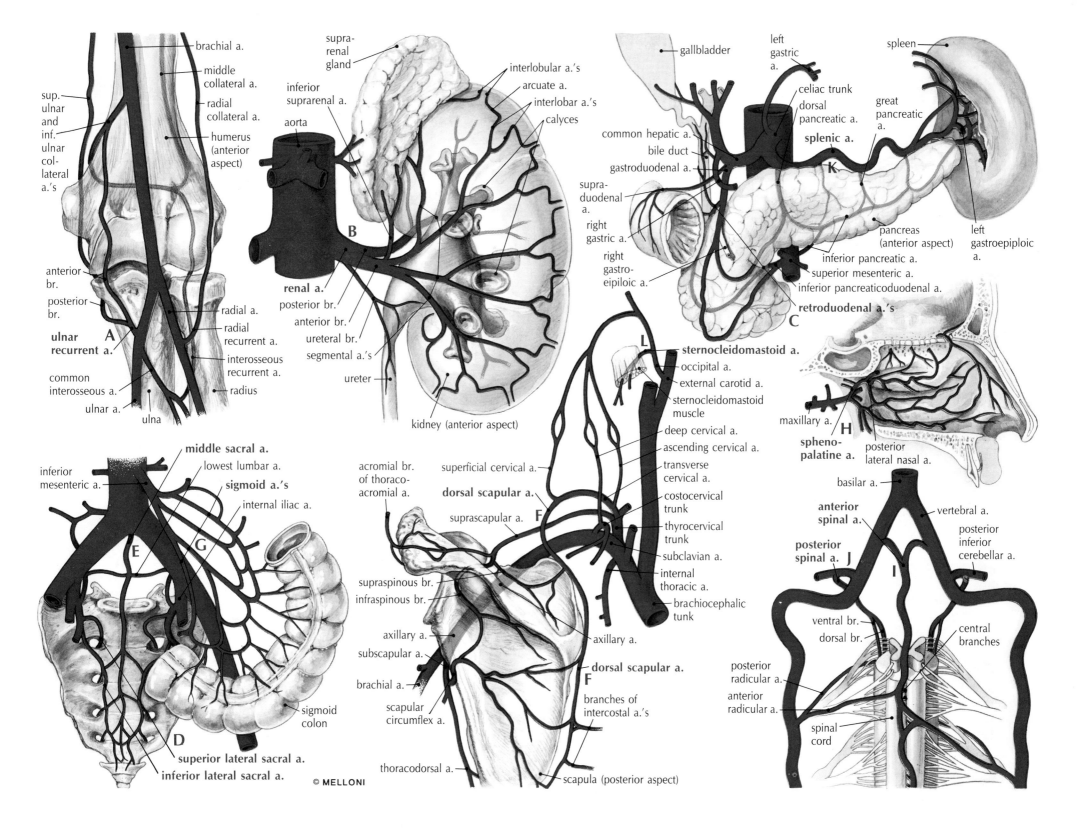

A

brachial a.
middle collateral a.
radial collateral a.
humerus (anterior aspect)
sup. ulnar and inf. ulnar collateral a.'s
anterior br.
posterior br.
ulnar recurrent a.
common interosseous a.
ulnar a.
ulna
radial a.
radial recurrent a.
interosseous recurrent a.
radius

B

supra-renal gland
inferior suprarenal a.
aorta
interlobular a.'s
arcuate a.
interlobar a.'s
calyces
renal a.
posterior br.
anterior br.
ureteral br.
segmental a.'s
ureter
kidney (anterior aspect)

C

gallbladder
left gastric a.
celiac trunk
dorsal pancreatic a.
spleen
great pancreatic a.
common hepatic a.
bile duct
gastroduodenal a.
supra-duodenal a.
right gastric a.
right gastro-eipiloic a.
splenic a.
K
left gastroepiploic a.
pancreas (anterior aspect)
inferior pancreatic a.
superior mesenteric a.
inferior pancreaticoduodenal a.
retroduodenal a.'s

H
maxillary a.
spheno-palatine a.
posterior lateral nasal a.

D / E / G

inferior mesenteric a.
middle sacral a.
lowest lumbar a.
sigmoid a.'s
internal iliac a.
sigmoid colon
superior lateral sacral a.
inferior lateral sacral a.

© MELLONI

F

acromial br. of thoraco-acromial a.
superficial cervical a.
dorsal scapular a.
suprascapular a.
supraspinous br.
infraspinous br.
axillary a.
subscapular a.
brachial a.
scapular circumflex a.
thoracodorsal a.
axillary a.
dorsal scapular a.
branches of intercostal a.'s
scapula (posterior aspect)

L

sternocleidomastoid a.
occipital a.
external carotid a.
sternocleidomastoid muscle
deep cervical a.
ascending cervical a.
transverse cervical a.
costocervical trunk
thyrocervical trunk
subclavian a.
internal thoracic a.
brachiocephalic tunk

I / J

basilar a.
anterior spinal a.
vertebral a.
posterior inferior cerebellar a.
posterior spinal a.
ventral br.
dorsal br.
central branches
posterior radicular a.
anterior radicular a.
spinal cord

	ARTERY	ORIGIN	BRANCHES	DISTRIBUTION
A	**a. stylomastoidea** *stylomastoid a.*	posterior auricular artery	posterior tympanic, mastoid, stapedial	tympanic cavity, stapedius muscle, mastoid air cells, semicircular canals
B	**a. subclavia** *subclavian a.*	right side: brachiocephalic trunk left side: arch of aorta	vertebral, internal thoracic, thyrocervical, costocervical, dorsal scapular; continues as axillary artery at the outer border of the first rib	neck, thoracic wall, muscles of upper limb, spinal cord and brain
C	**a. subcostalis** *subcostal a.*	thoracic aorta	dorsal, spinal	upper abdominal wall below twelfth rib, spinal cord
D	**a. sublingualis** *sublingual a.*	lingual artery	gingival, submental	sublingual gland, mylohyoid and geniohyoid muscles; mucous membrane of mouth and gums
E	**a. submentalis** *submental a.*	facial artery	superficial, deep	muscles in the region of the chin and lower lip, submandibular gland
F	**a. subscapularis** *subscapular a.*	axillary artery	circumflex scapular, thoracodorsal	subscapularis muscle and muscles of shoulder
G	**a. supraorbitalis** *supraorbital a.*	ophthalmic artery as it crosses the optic nerve	superficial, deep	forehead, rectus superior and levator palpebrae muscles, diploe
H	**a. suprarenalis inferior** *suprarenal a., inferior*	renal artery	none	adrenal gland
I	**a. suprarenalis media** *suprarenal a., middle*	abdominal aorta	none	adrenal gland
J	**aa. suprarenales superiores** *suprarenal a.'s, superior*	inferior phrenic artery	none	adrenal gland
K	**a. suprascapularis** *suprascapular a.* *transverse scapular a.*	thyrocervical trunk	suprasternal, articular, acromial, nutrient, supraspinous, infraspinous	clavicle, scapula, skin of chest, muscles of scapula region, acromioclavicular and shoulder joints
L	**a. supratrochlearis** *supratrochlear a.* *frontal a.*	ophthalmic artery	none	scalp

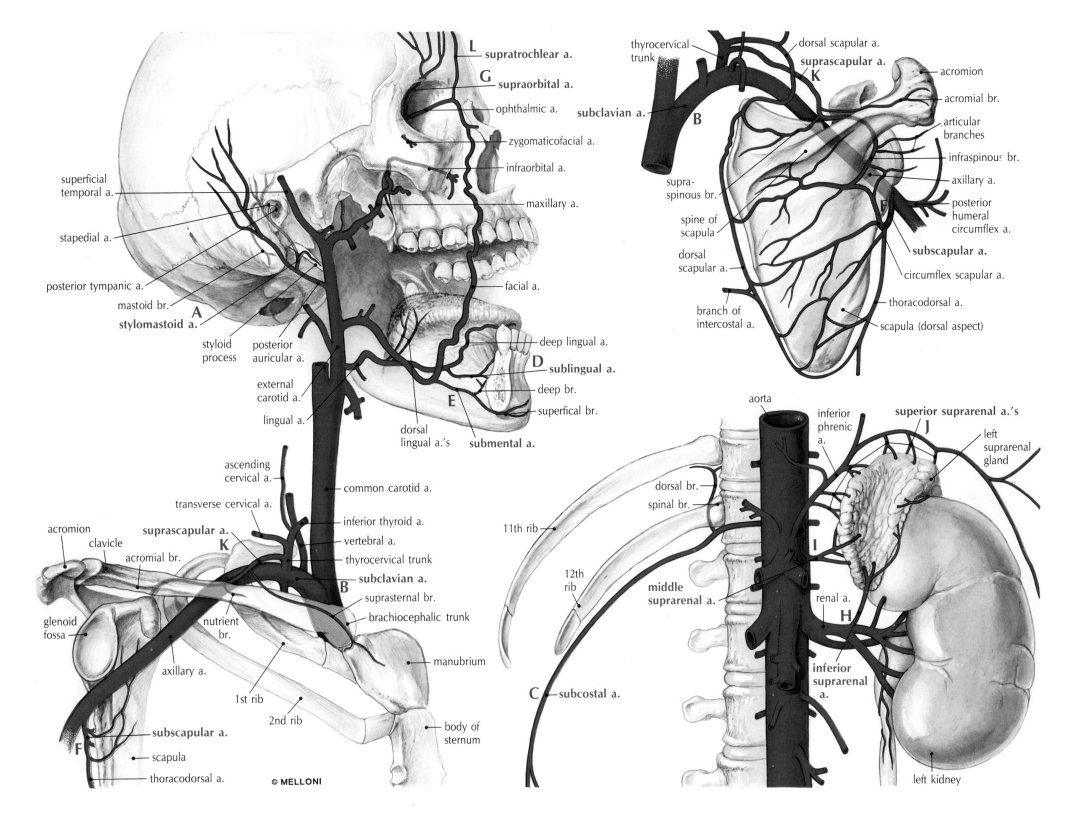

supratrochlear a. L

supraorbital a. G

ophthalmic a.

zygomaticofacial a.

infraorbital a.

superficial
temporal a.

maxillary a.

stapedial a.

posterior tympanic a.

mastoid br.

stylomastoid a. A

styloid
process

posterior
auricular a.

external
carotid a.

lingual a.

facial a.

deep lingual a.

sublingual a. D

deep br.

superfical br. E

dorsal
lingual a.'s

submental a.

ascending
cervical a.

common carotid a.

transverse cervical a.

inferior thyroid a.

suprascapular a. K

vertebral a.

acromial br.

thyrocervical trunk

subclavian a. B

suprasternal br.

brachiocephalic trunk

acromion

clavicle

nutrient
br.

manubrium

glenoid
fossa

axillary a.

1st rib

2nd rib

body of
sternum

subscapular a. F

scapula

thoracodorsal a.

© MELLONI

thyrocervical
trunk

dorsal scapular a.

suprascapular a. K

acromion

acromial br.

subclavian a. B

articular
branches

supra-
spinous br.

infraspinous br.

axillary a.

spine of
scapula

posterior
humeral
circumflex a.

dorsal
scapular a.

subscapular a. F

circumflex scapular a.

branch of
intercostal a.

thoracodorsal a.

scapula (dorsal aspect)

aorta

inferior
phrenic
a.

superior suprarenal a.'s J

left
suprarenal
gland

dorsal br.

spinal br.

11th rib

12th
rib

**middle
suprarenal a.** I

renal a.

H

**inferior
suprarenal
a.**

subcostal a. C

left kidney

	ARTERY	ORIGIN	BRANCHES	DISTRIBUTION
A	**aa. surales** *sural a.'s*	popliteal artery	none	gastrocnemius, plantaris, and soleus muscles
B	**a. tarsalis lateralis** *tarsal a., lateral*	dorsal artery of foot	none	extensor digitorum brevis muscle and tarsal articulations
C	**aa. tarsales mediales** *tarsal a.'s medial*	dorsal artery of foot	none	medial aspect of foot
D	**a. temporalis media** *temporal a., middle*	superficial temporal artery just above zygomatic arch	none	temporalis muscle
E	**aa. temporales profundae** *temporal a.'s, deep*	maxillary artery	none	temporalis muscle
F	**a. temporalis superficialis** *temporal a., superficial*	external carotid artery	anterior auricular, frontal, transverse facial, middle temporal, zygomatico-orbital, parietal, parotid	parotid gland, temporomandibular joint, masseter and temporalis muscles, orbit, auricle, external acoustic meatus
G	**a. testicularis** *testicular a.* *spermatic a., internal* *gonadal a.*	abdominal aorta about level of L2	capsular, ureteric, epididymal, cremasteric	testis, epididymis, ureter, cremaster muscle
H	**a. thoracica interna** *thoracic a., internal* *mammary a., internal*	subclavian artery	pericardiacophrenic, mediastinal, sternal, perforating, anterior intercostal, musculophrenic, superior epigastric, thymic	anterior thoracic wall, structures in mediastinum such as lymph nodes, diaphragm
I	**a. thoracica lateralis** *thoracic a., lateral* *long thoracic a.* *external mammary a.*	axillary artery	lateral mammary (in female)	pectoralis major and minor, serratus anterior and subscapularis muscles; mammary gland (in female), axillary lymph nodes

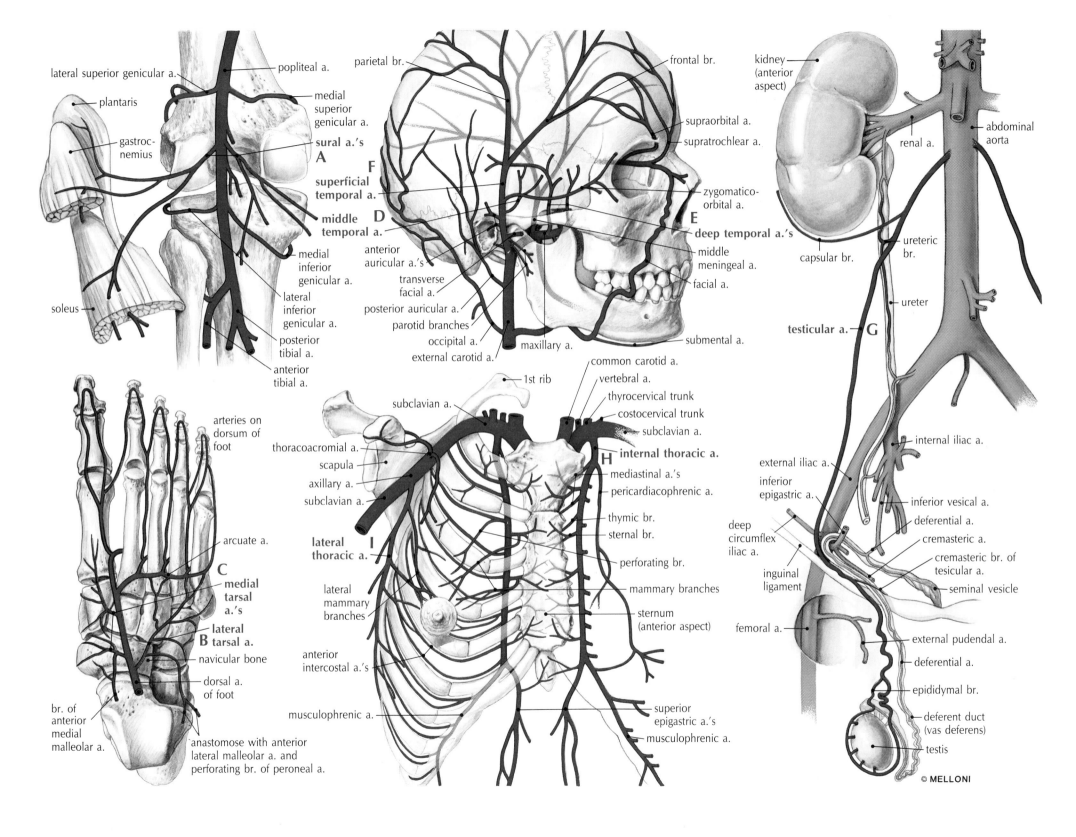

lateral superior genicular a.

plantaris

gastroc-
nemius

soleus

popliteal a.

medial
superior
genicular a.

sural a.'s

A

medial
inferior
genicular a.

lateral
inferior
genicular a.

posterior
tibial a.

anterior
tibial a.

arteries on
dorsum of
foot

arcuate a.

C

**medial
tarsal
a.'s**

**lateral
tarsal a.**

B

navicular bone

dorsal a.
of foot

br. of
anterior
medial
malleolar a.

anastomose with anterior
lateral malleolar a. and
perforating br. of peroneal a.

parietal br.

frontal br.

supraorbital a.

supratrochlear a.

F

**superficial
temporal a.**

**middle
temporal a.**

D

zygomatico-
orbital a.

E

deep temporal a.'s

anterior
auricular a.'s

middle
meningeal a.

transverse
facial a.

facial a.

posterior auricular a.

parotid branches

occipital a.

maxillary a.

submental a.

external carotid a.

1st rib

common carotid a.

vertebral a.

subclavian a.

thyrocervical trunk

costocervical trunk

subclavian a.

thoracoacromial a.

scapula

axillary a.

subclavian a.

H

internal thoracic a.

mediastinal a.'s

pericardiacophrenic a.

thymic br.

sternal br.

perforating br.

mammary branches

**lateral
thoracic a.**

I

lateral
mammary
branches

anterior
intercostal a.'s

sternum
(anterior aspect)

musculophrenic a.

superior
epigastric a.'s

musculophrenic a.

kidney
(anterior
aspect)

renal a.

abdominal
aorta

ureteric
br.

capsular br.

ureter

testicular a. **G**

internal iliac a.

external iliac a.

inferior
epigastric a.

inferior vesical a.

deferential a.

deep
circumflex
iliac a.

cremasteric a.

cremasteric br. of
tesicular a.

inguinal
ligament

seminal vesicle

femoral a.

external pudendal a.

deferential a.

epididymal br.

deferent duct
(vas deferens)

testis

© MELLONI

	ARTERY	ORIGIN	BRANCHES	DISTRIBUTION
A	**a. thoracica superior** *thoracic a., highest* *thoracic a., superior*	axillary artery	none	pectoralis major, pectoralis minor, anterior serratus, and intercostal muscles
B	**a. thoracoacromialis** *thoracoacromial a.* *acromiothoracic a.*	axillary artery	pectoral, acromial, deltoid, clavicular	pectoralis major and minor, subclavius, and deltoid muscles, sternoclavicular joint, acromion
C	**a. thoracodorsalis** *thoracodorsal a.*	subscapular artery	none	latissimus dorsi, subscapularis, and teres major muscles
D	**a. thyroidea ima** *thyroid ima a.* *thyroid a., lowest*	brachiocephalic trunk and occasionally arch of aorta or right common carotid artery	none	thyroid gland
E	**a. thyroidea inferior** *thyroid a., inferior*	thyrocervical trunk	ascending cervical, inferior laryngeal, tracheal, esophageal, pharyngeal, glandular	larynx, pharynx, trachea, esophagus, thyroid gland, and neighboring muscles of neck
F	**a. thyroidea superior** *thyroid a., superior*	external carotid artery	infrahyoid, sternocleidomastoid, superior laryngeal, cricothyroid, glandular	larynx, thyroid gland and neighboring muscles; cricothyroid ligament
G	**a. tibialis anterior** *tibial a., anterior*	popliteal artery	posterior tibial recurrent, anterior tibial recurrent, anterior medial malleolar, anterior lateral malleolar, continues as dorsal artery of foot	leg muscles, knee joint, ankle, foot
H	**a. tibialis posterior** *tibial a., posterior*	popliteal artery	medial plantar, lateral plantar, fibular circumflex, peroneal, medial malleolar, calcaneal, nutrient artery of tibia	muscles, bones, and articulations of leg; foot
I	**a. transversa cervicis** *transverse cervical a.*	thyrocervical trunk	superficial cervical, (occasionally) dorsal scapular	levator scapulae, trapezius, supraspinatus muscles

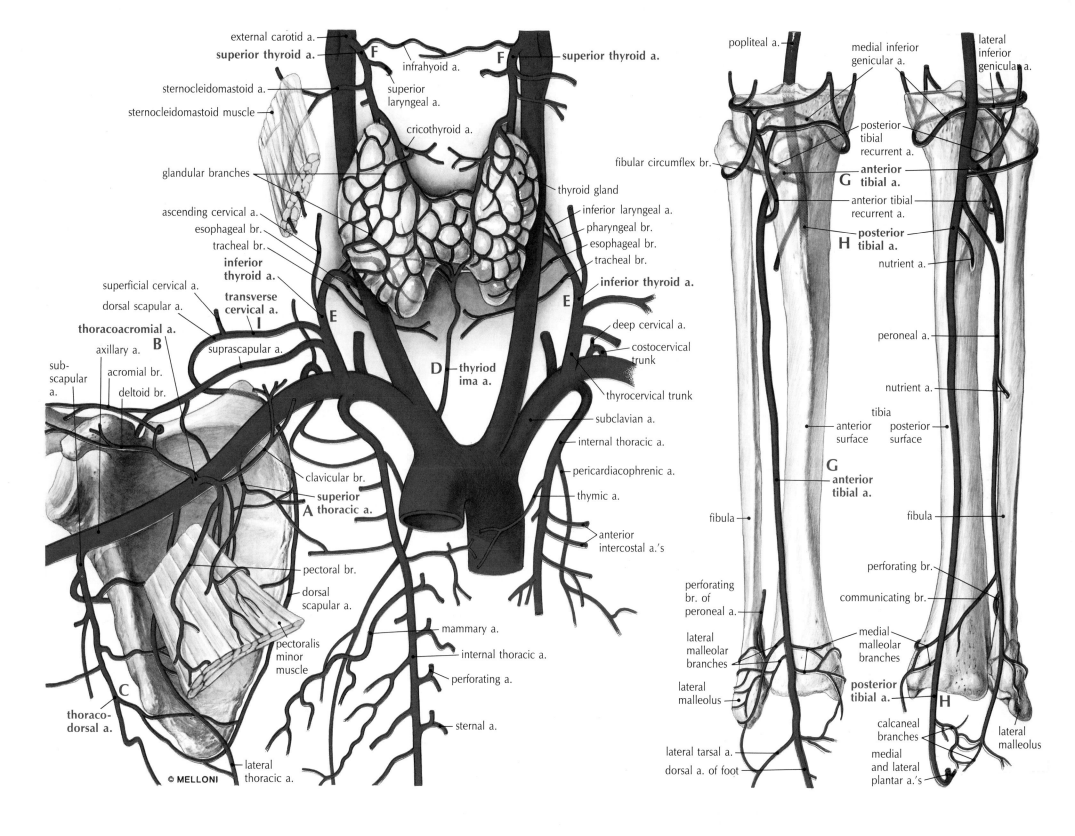

external carotid a.
superior thyroid a.
infrahyoid a.
F **F** **superior thyroid a.**
sternocleidomastoid a.
superior laryngeal a.
sternocleidomastoid muscle
cricothyroid a.
glandular branches
thyroid gland
inferior laryngeal a.
ascending cervical a.
pharyngeal br.
esophageal br.
esophageal br.
tracheal br.
tracheal br.
inferior thyroid a.
inferior thyroid a.
superficial cervical a.
E **E**
dorsal scapular a.
deep cervical a.
transverse cervical a.
I
costocervical trunk
thoracoacromial a.
suprascapular a.
axillary a.
B
D **thyriod ima a.**
thyrocervical trunk
acromial br.
sub-scapular a.
deltoid br.
subclavian a.
internal thoracic a.
clavicular br.
pericardiacophrenic a.
A **superior thoracic a.**
thymic a.
pectoral br.
dorsal scapular a.
anterior intercostal a.'s
pectoralis minor muscle
C
mammary a.
internal thoracic a.
perforating a.
thoraco-dorsal a.
sternal a.
lateral thoracic a.
© MELLONI

popliteal a.
medial inferior genicular a.
lateral inferior genicular a.
posterior tibial recurrent a.
fibular circumflex br.
G **anterior tibial a.**
anterior tibial recurrent a.
H **posterior tibial a.**
nutrient a.
peroneal a.
nutrient a.
tibia
anterior surface
posterior surface
G
anterior tibial a.
fibula
fibula
perforating br.
communicating br.
perforating br. of peroneal a.
medial malleolar branches
lateral malleolar branches
lateral malleolus
posterior tibial a. **H**
lateral tarsal a.
calcaneal branches
lateral malleolus
dorsal a. of foot
medial and lateral plantar a.'s

	ARTERY	ORIGIN	BRANCHES	DISTRIBUTION
A	**a. transversa faciei** *facial a., transverse*	superficial temporal artery before emerging from parotid gland	none	parotid gland and duct, messeter muscle, skin of face
B	**truncus brachiocephalicus** *brachiocephalic trunk* *innominate a.*	aortic arch	right common carotid, right subclavian, occasionally thyroid ima, thymic, and bronchial	right side of head and neck, sometimes thyroid, thymus, and bronchus
C	**truncus celiacus** *celiac trunk*	abdominal aorta just below aortic hiatus of diaphragm	left gastric, common hepatic, splenic	stomach, duodenum, pancreas, spleen, greater omentum, liver, common bile duct, hepatic ducts
D	**truncus costocervicalis** *costocervical trunk*	subclavian artery	deep cervical, highest intercostal	deep neck muscles, muscles of upper back, first and second intercostal spaces, vertebral column
E	**truncus pulmonalis** *pulmonary trunk*	right ventricle	right pulmonary, left pulmonary	lungs
F	**truncus thyrocervicalis** *thyrocervical trunk*	subclavian artery	inferior thyroid, suprascapular, transverse cervical	thyroid gland, scapular region, muscles of neck
G	**a. tympanica anterior** *tympanic a., anterior* *glaserian a.*	maxillary artery	none	tympanic membrane, middle ear
H	**a. tympanica inferior** *tympanic a., inferior*	ascending pharyngeal artery	none	middle ear
I	**a. tympanica posterior** *tympanic a., posterior*	stylomastoid artery	none	tympanic membrane, middle ear
J	**a. tympanica superior** *tympanic a., superior*	middle meningeal artery	none	tensor tympani muscle, middle ear

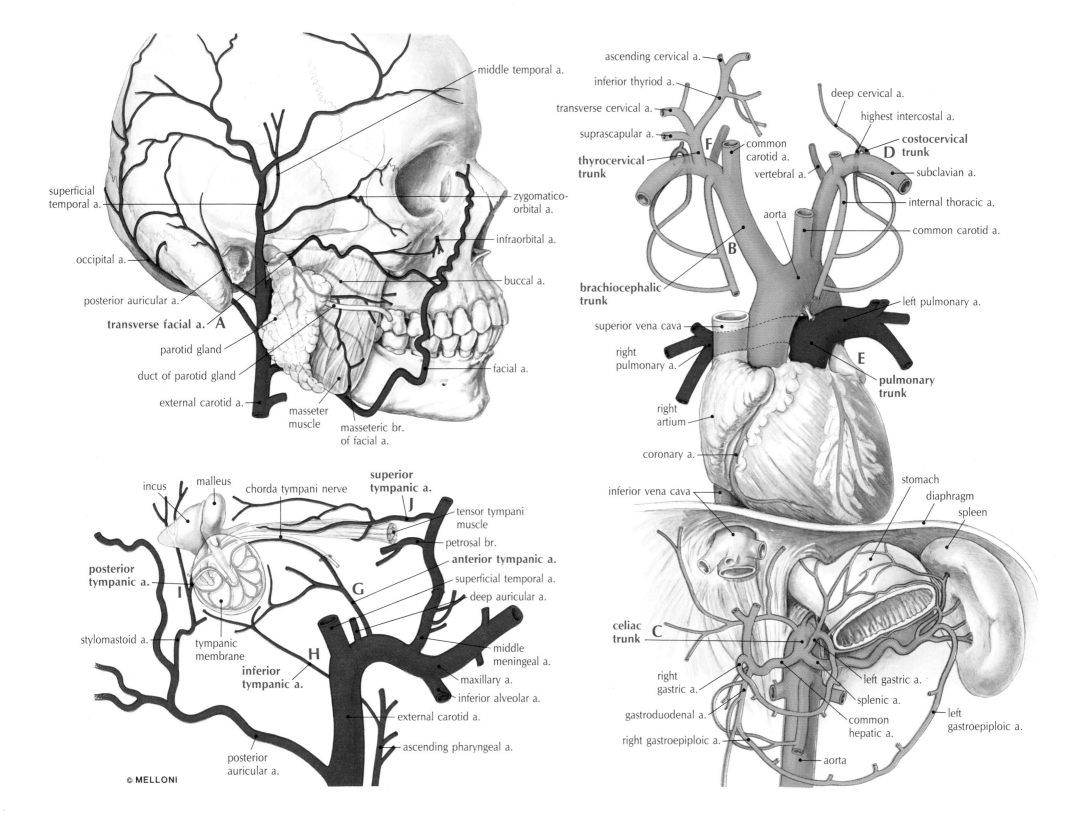

middle temporal a.

superficial temporal a.

occipital a.

posterior auricular a.

transverse facial a. A

parotid gland

duct of parotid gland

external carotid a.

masseter muscle

masseteric br. of facial a.

zygomatico-orbital a.

infraorbital a.

buccal a.

facial a.

ascending cervical a.

inferior thyriod a.

transverse cervical a.

suprascapular a.

thyrocervical trunk

F

common carotid a.

deep cervical a.

highest intercostal a.

costocervical trunk D

subclavian a.

vertebral a.

internal thoracic a.

aorta

common carotid a.

brachiocephalic trunk

B

superior vena cava

right pulmonary a.

left pulmonary a.

E

pulmonary trunk

right artium

coronary a.

inferior vena cava

stomach

diaphragm

spleen

incus

malleus

chorda tympani nerve

superior tympanic a.

J

tensor tympani muscle

petrosal br.

anterior tympanic a.

superficial temporal a.

deep auricular a.

posterior tympanic a.

I

G

stylomastoid a.

tympanic membrane

inferior tympanic a.

H

middle meningeal a.

maxillary a.

inferior alveolar a.

external carotid a.

ascending pharyngeal a.

posterior auricular a.

celiac trunk C

right gastric a.

gastroduodenal a.

right gastroepiploic a.

left gastric a.

splenic a.

common hepatic a.

left gastroepiploic a.

aorta

© MELLONI

	ARTERY	ORIGIN	BRANCHES	DISTRIBUTION
A	**a. ulnaris** *ulnar a.*	brachial artery slightly below elbow	anterior ulnar recurrent, posterior ulnar recurrent, common interosseous, palmar carpal, dorsal carpal, deep palmar, superficial palmar arch	muscles of forearm, wrist, and hand
B	**a. umbilicalis** *umbilical a.*	internal iliac artery	patent part: artery of the ductus deferens, superior vesical occluded part: umbilical ligament	ductus deferens, seminal vesicles, bladder
C	**a. urethralis** *urethral a.*	internal pudendal artery	none	urethra
D	**a. uterina** *uterine a.*	internal iliac artery	vaginal, ovarian, tubal, helicine	uterus, upper part of vagina, round ligament of uterus, cervix, uterine tube
E	**a. vaginalis** *vaginal a.*	internal iliac artery or uterine artery	none	vagina, fundus of urinary bladder, rectum
F	**a. vertebralis** *vertebral a.*	subclavian artery	cervical part: spinal, muscular cranial part: meningeal, posterior spinal, anterior spinal, posterior inferior cerebellar, medial and lateral medullary	vertebrae, deep muscles of neck, spinal cord cerebellum, medulla oblongata
G	**a. vesicalis inferior** *vesical a., inferior*	internal iliac artery	prostatic in males	fundus of urinary bladder, and (in male) prostate and seminal vesicles
H	**aa. vesicales superiores** *vesical a.'s, superior*	umbilical artery	ureteric	ureter, upper part of urinary bladder
I	**a. zygomaticoorbitalis** *zygomatico-orbital a.*	superficial temporal artery and occasionally middle temporal artery	none	orbicularis oculi muscle and lateral portion of orbit

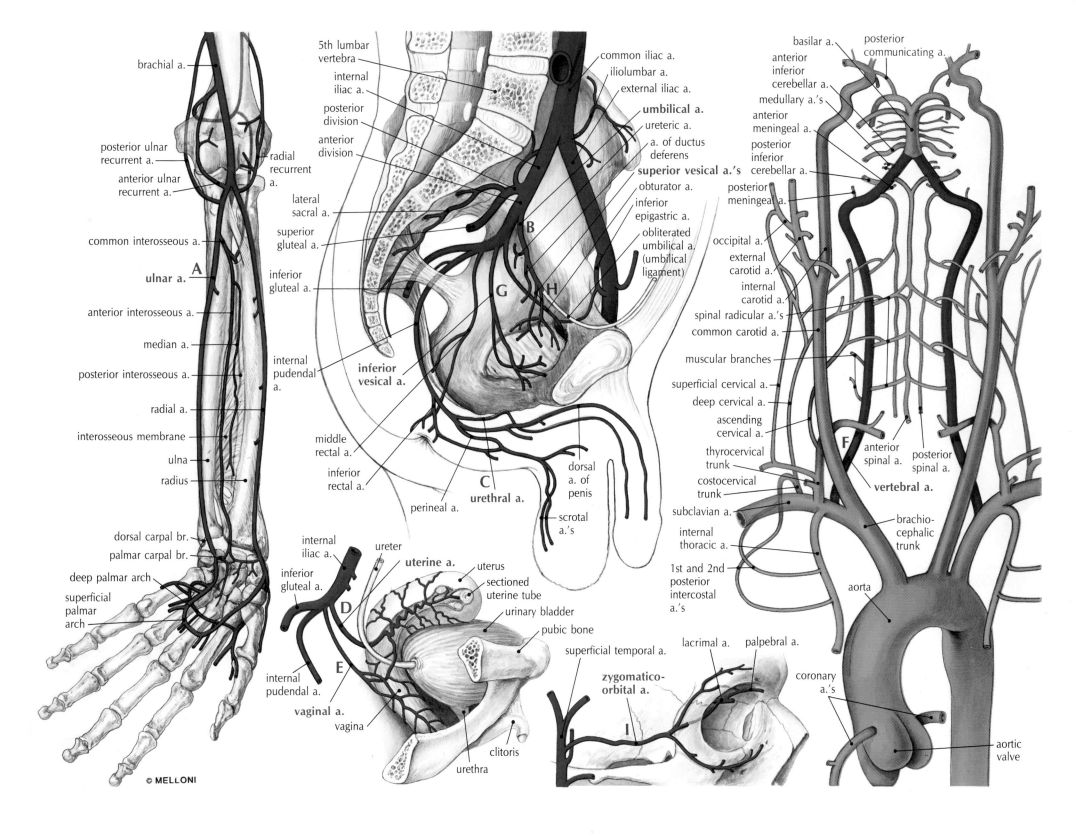

brachial a.

posterior ulnar recurrent a.

anterior ulnar recurrent a.

radial recurrent a.

common interosseous a.

ulnar a. **A**

anterior interosseous a.

median a.

posterior interosseous a.

radial a.

interosseous membrane

ulna

radius

dorsal carpal br.

palmar carpal br.

deep palmar arch

superficial palmar arch

© MELLONI

5th lumbar vertebra

internal iliac a.

posterior division

anterior division

lateral sacral a.

superior gluteal a.

inferior gluteal a.

internal pudendal a.

middle rectal a.

inferior rectal a.

inferior vesical a.

perineal a.

urethral a. **C**

B

G **H**

common iliac a.

iliolumbar a.

external iliac a.

umbilical a.

ureteric a.

a. of ductus deferens

superior vesical a.'s

obturator a.

inferior epigastric a.

obliterated umbilical a. (umbilical ligament)

dorsal a. of penis

scrotal a.'s

internal iliac a.

inferior gluteal a.

D

E

internal pudendal a.

vaginal a.

ureter

uterine a.

uterus

sectioned uterine tube

urinary bladder

pubic bone

vagina

clitoris

urethra

superficial temporal a.

zygomatico-orbital a.

I

lacrimal a.

palpebral a.

basilar a.

anterior inferior cerebellar a.

medullary a.'s

anterior meningeal a.

posterior inferior cerebellar a.

posterior meningeal a.

occipital a.

external carotid a.

internal carotid a.

spinal radicular a.'s

common carotid a.

muscular branches

superficial cervical a.

deep cervical a.

ascending cervical a.

thyrocervical trunk

costocervical trunk

subclavian a.

internal thoracic a.

1st and 2nd posterior intercostal a.'s

posterior communicating a.

F

anterior spinal a.

posterior spinal a.

vertebral a.

brachio-cephalic trunk

aorta

coronary a.'s

aortic valve

BONES

	BONE	LOCATION	DESCRIPTION	ARTICULATION	MUSCLE/TENDON ATTACHMENTS
A	**atlas** *atlas* *1st cervical vertebra*	neck, between skull and axis (2nd cervical vertebra)	ringlike vertebra lacking a body and a true spinous process; composed of: ANTERIOR ARCH (with tubercle and articular facet), POSTERIOR ARCH (with tubercle), two LATERAL MASSES (each with one superior and one inferior articular facets), and two TRANSVERSE PROCESSES. Rotates on dens (odontoid process) of axis	cranially: with occipital condyles on both sides of foramen magnum caudally: with superior articular facets of axis and dens of axis (anterior aspect)	anterior tubercle: longus colli (superior oblique part) posterior tubercle: rectus capitis posterior minor lateral mass: rectus capitis anterior transverse process: rectus capitis lateralis, obliquus capitis superior, obliquus capitis inferior, levator scapulae, splenius cervicis, scalenus medius
B	**axis** *axis* *2nd cervical vertebra*	neck, between atlas (1st cervical vertebra) and 3rd cervical vertebra	vertebra composed of: DENS, a peglike process on which the head rotates via the atlas (with apex and anterior articular facet), small BODY (with two superior articular facets), two PEDICLES, two TRANSVERSE PROCESSES (each with a tubercle), two ANTERIOR TUBERCLES, two INFERIOR ARTICULAR PROCESSES (with articular facets), two LAMINAE and a bifid SPINOUS PROCESS	cranially: with facet on anterior arch of atlas; inferior articular facets of atlas caudally: with superior articular facets of 3rd cervical vertebra	body: vertical part of longus colli transverse process: levator scapulae, scalenus medius, splenius cervicis spinous process: spinalis cervicis, semispinalis cervicis, rectus capitis posterior major, obliquus capitis inferior
C	**calcaneus** *calcaneus* *heel bone*	back of foot	largest bone of tarsus; projects backwards forming heel; has six SURFACES: posterior, anterior, superior (with sulcus calcanei), plantar (with tuberosity, two processes, and tubercle), medial (with sustentaculum tali, and groove for tendon of flexor hallucis longus muscle), lateral (with two grooves for tendons of peroneus muscles, and peroneal trochlea)	superior surface: with posterior, middle and anterior facets of talus anterior surface: with proximal surface of cuboid bone	plantar surface: abductor hallucis, abductor digiti minimi, flexor digitorum brevis, quadratus plantae (flexor digitorum accessorius) dorsolateral surface: extensor digitorum brevis, extensor hallucis brevis posterior surface: gastrocnemius in common with soleus via calcaneal tendon (tendo calcaneus)
D	**carpalia** *carpus*	hand	the eight bones of the wrist; arranged in two rows: PROXIMAL ROW (with scaphoid, lunate, triquetral, and pisiform bones) and DISTAL ROW (with trapezium, trapezoid, capitate, and hamate bones)	proximal row (lunate and scaphoid): with radius distal row: with metacarpal bones	see individual bones

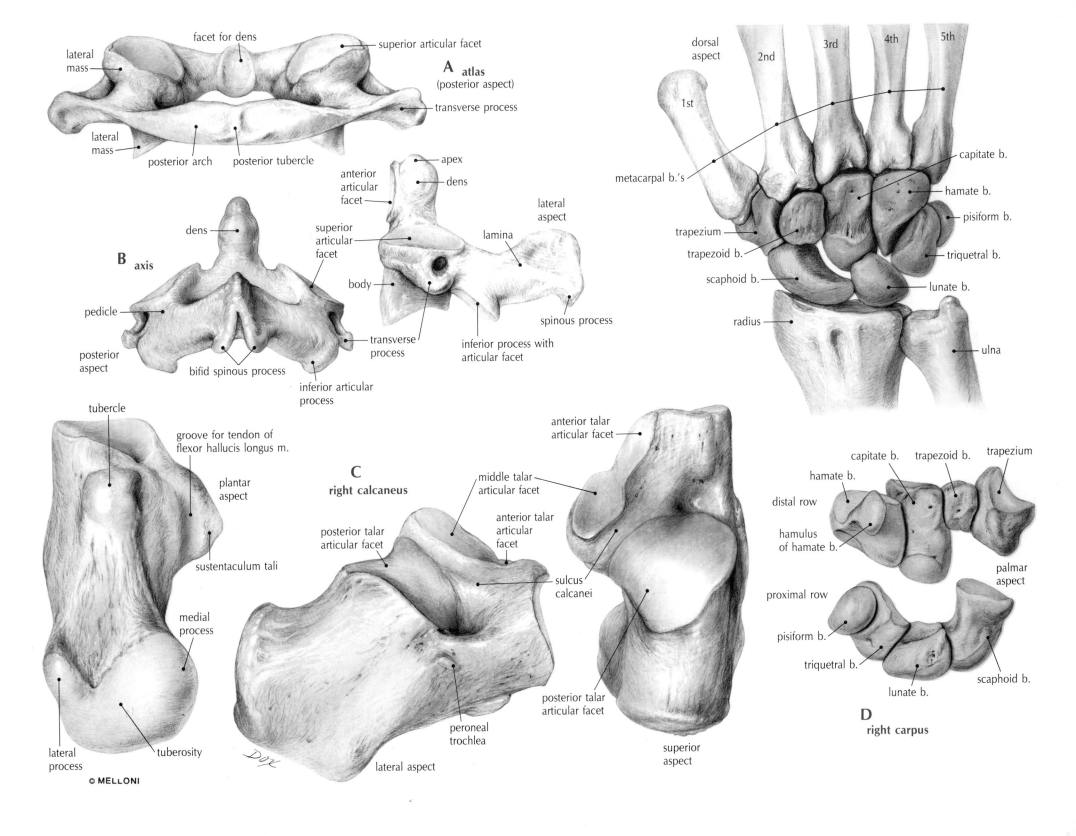

A atlas (posterior aspect)

facet for dens

superior articular facet

lateral mass

transverse process

lateral mass

posterior arch

posterior tubercle

apex

dens

anterior articular facet

lateral aspect

B axis

dens

superior articular facet

lamina

pedicle

body

posterior aspect

bifid spinous process

transverse process

inferior process with articular facet

spinous process

inferior articular process

tubercle

groove for tendon of flexor hallucis longus m.

plantar aspect

sustentaculum tali

medial process

lateral process

tuberosity

C right calcaneus

anterior talar articular facet

middle talar articular facet

posterior talar articular facet

anterior talar articular facet

sulcus calcanei

posterior talar articular facet

peroneal trochlea

lateral aspect

superior aspect

© MELLONI

dorsal aspect

2nd

3rd

4th

5th

1st

metacarpal b.'s

capitate b.

hamate b.

pisiform b.

trapezium

trapezoid b.

triquetral b.

scaphoid b.

lunate b.

radius

ulna

capitate b.

trapezoid b.

trapezium

hamate b.

distal row

hamulus of hamate b.

palmar aspect

proximal row

pisiform b.

triquetral b.

lunate b.

scaphoid b.

D right carpus

	BONE	LOCATION	DESCRIPTION	ARTICULATION	MUSCLE/TENDON ATTACHMENTS
A	**clavicula** *clavicle*	uppermost part of chest, from root of neck to point of shoulder	long, curved bone forming anterior (ventral) portion of pectoral girdle; composed of: STERNAL END (with articular surface and impression for costoclavicular ligament), BODY (with subclavian groove), and ACROMIAL END (with articular facet, deltoid tubercle, trapezoid line, and conoid tubercle)	sternal end: with clavicular notch of manubrium of sternum, and cartilage of 1st rib acromial end: with medial side of acromion	medial 2/3 of bone: sternohyoid, sternocleidomastoid, pectoralis major, subclavius lateral 1/3 of bone: deltoid, trapezius
B	**coccyx** *coccyx*	inferior end of spinal column	small triangular bone; composed of from three to five VERTEBRAE (usually fused together), rudimentary TRANSVERSE PROCESSES, two coccygeal CORNUA, and two SURFACES (pelvic and dorsal)	with apex of sacrum	pelvic surface: levator ani, coccygeus dorsal surface: gluteus maximus, sphincter ani externus
C	**columna vertebralis** *vertebral column* *spine*	midline of back, from skull to pelvis	part of axial skeleton composed of 32 to 34 VERTEBRAE (7 cervical, 12 thoracic, 5 lumbar, 5 fused sacral, 3 to 5 fused coccygeal); contains VERTEBRAL CANAL; has three CURVATURES: cervical (convex anteriorly), thoracic (concave anteriorly), and lumbar (convex anteriorly)	atlas (1st cervical): with occipital condyles thoracic (1 to 10): with tubercles of ribs thoracic (12): with heads of ribs sacrum: with auricular surface of ilium	see: vertebrae, atlas, axis, sacrum, coccyx
D	**concha nasalis inferior** *inferior nasal concha*	nasal cavity; extends horizontally on lower outer wall of cavity	thin, spongy, scroll-shaped bone; composed of three PROCESSES (ethmoidal, lacrimal, and maxillary), two SURFACES (medial and lateral), two BORDERS (superior and inferior), and two ENDS (anterior and posterior)	with ethmoid, maxilla, palatine bone, and lacrimal bone	none

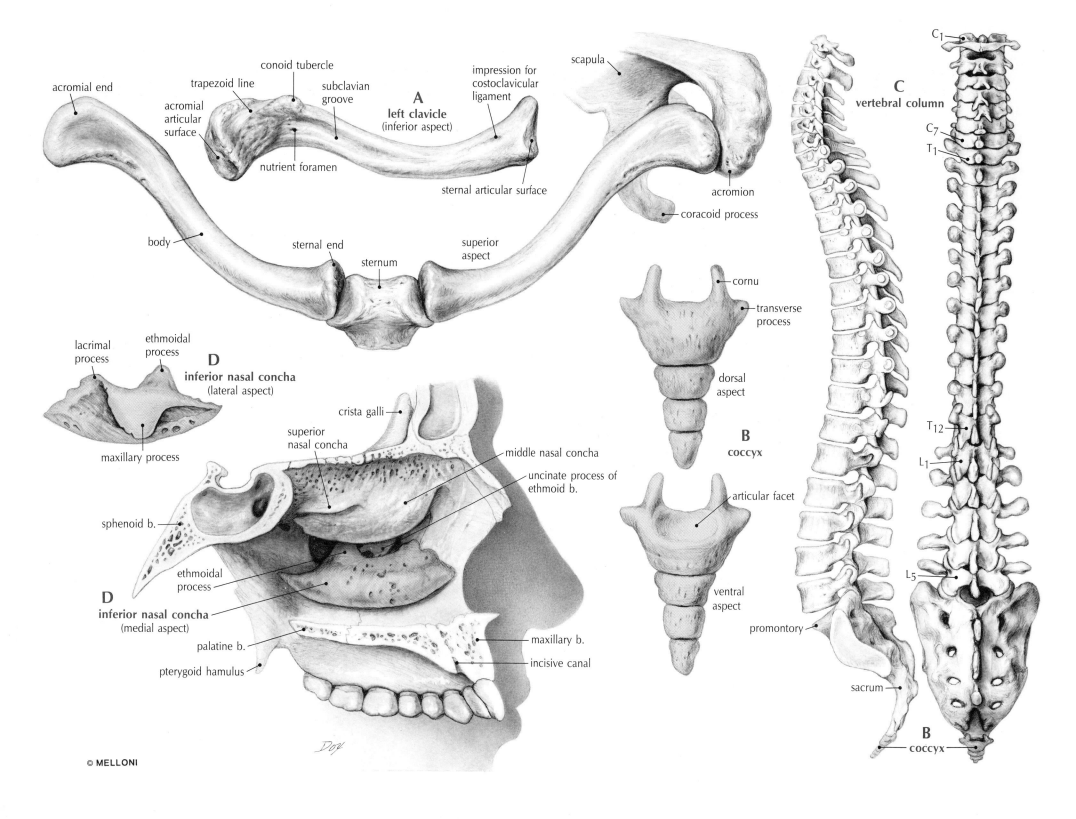

acromial end

conoid tubercle
trapezoid line
acromial
articular
surface
subclavian
groove

A
left clavicle
(inferior aspect)

impression for
costoclavicular
ligament

scapula

C
vertebral column

C₁

nutrient foramen

sternal articular surface

C₇

T₁

acromion

coracoid process

body

sternal end

sternum

superior
aspect

cornu

transverse
process

dorsal
aspect

B
coccyx

T₁₂

L₁

lacrimal
process

ethmoidal
process

D
inferior nasal concha
(lateral aspect)

crista galli

superior
nasal concha

middle nasal concha

uncinate process of
ethmoid b.

articular facet

maxillary process

sphenoid b.

ethmoidal
process

D
inferior nasal concha
(medial aspect)

palatine b.

pterygoid hamulus

maxillary b.

incisive canal

ventral
aspect

L₅

promontory

sacrum

B
coccyx

© MELLONI

BONE	LOCATION	DESCRIPTION	ARTICULATION	MUSCLE/TENDON ATTACHMENTS
costae *ribs*	thorax	24 (12 on each side) flat, narrow curved bones forming walls of thorax; known as TRUE RIBS (upper seven pairs) and FALSE RIBS (lower five pairs) of which the last two pairs are called FLOATING RIBS; typical rib composed of: POSTERIOR END (with head, neck, tubercle, and three articular facets), BODY (with costal groove and angle of rib), and ANTERIOR END Heads of atypical ribs have only one articular facet; 1st rib: shortest with two shallow grooves and scalene tubercle on body; 2nd rib: transition between 1st and typical rib; 10th rib: like typical rib but smaller; 11th and 12th rib: no neck, no tubercle	head: with bodies of adjoining vertebrae and intervertebral disk tubercle: with transverse process of corresponding thoracic vertebra anteriorly: with sternum (upper seven pairs via individual cartilages; each cartilage of ribs 8, 9, and 10 fuse with cartilage of rib above)	at different levels: intercostales (externi, interni, and intimi), levatores costarum, subcostales, iliocostalis (cervicis, thoracis, and lumborum), longissimus thoracis, quadratus lumborum, serratus posterior (superior and inferior), serratus anterior, scalenus (posterior, medius, anterior, and minimus), subclavius, obliquus abdominis (externus and internus), pectoralis (major and minor), diaphragm
cranium *skull*	head	superior end of axial skeleton; composed of: CALVARIA and FACIAL SKELETON; has six unpaired bones (frontal, occipital, mandible, ethmoid, sphenoid, vomer) and eight paired bones (parietal, temporal, maxillae, nasal, lacrimal, zygomatic, inferior nasal conchae, palatine); contains: CAVITIES (nasal, oral, orbital, cranial with three fossae); MIDDLE EAR CHAMBER; ear OSSICLES; INTERNAL EAR; SINUSES (frontal, sphenoidal, ethmoidal, maxillary)	occipital condyles: with superior articular facets of atlas (1st cervical vertebra)	see individual bones

A

B

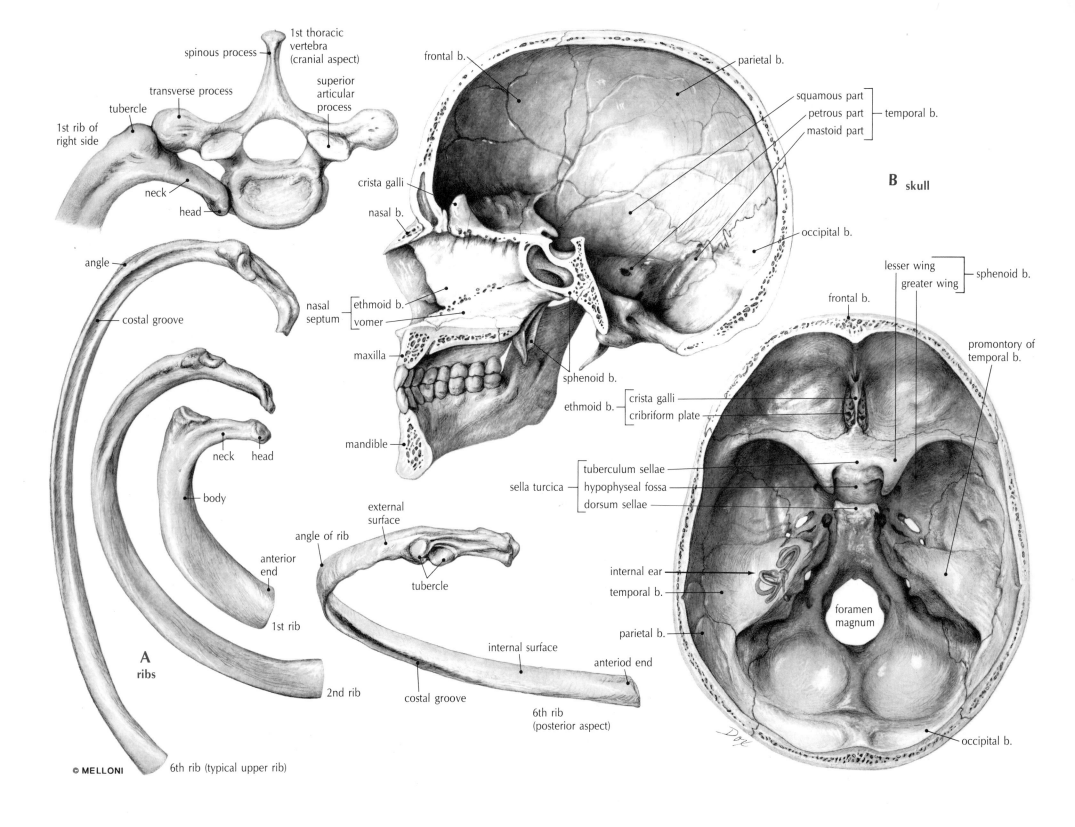

spinous process

1st thoracic vertebra (cranial aspect)

transverse process

superior articular process

tubercle

1st rib of right side

neck

head

frontal b.

parietal b.

squamous part
petrous part — temporal b.
mastoid part

crista galli

nasal b.

occipital b.

angle

costal groove

nasal septum — ethmoid b.
vomer

maxilla

sphenoid b.

lesser wing
greater wing — sphenoid b.

frontal b.

promontory of temporal b.

B skull

neck head

body

external surface

angle of rib

tubercle

ethmoid b. — crista galli
cribriform plate

tuberculum sellae
sella turcica — hypophyseal fossa
dorsum sellae

anterior end

1st rib

mandible

internal ear

temporal b.

parietal b.

foramen magnum

internal surface

anteriod end

A
ribs

2nd rib

costal groove

6th rib (posterior aspect)

© MELLONI

6th rib (typical upper rib)

occipital b.

BONE	LOCATION	DESCRIPTION	ARTICULATION	MUSCLE/TENDON ATTACHMENTS
femur *femur*	thigh, between hip and knee	longest, strongest, heaviest bone in body; composed of: PROXIMAL END (with head, fovea, anatomical neck, surgical neck, greater and lesser trochanters, trochanteric fossa, intertrochanteric crest, inter-trochanteric line, and quadrate tubercle); SHAFT (with gluteal tuberosity, linea aspera, pectineal line, lateral and medial supra-condylar lines, and popliteal surface); and DISTAL END (with lateral and medial condyles, lateral and medial epicondyles, intercondy-lar fossa, intercondylar line, patellar surface, and adductor tubercle)	PROXIMAL END head: with acetabulum of hipbone DISTAL END patellar surface: with articular (posterior) surface of patella condyles: with superior articular surface of tibia	greater trochanter: gluteus (medius and minimus), piriformis, common tendon of obturator internus and gemellus (superior and inferior) trochanteric fossa: obturator externus quadrate tubercle: quadratus femoris lesser trochanter: psoas major, iliacus shaft: pectineus; gluteus maximus; vastus (lateralis, intermedius, and medialis); adductor (brevis, magnus, and longus); articularis genu; biceps femoris (short head); plantaris; gastrocnemius (medial head) lateral condyle: gastrocnemius (lateral head), popliteus medial condyle: adductor magnus
fibula *fibula*	lateral aspect of leg; between the knee and ankle	slender lateral bone of leg; composed of: PROXIMAL END (with head, articular surface, apex, and neck); SHAFT with medial crest, three surfaces (medial, posterior, lateral), three borders (anterior, interosseous, posterior); and DISTAL END (with lateral malleolus, articular surface, malleolar fossa, and groove)	PROXIMAL END head: with inferior surface of lateral epicondyle of tibia DISTAL END lateral malleolus: with lateral surface of talus at the ankle	head: biceps femoris, peroneus longus, extensor digitorum longus medial surface of shaft: extensor digitorum longus, extensor hallucis longus, peroneus tertius posterior surface of shaft: soleus, flexor hallucis longus, tibialis posterior lateral surface of shaft: peroneus (longus, brevis)
humerus *humerus*	arm, between shoulder and elbow	largest and longest bone of upper extremity; composed of: PROXIMAL END (with head, anatomical neck, surgical neck, greater and lesser tubercles, intertubercular sulcus, and crests of greater and lesser tubercles); SHAFT (with lateral and medial borders, anterolateral, anteromedial and posterior surfaces, deltoid tuberosity, sulcus for radial nerve); and DISTAL END (with medial epicondyle, trochlea, capitulum, lateral epicondyle, olecranon fossa, ulnar sulcus, coronoid fossa, lateral and medial supracondylar ridges)	PROXIMAL END head: with glenoid fossa of scapula DISTAL END trochlea: with trochlear notch of ulna capitulum: with head of radius	greater tubercle: supraspinatus, teres minor, infraspinatus lesser tubercle: subscapularis shaft: pectoralis major, latissimus dorsi, brachialis, coracobrachialis, triceps (medial and lateral heads), teres major, deltoid, brachioradialis, extensor carpi radialis longus lateral epicondyle: anconeus, extensor digitorum, extensor carpi radialis brevis, extensor carpi ulnaris medial epicondyle: pronator teres, flexor carpi radialis, flexor carpi ulnaris, palmaris longus

A

B

C

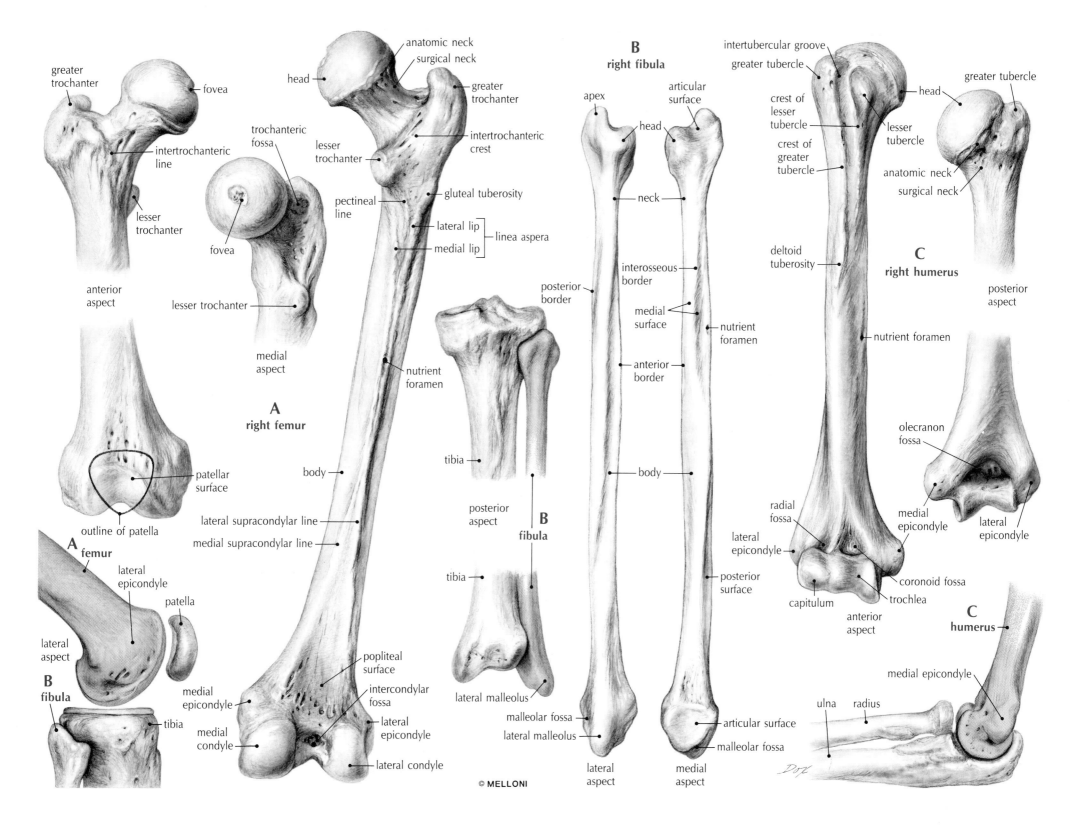

greater trochanter

fovea

intertrochanteric line

lesser trochanter

anterior aspect

trochanteric fossa

fovea

lesser trochanter

medial aspect

patellar surface

outline of patella

A femur

lateral epicondyle

lateral aspect

B fibula

tibia

patella

medial epicondyle

medial condyle

anatomic neck

surgical neck

head

greater trochanter

lesser trochanter

pectineal line

intertrochanteric crest

gluteal tuberosity

lateral lip ⎤
          ⎬ linea aspera
medial lip ⎦

nutrient foramen

A
right femur

body

lateral supracondylar line

medial supracondylar line

popliteal surface

intercondylar fossa

lateral epicondyle

lateral condyle

posterior border

tibia

posterior aspect

B
fibula

tibia

lateral malleolus

B
right fibula

apex

head

neck

articular surface

interosseous border

medial surface

anterior border

nutrient foramen

body

malleolar fossa

lateral malleolus

lateral aspect

posterior surface

articular surface

malleolar fossa

medial aspect

intertubercular groove

greater tubercle

crest of lesser tubercle

crest of greater tubercle

deltoid tuberosity

head

lesser tubercle

anatomic neck

surgical neck

greater tubercle

C
right humerus

posterior aspect

nutrient foramen

olecranon fossa

medial epicondyle

lateral epicondyle

radial fossa

lateral epicondyle

capitulum

coronoid fossa

trochlea

anterior aspect

C
humerus

medial epicondyle

ulna

radius

© MELLONI

	BONE	LOCATION	DESCRIPTION	ARTICULATION	MUSCLE/TENDON ATTACHMENTS
A	**incus** *incus*	middle ear, between stapes and malleus	one of three ear ossicles; composed of: BODY (with articular facet), LONG PROCESS, SHORT PROCESS and LENTIFORM PROCESS (with articular facet)	body: with head of malleus lentiform process: with head of stapes	none
B	**malleus** *malleus*	middle ear, between tympanic membrane and incus	mallet-shaped, largest and most lateral of ear ossicles; composed of: HEAD (with articular facet), NECK, MANUBRIUM, ANTERIOR PROCESS, and LATERAL PROCESS	posterior aspect of head: with anterior surface of body of incus	tensor tympani
C	**mandible** *mandible*	lowest portion of face	the lower jaw; horseshoe-shaped and strongest bone of face containing sockets for 16 teeth; composed of: BODY (with two mental tubercles, two mental foramina, two oblique lines and mental protuberance on external surface; two digastric fossae, mental spine, two mylohyoid lines, two submandibular fossae and two sublingual fossae on internal surface), a RAMUS on either side of bone (each with condylar process, pterygoid fovea, neck, mandibular notch, and coronoid process; on internal surface of ramus: mandibular foramen, lingula, and mylohyoid groove)	condylar process: with mandibular fossa of the squamous part of both temporal bones	body: mentalis, orbicularis oris (incisivus labii inferioris), depressor labii inferioris, depressor anguli oris, buccinator, platysma, genioglossus, geniohyoid, digastric (anterior belly), mylohyoid ramus: superior constrictor of pharynx, medial pterygoid, masseter coronoid process: temporalis neck: lateral pterygoid (lower head)
D	**maxilla** *maxilla*	middle of face	bone which, united with its opposite, forms the upper jaw and most of the roof of the mouth, also forms the floor and lateral wall of the nasal cavity, and part of the orbit; encloses the maxillary sinus and houses the upper teeth; composed of: BODY (with four SURFACES—orbital, anterior, infratemporal, and nasal) and four PROCESSES (zygomatic, frontal, palatine, and alveolar)	body: with maxilla of opposite side, lacrimal bone, orbital plate of ethmoid, orbital and pyramidal processes of palatine bone, perpendicular plate of ethmoid bone, and inferior nasal concha zygomatic process: with zygomatic bone frontal process: with frontal, nasal, and lacrimal bones palatine process: with palatine process of opposite bone, vomer, and horizontal plate of palatine bone	body: orbicularis oris (incisivus labii superioris), levator anguli oris, nasalis, depressor septinasi, medial pterygoid, obliquus inferior (of eyeball) frontal process: orbicularis oculi, levator labii superioris alaeque nasi alveolar process: buccinator zygomatic process: levator labii superioris

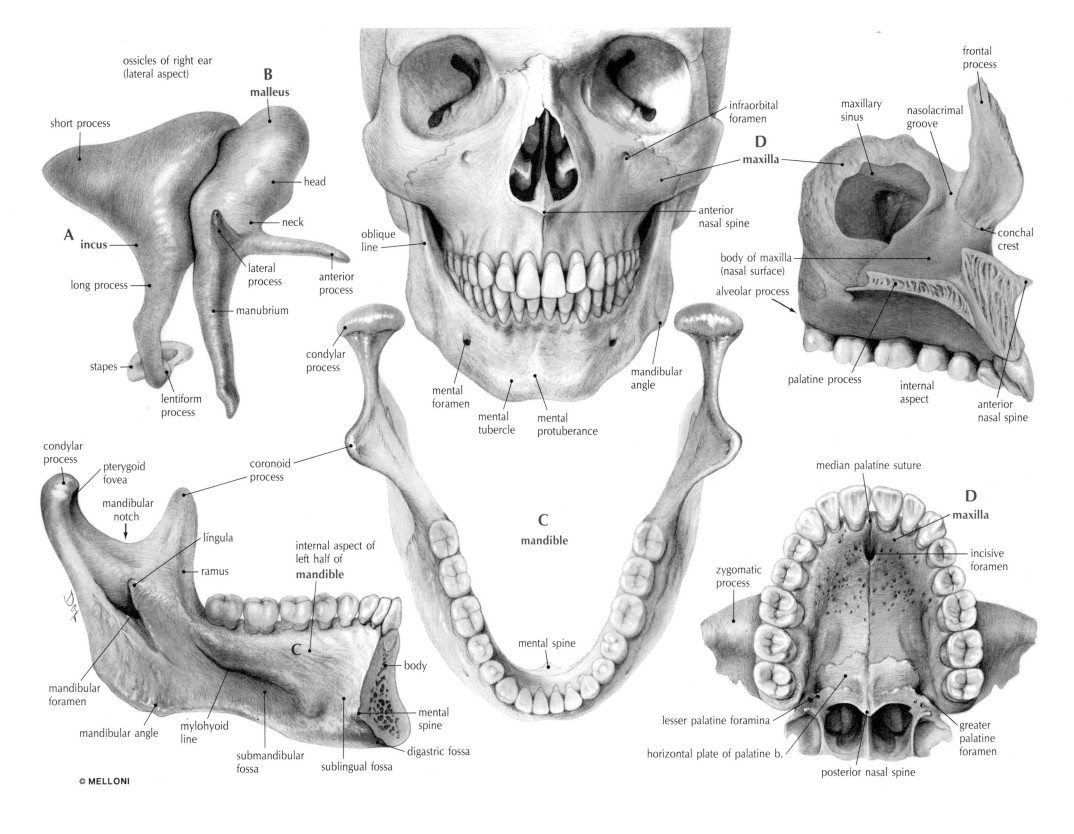

ossicles of right ear
(lateral aspect)

B
malleus

short process

head

neck

A **incus**

lateral
process

anterior
process

long process

manubrium

stapes

lentiform
process

condylar
process

pterygoid
fovea

mandibular
notch

lingula

ramus

coronoid
process

condylar
process

internal aspect of
left half of
mandible

C

mandibular
foramen

mandibular angle

mylohyoid
line

submandibular
fossa

sublingual fossa

body

mental
spine

digastric fossa

infraorbital
foramen

oblique
line

anterior
nasal spine

condylar
process

mental
foramen

mandibular
angle

mental
tubercle

mental
protuberance

C
mandible

mental spine

frontal
process

maxillary
sinus

nasolacrimal
groove

D
maxilla

conchal
crest

body of maxilla
(nasal surface)

alveolar process

palatine process

internal
aspect

anterior
nasal spine

median palatine suture

D

maxilla

incisive
foramen

zygomatic
process

lesser palatine foramina

horizontal plate of palatine b.

posterior nasal spine

greater
palatine
foramen

© MELLONI

BONE	LOCATION	DESCRIPTION	ARTICULATION	MUSCLE/TENDON ATTACHMENTS
metacarpalia *metacarpus*	hand, between wrist and fingers	5 miniature long bones; each consisting of: BASE, SHAFT, and HEAD; numbered from 1st to 5th starting from side of thumb	head of each bone: with proximal phalanx of corresponding finger 1st metacarpal: with trapezium 2nd metacarpal: with 3rd metacarpal, trapezium, trapezoid, and capitate bones 3rd metacarpal: with 2nd and 4th metacarpal and capitate bones 4th metacarpal: with 3rd and 5th metacarpal, capitate, and hamate bones 5th metacarpal: with 4th metacarpal and hamate bones	1st metacarpal: opponens pollicis, abductor pollicis longus, radial head of 1st dorsal interosseous, 1st palmar interosseous 2nd metacarpal: extensor carpi radialis longus and brevis, flexor carpi radialis, ulnar head of 1st dorsal interosseous, 2nd palmar interosseous, radial head of 2nd dorsal interosseous 3rd metacarpal: flexor carpi radialis, extensor carpi radialis brevis, ulnar head of 2nd dorsal interosseous, radial head of 3rd dorsal interosseous, transverse head of adductor pollicis 4th metacarpal: 3rd palmar interosseous, ulnar head of 3rd dorsal interosseous, radial head of 4th dorsal interosseous 5th metacarpal: extensor carpi ulnaris, opponens digiti minimi, 4th palmar interosseous, ulnar head of 4th dorsal interosseous
metatarsalia *metatarsus*	foot; between distal row of tarsal bones and 1st phalanges of toes	five miniature bones, each consisting of: BASE, SHAFT, and HEAD; numbered 1st to 5th, from medial to lateral side	head of each bone: with proximal phalanx of corresponding toe 1st metatarsal: with 2nd metatarsal and 2nd cuneiform bones 2nd metatarsal: with 1st and 3rd metatarsal bones and cuneiform bones (medial, intermediate, lateral) 3rd metatarsal: with 2nd and 4th metatarsal bones and lateral cuneiform bone 4th metatarsal: with 3rd and 5th metatarsal bones and cuboid bone 5th metatarsal: with 4th metatarsal bone and cuboid bone	1st metatarsal: tibialis anterior, 1st dorsal interosseous 2nd metatarsal: lateral head of 1st dorsal interosseous, medial head of 2nd dorsal interosseous 3rd metatarsal: lateral head of 2nd dorsal interosseous, 1st plantar medial head of 3rd dorsal interosseous 4th metatarsal: lateral head of 3rd dorsal, 2nd plantar interosseous, medial head of 4th dorsal interosseous 5th metatarsal: peroneus tertius, peroneus brevis, flexor digiti minimi brevis, lateral head of 4th dorsal interosseous, 3rd plantar interosseous

A

B

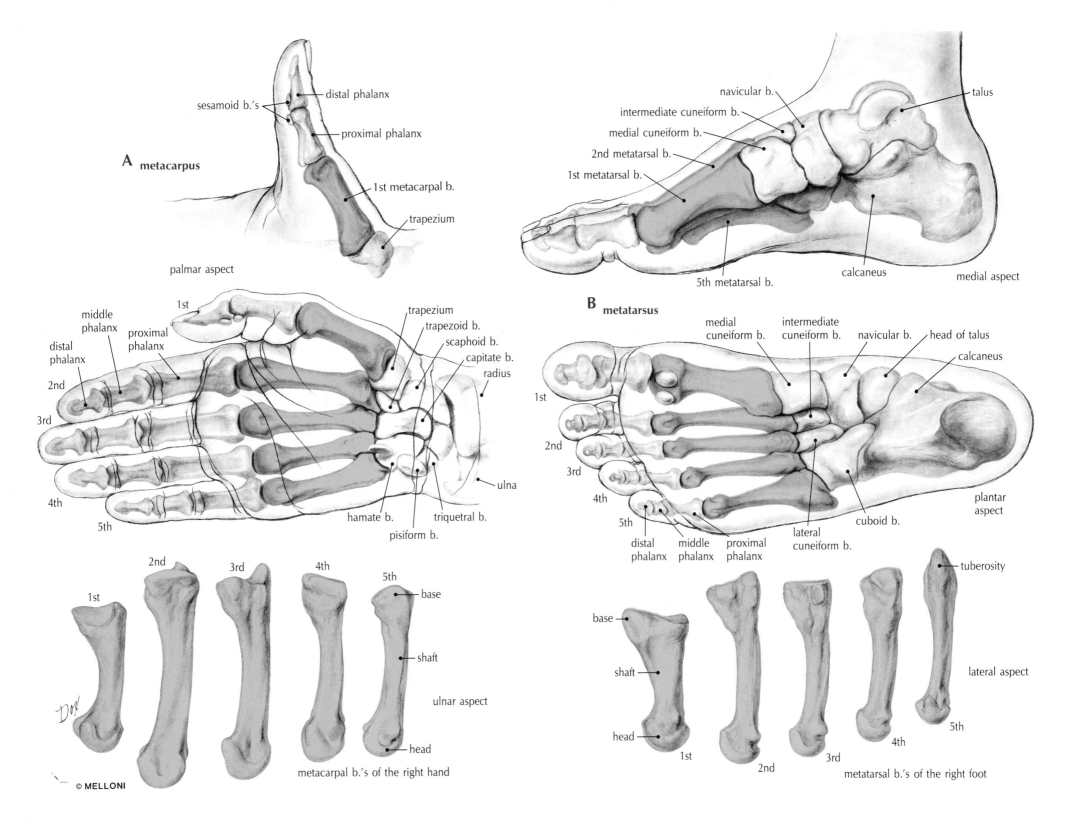

A metacarpus

sesamoid b.'s — distal phalanx

proximal phalanx

1st metacarpal b.

trapezium

palmar aspect

navicular b.

intermediate cuneiform b. — talus

medial cuneiform b.

2nd metatarsal b.

1st metatarsal b.

5th metatarsal b.

calcaneus

medial aspect

B metatarsus

middle phalanx

proximal phalanx

distal phalanx

2nd

3rd

4th

5th

1st

trapezium

trapezoid b.

scaphoid b.

capitate b.

radius

ulna

hamate b.

pisiform b.

triquetral b.

medial cuneiform b.

intermediate cuneiform b.

navicular b.

head of talus

calcaneus

1st

2nd

3rd

4th

5th

distal phalanx

middle phalanx

proximal phalanx

lateral cuneiform b.

cuboid b.

plantar aspect

1st

2nd

3rd

4th

5th

base

shaft

head

metacarpal b.'s of the right hand

ulnar aspect

© MELLONI

tuberosity

base

shaft

head

1st

2nd

3rd

4th

5th

lateral aspect

metatarsal b.'s of the right foot

BONE	LOCATION	DESCRIPTION	ARTICULATION	MUSCLE/TENDON ATTACHMENTS
os capitatum *capitate bone*	wrist; center of distal row of carpal bones	largest bone of carpus with six SURFACES (distal, proximal, medial, lateral, dorsal, and palmar)	distal surface: with 2nd, 3rd, and 4th metacarpal bones proximal surface: with lunate bone medial surface: with hamate bone lateral surface: with scaphoid bone	palmar surface: adductor pollicis (oblique head), flexor pollicis brevis (deep head)
os coxae *hipbone* *innominate bone*	hip and pelvis	large, irregularly shaped, paired bone, which, with sacrum and opposite hipbone, forms the pelvis; composed of: PUBIS, ISCHIUM, and ILIUM; contains the OBTURATOR FORAMEN and ACETABULUM (formed superiorly by ilium, anteroinferiorly by pubis, and posteroinferiorly by ischium)	anteriorly: with bone of opposite side (through pubic symphysis) posteriorly: with sacrum laterally: with head of femur	see ilium, pubis, and ischium
os cuboideum *cuboid bone*	lateral side of foot, between calcaneus and 4th and 5th metatarsal bones	short bone with: PROCESS; TUBEROSITY; GROOVE for tendon of peroneus longus muscle; six SURFACES (dorsal, lateral, plantar, medial, distal, and proximal)	medial surface: with lateral cuneiform bone and navicular bone (occasionally) distal surface: with 4th and 5th metatarsal bones proximal surface: with calcaneus plantar surface: with sesamoid bone	plantar surface: tibialis posterior, flexor hallucis brevis
os cuneiforme intermedium *intermediate cuneiform bone*	foot, at base of 2nd toe; distal row of tarsus, between medial and lateral cuneiform bones	short wedge-shaped bone; smallest of cuneiform bones; has six SURFACES (dorsal, plantar, proximal, distal, lateral, medial)	distal surface: with 2nd metatarsal bone proximal surface: with navicular bone medial surface: with medial cuneiform bone lateral surface: with lateral cuneiform bone	plantar surface: tibialis posterior

A
B
C
D

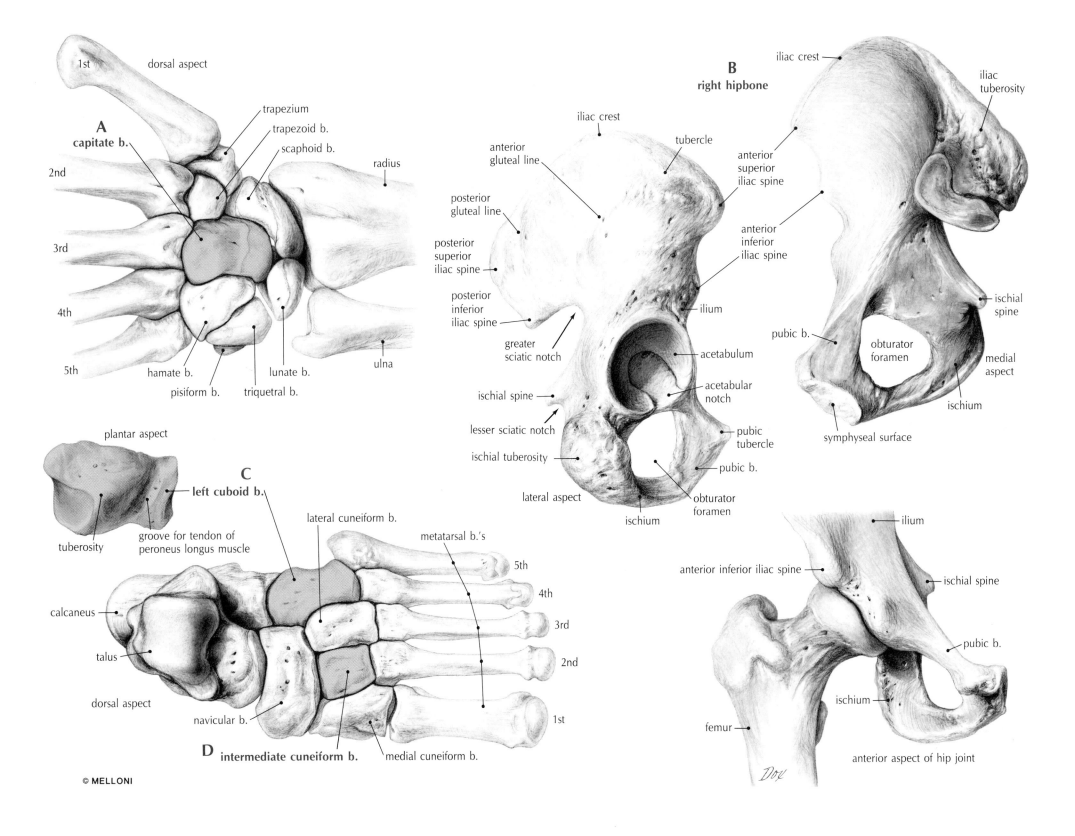

A

1st
dorsal aspect
trapezium
trapezoid b.
capitate b.
scaphoid b.
radius
2nd
3rd
4th
5th
hamate b.
pisiform b.
triquetral b.
lunate b.
ulna

B
right hipbone

iliac crest
iliac crest
iliac tuberosity
tubercle
anterior gluteal line
anterior superior iliac spine
posterior gluteal line
anterior inferior iliac spine
posterior superior iliac spine
posterior inferior iliac spine
greater sciatic notch
ilium
pubic b.
ischial spine
acetabulum
obturator foramen
acetabular notch
medial aspect
ischial spine
lesser sciatic notch
ischium
ischial tuberosity
pubic tubercle
symphyseal surface
lateral aspect
pubic b.
ischium
obturator foramen

C

plantar aspect
left cuboid b.
lateral cuneiform b.
metatarsal b.'s
tuberosity
groove for tendon of peroneus longus muscle
5th
4th
3rd
2nd
calcaneus
talus
dorsal aspect
navicular b.
1st
D   intermediate cuneiform b.
medial cuneiform b.

ilium
anterior inferior iliac spine
ischial spine
pubic b.
ischium
femur
anterior aspect of hip joint

© MELLONI

Dox

BONE	LOCATION	DESCRIPTION	ARTICULATION	MUSCLE/TENDON ATTACHMENTS
os cuneiform laterale *lateral cuneiform bone*	foot, at base of 3rd toe; distal row of tarsus, between intermediate and cuneiform and cuboid bones	short wedge-shaped bone with six SURFACES (dorsal, plantar, medial, distal, proximal, and lateral)	medial surface: with intermediate cuneiform and 2nd metatarsal bones distal surface: with 3rd metatarsal bone lateral surface: with cuboid and 4th metatarsal bones proximal surface: with navicular bone	plantar surface: tibialis posterior, flexor hallucis brevis (occasionally)
os cuneiforme mediale *medial cuneiform bone*	medial side of foot, at base of big toe; distal row of tarsal bones	short wedge-shaped bone; largest of cuneiform bones; has six SURFACES (dorsal, plantar, distal, proximal, medial, and lateral)	distal surface: with 1st metatarsal bone proximal surface: with navicular bone lateral surface: with 2nd metatarsal and intermediate cuneiform bones	plantar surface: tibialis posterior medial surface: tibialis anterior
ossa digitorum [phalanges] manus *phalanges of hand*	fingers	14 bones of fingers, three in each finger (proximal, middle, and distal) and two in thumb (proximal and distal); each bone consists of BASE, BODY, and HEAD	thumb—proximal phalanx: with 1st metacarpal bone and distal phalanx; distal phalanx: with proximal phalanx fingers 2, 3, 4, 5—proximal phalanx: with corresponding metacarpal bone and middle phalanx; middle phalanx: with proximal and distal phalanges; distal phalanx: with middle phalanx	thumb—proximal phalanx: extensor pollicis brevis, flexor pollicis brevis, abductor pollicis brevis, adductor pollicis; distal phalanx: extensor pollicis longus, flexor pollicis longus fingers 2, 3, 4—proximal phalanx: extensor indicis (finger 2), lumbricalis, interosseous dorsalis, interosseous palmaris (fingers 2 and 4); middle phalanx: extensor digitorum, flexor digitorum superficialis; distal phalanx: extensor digitorum, flexor digitorum profundus little finger—proximal phalanx: flexor digiti minimi, flexor digiti minimi brevis, abductor digiti minimi, lumbricalis, interosseous palmaris; middle phalanx: extensor digitorum, extensor digiti minimi, flexor digitorum superficialis; distal phalanx: extensor digitorum, extensor digiti minimi, flexor digitorum profundus

A

B

C

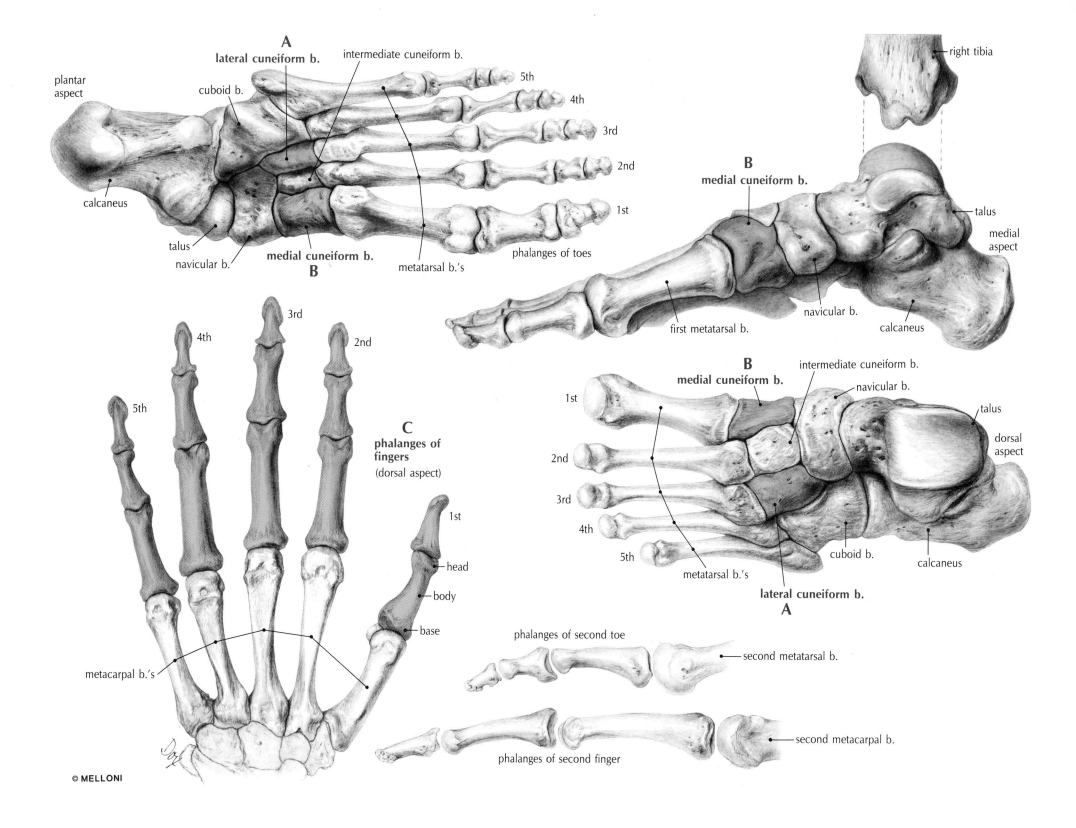

A

lateral cuneiform b.

intermediate cuneiform b.

plantar aspect

cuboid b.

5th

4th

3rd

2nd

1st

calcaneus

talus

navicular b.

medial cuneiform b.

B

metatarsal b.'s

phalanges of toes

right tibia

B

medial cuneiform b.

talus

medial aspect

navicular b.

calcaneus

first metatarsal b.

B

intermediate cuneiform b.

medial cuneiform b.

navicular b.

1st

talus

dorsal aspect

2nd

3rd

4th

5th

metatarsal b.'s

cuboid b.

calcaneus

lateral cuneiform b.

A

C

phalanges of fingers

(dorsal aspect)

3rd

4th

2nd

5th

1st

head

body

base

metacarpal b.'s

phalanges of second toe

second metatarsal b.

phalanges of second finger

second metacarpal b.

© MELLONI

BONE	LOCATION	DESCRIPTION	ARTICULATION	MUSCLE/TENDON ATTACHMENTS
ossa digitorum [phalanges] pedis *phalanges of foot*	toes	14 bones of toes, three in each toe (proximal, middle and distal) and 2 in big toe (proximal and distal); each bone consists of BASE, BODY, and HEAD	big toe—proximal phalanx: with 1st metatarsal bone and distal phalanx toes 2, 3, 4, 5—proximal phalanx: with corresponding metatarsal bone and middle phalanx; middle phalanx: with proximal and distal phalanges; distal phalanx: with proximal phalanx	big toe—proximal phalanx: extensor hallucis brevis, flexor hallucis brevis, abductor hallucis, adductor hallucis; distal phalanx: extensor hallucis longus, flexor hallucis longus toes 2, 3, 4—proximal phalanx: lumbricalis, interosseous dorsalis, interosseous plantaris (toes 3 and 4); middle phalanx: extensor digitorum longus, extensor digitorum brevis, flexor digitorum brevis; distal phalanx: extensor digitorum longus, extensor digitorum brevis, flexor digitorum longus little toe—proximal phalanx: flexor digiti minimi brevis, abductor digiti minimi, lumbricalis, interosseous plantaris; middle phalanx: extensor digitorum longus, extensor digitorum brevis, flexor digitorum brevis; distal phalanx: extensor digitorum longus, flexor digitorum longus, abductor digiti minimi
os ethmoidale *ethmoid bone*	anterior portion of skull, below frontal bone, anterior to sphenoid bone	unpaired bone forming part of orbits, posterosuperior part of nasal septum, and roof and lateral walls of nasal cavity; composed of: CRIBRIFORM PLATE, CRISTA GALLI (with two alar processes), PERPENDICULAR PLATE and two LABYRINTHS (each with ethmoidal cells, superior and middle nasal conchae, orbital plate, and uncinate process)	cribriform plate: with frontal bone perpendicular plate: with nasal spine of frontal bone, nasal bones, sphenoid, and vomer labyrinths: with maxilla; frontal, palatine, lacrimal, and sphenoid bones; and inferior nasal concha	none
os frontale *frontal bone*	anterosuperior part of skull	flat, unpaired bone of forehead forming part of roof of orbits and nasal cavity; composed of: EXTERNAL SURFACE (either side of midline with a frontal eminence, superciliary arch, supraorbital margin, and supraorbital notch), two TEMPORAL SURFACES (each with zygomatic process, temporal line, parietal margin, and part of temporal fossa), INTERNAL SURFACE (with frontal crest and foramen cecum), two ORBITAL PORTIONS (each with an orbital plate, fossa for lacrimal gland, and ethmoidal notch), and NASAL PORTION (with nasal spine); contains FRONTAL SINUSES	zygomatic processes: with zygomatic bones nasal part: with nasal bones and perpendicular plate of ethmoid bone parietal margins: with greater wings of sphenoid bones and parietal bones ethmoidal notch: with cribriform plate of ethmoid bone orbital plates: with greater and lesser wings of sphenoid bone	temporal surface: temporal supraorbital margin: superciliary corrugator

A

B

C

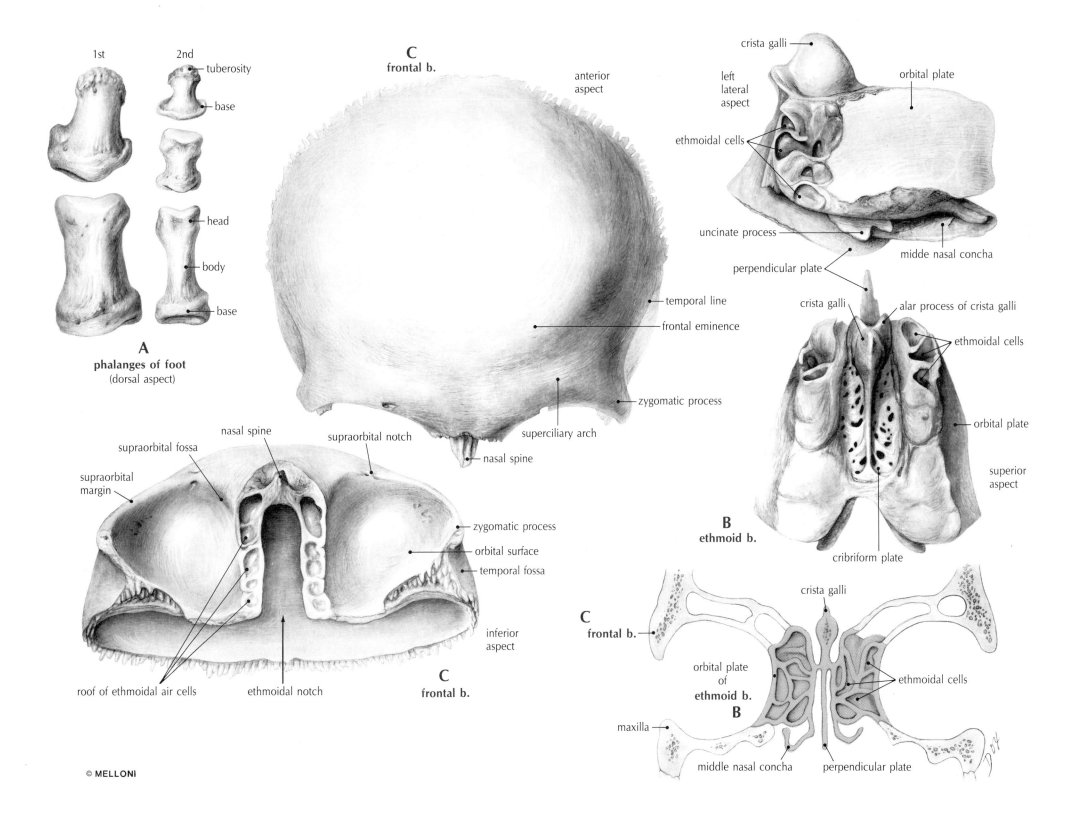

1st 2nd

tuberosity

base

head

body

base

A

phalanges of foot
(dorsal aspect)

C
frontal b.

anterior
aspect

temporal line

frontal eminence

zygomatic process

superciliary arch

nasal spine

supraorbital fossa

nasal spine

supraorbital notch

supraorbital
margin

zygomatic process

orbital surface

temporal fossa

inferior
aspect

roof of ethmoidal air cells

ethmoidal notch

C
frontal b.

crista galli

left
lateral
aspect

orbital plate

ethmoidal cells

uncinate process

midde nasal concha

perpendicular plate

crista galli

alar process of crista galli

ethmoidal cells

orbital plate

superior
aspect

B
ethmoid b.

cribriform plate

C
frontal b.

crista galli

orbital plate
of
ethmoid b.

ethmoidal cells

B

maxilla

middle nasal concha

perpendicular plate

© MELLONI

	BONE	LOCATION	DESCRIPTION	ARTICULATION	MUSCLE/TENDON ATTACHMENTS
A	**os hamatum** *hamate bone*	wrist, most medial of distal row of carpal bones	wedge-shaped bone at the base of ring and little fingers; has HAMULUS (a hook-like process) on its palmar surface; 6 SURFACES (distal, proximal, medial, lateral, dorsal, and palmar)	distal surface: with 4th and 5th metacarpal bones proximal surface: with lunate bone medial surface: with triquetral bone lateral surface: with capitate bone	palmar surface: flexor digiti minimi, opponens digiti minimi
B	**os hyoideum** *hyoid bone*	anterior part of neck	small unpaired U-shaped bone; composed of: BODY and four CORNUA (two greater, two lesser)	none	body: geniohyoid, hyoglossus, mylohyoid, sternohyoid, omohyoid, genioglossus, sternohyoid, thyrohyoid, levator glandulae thyroideae, chondroglossus greater cornu: middle constrictor of pharynx, hyoglossus, stylohyoid, thyrohyoid lesser cornu: middle constrictor of pharynx, chondroglossus
C	**os illi [ilium]** *ilium*	pelvis	superior portion of hipbone: forms superior portion of acetabulum; composed of: BODY, ALA with iliac crest, four SPINES (anterior superior, anterior inferior, posterior superior, and posterior inferior), GLUTEAL SURFACE (with anterior, posterior, and inferior gluteal lines), MEDIAL SURFACE (with arcuate line and iliac fossa), SACROPELVIC SURFACE (with auricular surface, pelvic surface and iliac tuberosity), two LIPS (internal and external), TUBERCLE, INTERMEDIATE LINE, and upper portion of GREATER SCIATIC NOTCH	body: with pubis, ischium, and head of femur	iliac crest: obliquus abdominis (internus and externus), latissimus dorsi, tensor fasciae latae, transversus abdominis, quadratus lumborum, erector spinae anterior superior spine: sartorius gluteal surface: piriformis, gluteus (maximus, medius, and minimus), rectus femoris iliac fossa: iliacus, psoas major pelvic surface: superior part of obturator internus

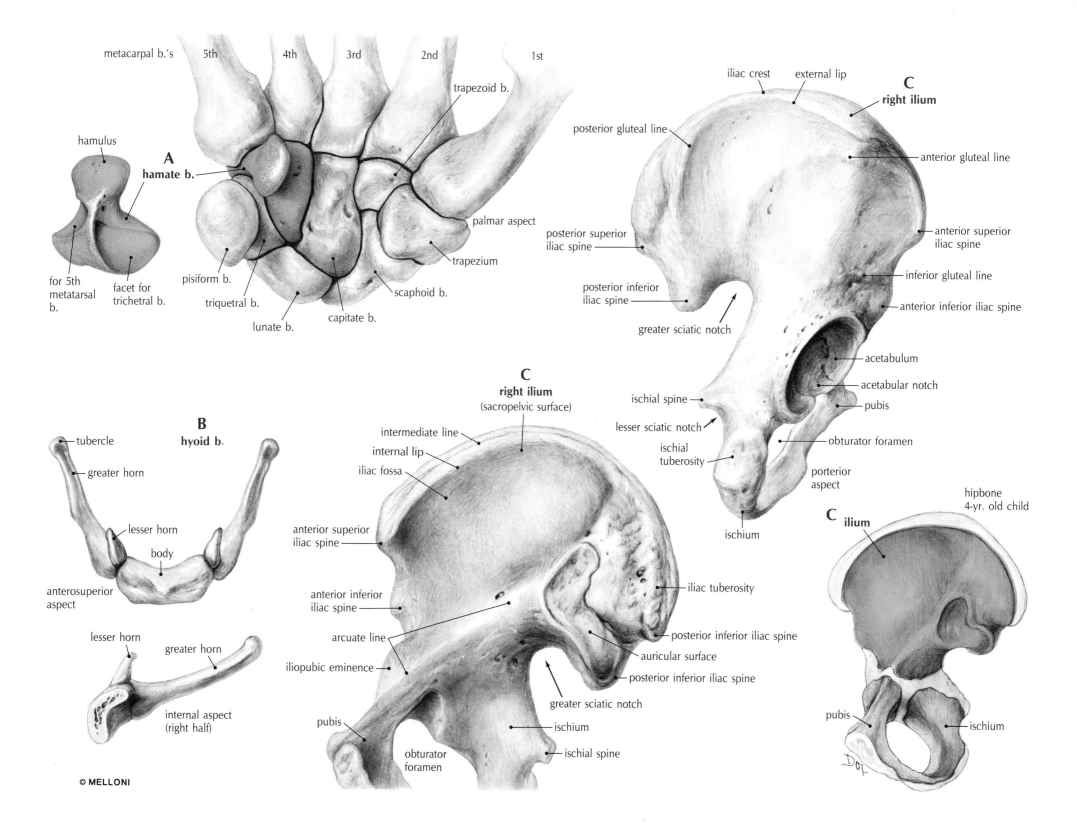

metacarpal b.'s 5th 4th 3rd 2nd 1st

hamulus

A
hamate b.

for 5th metatarsal b.

facet for trichetral b.

trapezoid b.

palmar aspect

trapezium

pisiform b.

scaphoid b.

triquetral b.

lunate b.

capitate b.

B
hyoid b.

tubercle

greater horn

lesser horn

body

anterosuperior aspect

lesser horn

greater horn

internal aspect (right half)

© MELLONI

C
right ilium
(sacropelvic surface)

intermediate line

internal lip

iliac fossa

anterior superior iliac spine

anterior inferior iliac spine

arcuate line

iliopubic eminence

pubis

obturator foramen

iliac tuberosity

posterior inferior iliac spine

auricular surface

posterior inferior iliac spine

greater sciatic notch

ischium

ischial spine

C
right ilium

iliac crest

external lip

posterior gluteal line

anterior gluteal line

anterior superior iliac spine

posterior superior iliac spine

inferior gluteal line

posterior inferior iliac spine

anterior inferior iliac spine

greater sciatic notch

acetabulum

acetabular notch

ischial spine

pubis

lesser sciatic notch

ischial tuberosity

obturator foramen

porterior aspect

ischium

hipbone
4-yr. old child

C **ilium**

pubis

ischium

	BONE	LOCATION	DESCRIPTION	ARTICULATION	MUSCLE/TENDON ATTACHMENTS
A	**os ischii [ischium]** *ischium*	pelvis	posteroinferior part of hipbone; forms inferolateral border of obturator foramen and postero-inferior portion of acetabulum; composed of: BODY with two surfaces (femoral and dorsal), RAMUS (with anterior and posterior surfaces, and ischial tuberosity), ISCHIAL SPINE, LESSER SCIATIC NOTCH, and lower portion of GREATER SCIATIC NOTCH	body: with pubis, ilium, and head of femur ramus: with inferior ramus of pubis	body: obturator internus, obturator externus, quadratus femoris ramus: obturator externus, adductor magnus, gracilis, obturator internus, sphincter urethrae, ischiocavernosus, transversus perinei superficialis ischial tuberosity: semimembranosus, semitendinosus, biceps femoris (long head), adductor magnus, gemellus inferior ischial spine: coccygeus, levator ani, gemellus superior
B	**os lacrimale** *lacrimal bone*	anteromedial wall of orbit	paired, smallest, and most fragile bone of face; composed of: two SURFACES (orbital and nasal), four BORDERS (anterior, superior, posterior, and inferior), descending PROCESS, posterior lacrimal CREST, and lacrimal HAMULUS	anterior border: with frontal process of maxilla superior border: with frontal bone posterior border: with orbital plate of ethmoid bone inferior border: with orbital surface of maxilla descending process: with maxilla and lacrimal process of nasal concha	lacrimal part of orbicularis oculi
C	**os lunatum** *lunate bone* *semilunar bone*	wrist, in middle of proximal row of carpal bones	crescent-shaped with convexity toward radius; has six SURFACES (proximal, distal, lateral, medial, dorsal, and palmar)	proximal surface: with radius distal surface: with capitate bone medial surface: with triquetral bone lateral surface: with scaphoid bone	none
D	**os nasale** *nasal bone*	middle of face	small bone forming, with nasal bone of opposite side, the bridge of the nose; has two SURFACES (external and internal), four BORDERS (superior, inferior, lateral, and medial), and an ETHMOIDAL GROOVE	superior border: frontal bone lateral border: frontal process of maxilla medial border: opposite nasal bone, nasal spine of frontal bone, and perpendicular plate of ethmoid bone	none

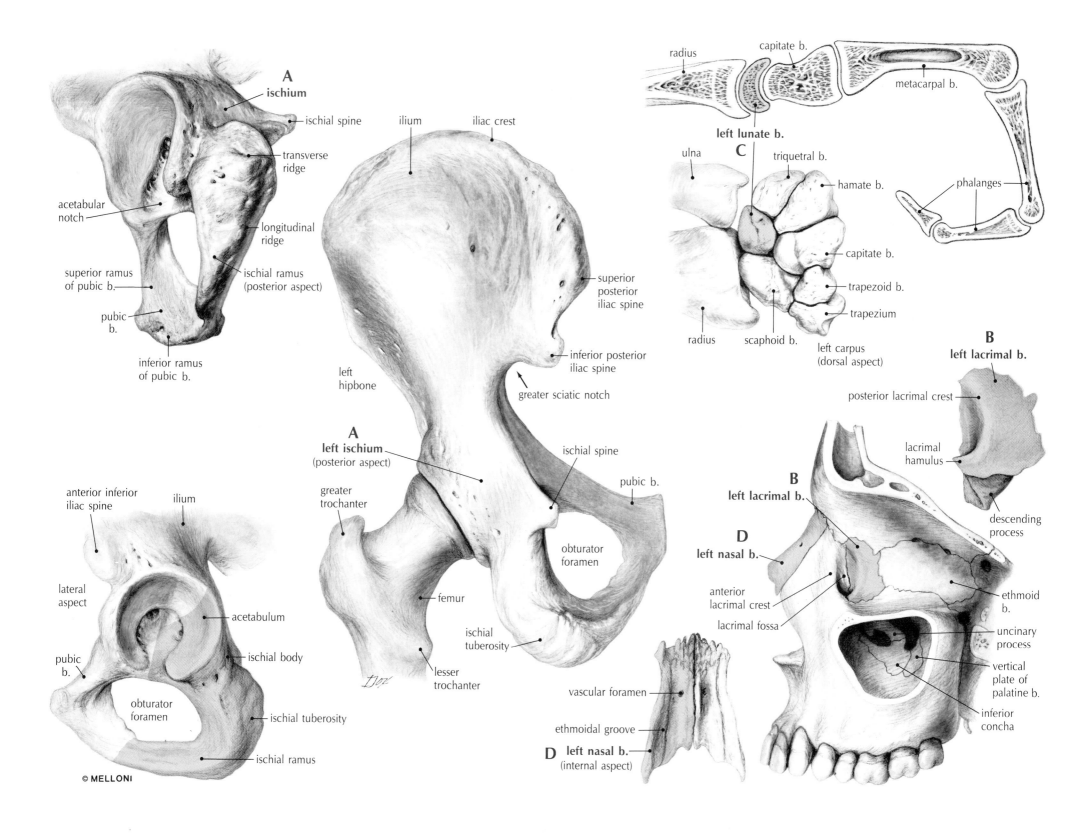

A

ischium

ischial spine

transverse ridge

acetabular notch

longitudinal ridge

superior ramus of pubic b.

ischial ramus (posterior aspect)

pubic b.

inferior ramus of pubic b.

ilium

iliac crest

left hipbone

superior posterior iliac spine

inferior posterior iliac spine

greater sciatic notch

A
left ischium
(posterior aspect)

greater trochanter

ischial spine

pubic b.

obturator foramen

femur

ischial tuberosity

lesser trochanter

anterior inferior iliac spine

ilium

lateral aspect

acetabulum

pubic b.

ischial body

obturator foramen

ischial tuberosity

ischial ramus

© MELLONI

radius

capitate b.

metacarpal b.

left lunate b.

ulna

C

triquetral b.

hamate b.

capitate b.

trapezoid b.

trapezium

radius

scaphoid b.

left carpus
(dorsal aspect)

phalanges

B
left lacrimal b.

posterior lacrimal crest

lacrimal hamulus

descending process

B
left lacrimal b.

D
left nasal b.

anterior lacrimal crest

lacrimal fossa

ethmoid b.

uncinary process

vertical plate of palatine b.

inferior concha

vascular foramen

ethmoidal groove

D **left nasal b.**
(internal aspect)

	BONE	LOCATION	DESCRIPTION	ARTICULATION	MUSCLE/TENDON ATTACHMENTS
A	**os naviculare** *navicular bone*	foot; medial aspect of tarsus between talus and 3 cuneiform bones	boat-shaped bone; shortest bone of tarsus; has TUBEROSITY on medial surface; six SURFACES (distal, proximal, medial, lateral, dorsal, and plantar)	proximal surface: with head of talus distal surface: with three cuneiform bones	tuberosity: tibialis posterior
B	**os occipitale** *occipital bone*	inferoposterior part of cranium	unpaired bone enclosing foramen magnum; composed of: SQUAMOUS PART, has external surface (with external occipital protuberance, highest nuchal line, superior nuchal line, inferior nuchal line); internal surface (with internal occipital protuberance, and sulci for superior sagittal sinus, transverse sinus, and sigmoid sinus); BASILAR PART, inferior surface (with pharyngeal tubercle); superior surface (with clivus); LATERAL PARTS, inferior surfaces (each with occipital condyle, hypoglossal canal, condylar canal, condylar fossa, jugular process, jugular notch, intrajugular process); superior surfaces (each with a jugular tubercle)	squamous part: with temporal bones (mastoid parts), parietal bones basilar part: with temporal bones (petrous parts), sphenoid bones occipital condyles: with atlas (superior facets)	squamous part: semispinalis capitis, obliquus capitis superior, rectus capitis posterior (major and minor), splenius capitis, sternocleidomastoideus, occipitofrontalis (occipital belly), and trapezius basilar part: longus capitis, rectus capitis anterior lateral part: rectus capitis lateralis
C	**os palatinum** *palatine bone*	posterior nasal cavity	L-shaped, paired bone; contributes to formation of hard palate, floor and lateral wall of nasal cavity, and floor of orbit; composed of: three PROCESSES (pyramidal, orbital, sphenoidal) and two PLATES (horizontal, perpendicular)	horizontal plate: palatine process of maxilla, opposite palatine bone, vomer perpendicular plate: inferior and middle nasal conchae; maxilla; sphenoid bone (medial pterygoid plate, body) pyramidal process: lateral and medial pterygoid plates, tuberosity of maxilla orbital process: maxilla, sphenoidal concha, labyrinth of ethmoid bone sphenoidal process: sphenoidal concha, medial pterygoid plate, ala of vomer	horizontal plate: tensor veli palatini, musculus uvulae pyramidal process: medial pterygoid

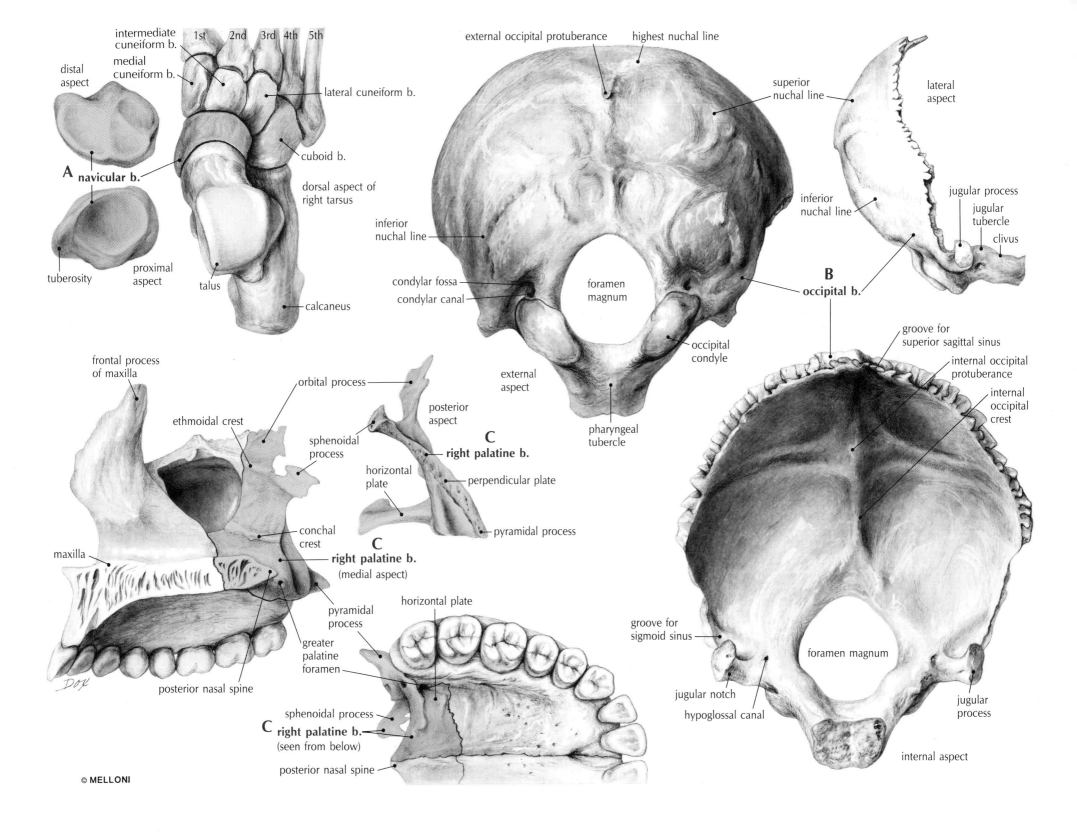

A

distal aspect

intermediate cuneiform b.

medial cuneiform b.

1st 2nd 3rd 4th 5th

lateral cuneiform b.

navicular b.

cuboid b.

dorsal aspect of right tarsus

tuberosity

proximal aspect

talus

calcaneus

frontal process of maxilla

orbital process

ethmoidal crest

sphenoidal process

posterior aspect

C

right palatine b.

horizontal plate

perpendicular plate

pyramidal process

conchal crest

C

right palatine b.
(medial aspect)

maxilla

pyramidal process

greater palatine foramen

posterior nasal spine

horizontal plate

sphenoidal process

C right palatine b.
(seen from below)

posterior nasal spine

external occipital protuberance

highest nuchal line

superior nuchal line

lateral aspect

inferior nuchal line

jugular process

jugular tubercle

clivus

inferior nuchal line

condylar fossa

condylar canal

foramen magnum

B

occipital b.

occipital condyle

external aspect

pharyngeal tubercle

groove for superior sagittal sinus

internal occipital protuberance

internal occipital crest

groove for sigmoid sinus

foramen magnum

jugular notch

hypoglossal canal

jugular process

internal aspect

© MELLONI

	BONE	LOCATION	DESCRIPTION	ARTICULATION	MUSCLE/TENDON ATTACHMENTS
A	**os parietale** *parietal bone*	laterosuperior part of cranium	paired quadrilateral bones; forms roof and sides of cranium with bone of opposite side; composed of: four BORDERS (frontal, sagittal, occipital, squamosal); two SURFACES, internal surface (with sulcus for sigmoid sinus, groove for superior sagittal sinus, granular foveolae), external surface (with superior temporal lines, parietal tuberosity)	frontal border: with frontal bone sagittal border: with parietal bone of opposite side occipital border: with squamous part of occipital bone squamous border: with sphenoid bone (greater wing), temporal bone (squamous and mastoid parts)	temporalis
B	**os pisiforme** *pisiform bone*	wrist; ulnar side of proximal row of carpal bones	smallest bone of carpus; somewhat spherical in shape with a flat articular facet on the DORSAL SURFACE	dorsal surface: with palmar surface of triquestral bone	palmar side: flexor carpi ulnaris, proximally; abductor digiti minimi, distally
C	**os pubis** *pubic bone* *pubis*	pelvis	anterior portion of hipbone: forms anterosuperior portions of acetabulum and obturator foramen; composed of: BODY (with anterior, posterior, and symphyseal surfaces, pubic crest, and pubic tubercle); SUPERIOR RAMUS (with pelvic, pectineal, and obturator surfaces, obturator groove, obturator crest, iliopubic eminence, and pecten pubis); and INFERIOR RAMUS with two surfaces (internal and external)	body: with bone of opposite side superior ramus: with ischium, ilium, and head of femur inferior ramus: with ramus of ischium	pectineal surface of superior ramus: pectineus pubic tubercle: cremaster (medial part) pubic crest: rectus abdominis, pyramidalis body (anterior surface): adductor (longus, and brevis), gracilis, obturator externus inferior ramus (external surface): gracilis, adductor brevis, obturator externus pecten pubis: psoas minor iliopubic eminence: psoas minor body (posterior surface): anterior fibers of levator ani, obturator internus inferior ramus (internal surface): sphincter urethrae, obturator internus
D	**os sacrum** **[sacrale]** *sacrum*	lower back	triangular bone forming posterior portion of pelvic girdle: formed by fusion of five vertebrae; contains sacral canal; composed of: BASE (with two superior articular processes and promontory), two LATERAL PARTS (each with auricular surface and sacral tuberosities), PELVIC SURFACE (with transverse lines, anterior sacral foramina, and intervertebral foramina), DORSAL SURFACE (with posterior sacral foramina, two cornua, sacral hiatus, and median, intermediate, and lateral sacral crests), and APEX (with articular facet)	base: with 5th lumbar vertebra auricular surface: with auricular surface of ilium apex: with base of coccyx	dorsal surface: multifidus, erector spinae, gluteus maximus pelvis surface: iliacus, pisiformis, coccygeus

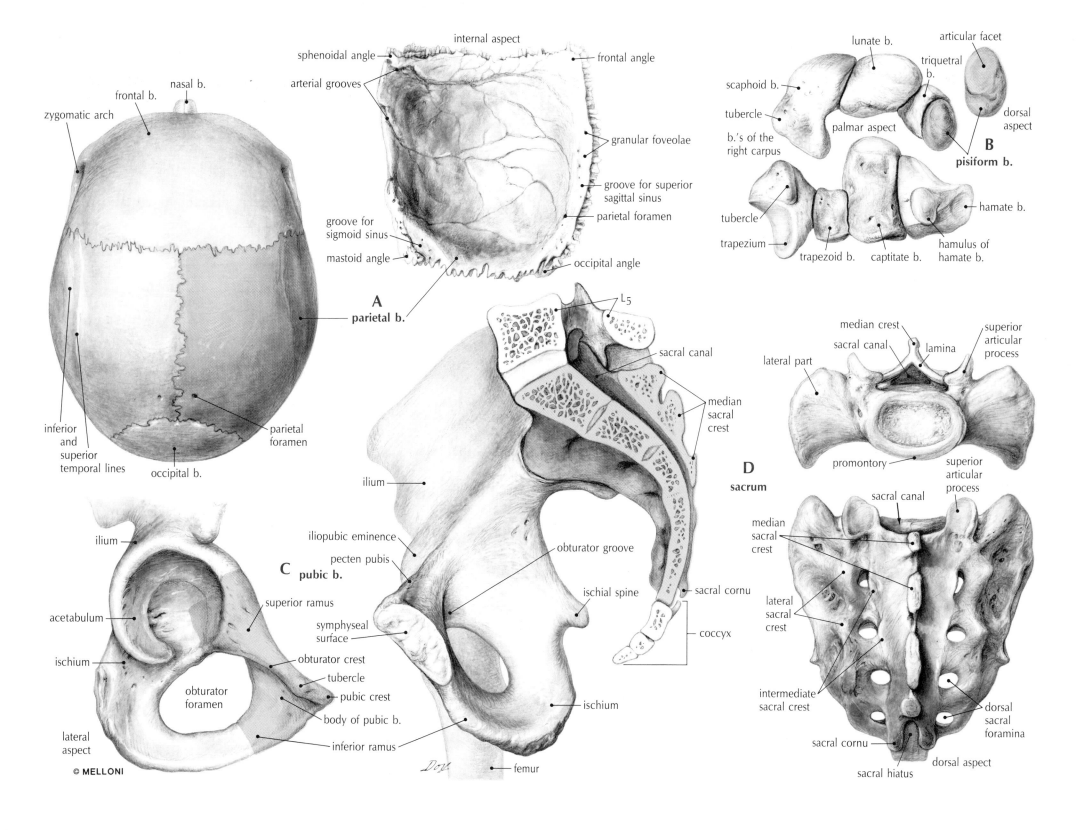

zygomatic arch

frontal b.

nasal b.

inferior and superior temporal lines

parietal foramen

occipital b.

A parietal b.

internal aspect

sphenoidal angle

arterial grooves

frontal angle

granular foveolae

groove for superior sagittal sinus

parietal foramen

groove for sigmoid sinus

mastoid angle

occipital angle

lunate b.

scaphoid b.

triquetral b.

articular facet

tubercle

palmar aspect

b.'s of the right carpus

dorsal aspect

B pisiform b.

tubercle

hamate b.

trapezium

hamulus of hamate b.

trapezoid b.

captitate b.

L5

sacral canal

median sacral crest

ilium

C pubic b.

iliopubic eminence

pecten pubis

obturator groove

ischial spine

sacral cornu

symphyseal surface

coccyx

ischium

femur

median crest

sacral canal

lamina

superior articular process

lateral part

promontory

superior articular process

D sacrum

sacral canal

median sacral crest

lateral sacral crest

intermediate sacral crest

dorsal sacral foramina

sacral cornu

dorsal aspect

sacral hiatus

ilium

acetabulum

ischium

obturator foramen

lateral aspect

superior ramus

obturator crest

tubercle

pubic crest

body of pubic b.

inferior ramus

© MELLONI

	BONE	LOCATION	DESCRIPTION	ARTICULATION	MUSCLE/TENDON ATTACHMENTS
A	**os scaphoideum** *scaphoid bone*	wrist; most lateral of proximal row of carpal bones	largest bone of proximal row; has TUBERCLE on its palmar surface; seven SURFACES (dorsal, palmar, lateral, distal, radial, lunate, and capitate)	distally: with trapezium; trapezoid bone medially: with capitate and lunate bones proximally: with radius	tubercle: abductor pollicis brevis
B	**ossa sesamoidea** *sesamoid bones*	usually within tendons, especially of extremities	small ovoid bones (patella is the largest sesamoid bone)	none	none
C	**os sphenoidale** *sphenoid bone*	base of skull	unpaired flat bone; composed of: a BODY (with sella turcica, sulcus prechiasmaticus, two carotid sulci, lingula, crest, sinus, two conchae, orbital surface, cerebral surface); two GREATER WINGS (each with foramina rotundum, ovale, and spinosum; infratemporal crest; sphenoidal spine); two LESSER WINGS (each with optical canal, anterior clinoid process, superior orbital fissure); two PTERYGOID PROCESSES (each with lateral and medial laminae, pterygoid and scaphoid fossae, pterygoid notch, vaginal process, pterygoid hamulus, pterygoid canal); four PTERYGOID PLATES (two lateral, two medial); two PTERYGOID PROCESSES	body: with ethmoid bone (cribriform plate, perpendicular plate, labyrinth, orbital plate); petrous part of temporal bone greater wing: with orbital plate of frontal bone, zygomatic bone, temporal bone (petrous and squamous parts), parietal bone lesser wing: with orbital plate of frontal bone pterygoid process: with pyramidal process of palatine bone lateral pterygoid plate: with palatine bone medial pterygoid plate: with palatine bone (sphenoidal process, perpendicular plate); ala of vomer sphenoidal conchae: with palatine bone (orbital process), ala of vomer, ethmoid bone (orbital plate), frontal bone	greater wing: temporalis, lateral pterygoid (upper head), common annular tendon (rectus muscles of eyeball) pterygoid process: tensor veli palatini lateral pterygoid plate: lateral pterygoid (lower head), medial pterygoid medial pterygoid plate: tensor veli palatini, superior constrictor (pharynx)
D	**ossa suturarum** *sutural bones* *wormian bones*	in sutures, of skull, especially lambdoid suture	small, irregular, infrequent	none	none

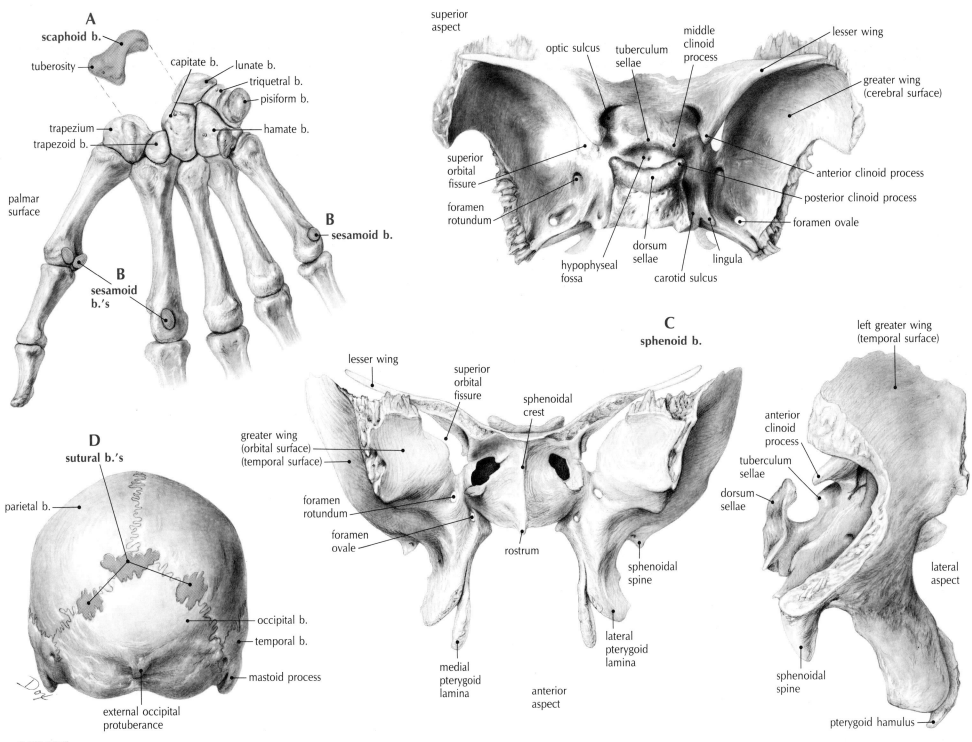

A

scaphoid b.

tuberosity

capitate b.

lunate b.

triquetral b.

pisiform b.

trapezium

trapezoid b.

hamate b.

palmar
surface

B sesamoid b.

B
**sesamoid
b.'s**

D

sutural b.'s

parietal b.

external occipital
protuberance

occipital b.

temporal b.

mastoid process

superior
aspect

optic sulcus

tuberculum
sellae

middle
clinoid
process

lesser wing

greater wing
(cerebral surface)

superior
orbital
fissure

foramen
rotundum

hypophyseal
fossa

dorsum
sellae

carotid sulcus

lingula

anterior clinoid process

posterior clinoid process

foramen ovale

C
sphenoid b.

lesser wing

superior
orbital
fissure

sphenoidal
crest

left greater wing
(temporal surface)

greater wing
(orbital surface)
(temporal surface)

foramen
rotundum

foramen
ovale

rostrum

sphenoidal
spine

lateral
pterygoid
lamina

medial
pterygoid
lamina

anterior
aspect

anterior
clinoid
process

tuberculum
sellae

dorsum
sellae

lateral
aspect

sphenoidal
spine

pterygoid hamulus

© MELLONI

BONE	LOCATION	DESCRIPTION	ARTICULATION	MUSCLE/TENDON ATTACHMENTS
os temporalis *temporal bone*	side of skull	paired bone composed of: SQUAMOUS PART, forms part of temporal fossa and external acoustic meatus; has posterior surface, temporal surface (with zygomatic process, mandibular fossa); MASTOID PART, contains middle ear chamber, antrum, and air cells; has outer surface (with mastoid process), inner surface (with sigmoid sulcus); PETROUS PART, contains labyrinth and internal acoustic meatus; has anterior surface (with arcuate eminence, tegmen tympani), inferior surface (with styloid process, jugular fossa), apex (with carotid canal, semicanals for auditory tube and tensor tympani muscle); TYMPANIC PART, forms part of external acoustic meatus and has tympanic sulcus for tympanic membrane	anteroinferior border: with greater wing of sphenoid bone posterosuperior border: with parietal bone posteroinferior border: with occipital bone zygomatic process: with zygomatic bone	temporal fossa: temporalis zygomatic process: masseter styloid process: styloglossus, stylopharyngeus, stylohoid mastoid process: sternocleidomastoid, splenius capitis, longissimus capitis, digastric posterior wall of middle ear chamber: stapedius semicanal in petrous part of temporal bone: tensor tympani
os trapezium *trapezium* *greater multangular bone*	wrist; distal row of carpal bones at base of thumb	roughly cuboid bone; has a TUBERCLE and a GROOVE on its palmar surface; six SURFACES (palmar, dorsal, proximal, distal, medial, and lateral)	proximal surface: with scaphoid bone distal surface: with 1st and 2nd metacarpal bones laterally and medially respectively medial surface: with trapezoid bone	tubercle: flexor pollicis brevis (superficial head), opponens pollicis, abductor pollicis brevis
os trapezoideum *trapezoid bone* *lesser multangular bone*	wrist; distal row of carpal bones at base of 2nd metacarpal bone (of index finger)	small bone, somewhat triangular or wedge-shaped; has six SURFACES (palmar, dorsal, distal, proximal, medial, and lateral)	distal surface: with 2nd metacarpal bone proximal surface: with scaphoid bone medial surface: with distal part of capitate bone lateral surface: with trapezium	palmar surface: flexor pollicis brevis (deep head)

A

B

C

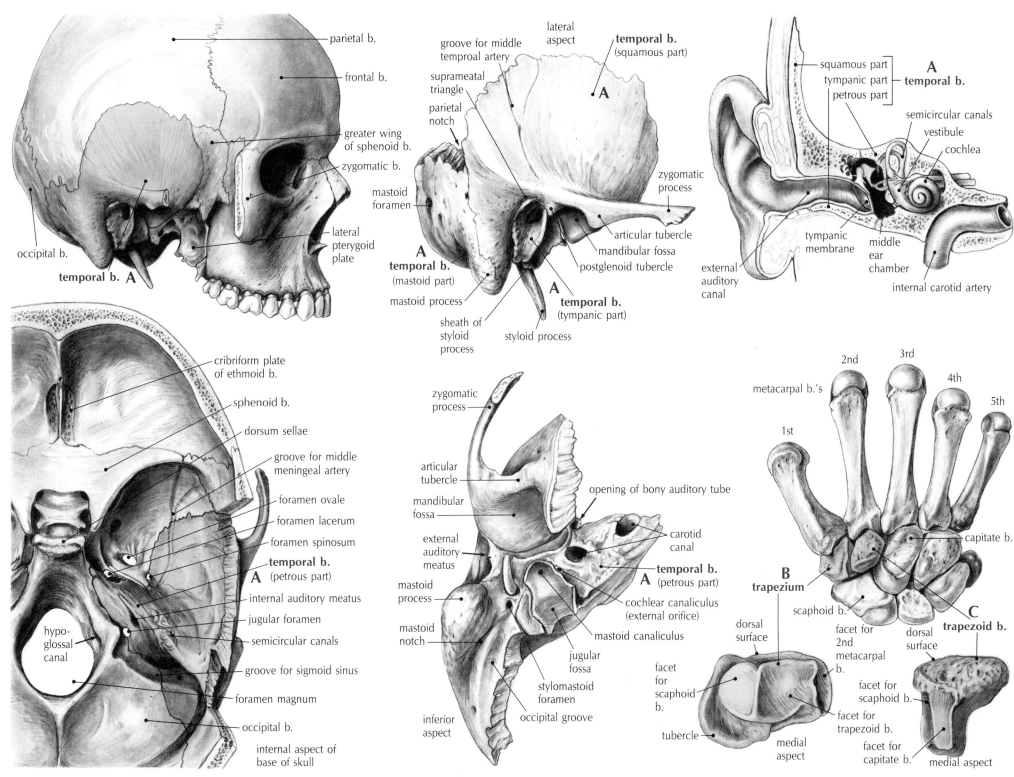

parietal b.

frontal b.

greater wing of sphenoid b.

zygomatic b.

lateral pterygoid plate

occipital b.

temporal b. A

lateral aspect

groove for middle temproal artery

suprameatal triangle

parietal notch

temporal b. (squamous part)

A

mastoid foramen

zygomatic process

articular tubercle

mandibular fossa

postglenoid tubercle

A

temporal b. (mastoid part)

mastoid process

sheath of styloid process

styloid process

A

temporal b. (tympanic part)

squamous part
tympanic part
petrous part

A

temporal b.

semicircular canals

vestibule

cochlea

tympanic membrane

middle ear chamber

external auditory canal

internal carotid artery

cribriform plate of ethmoid b.

sphenoid b.

dorsum sellae

groove for middle meningeal artery

foramen ovale

foramen lacerum

foramen spinosum

temporal b. **A** (petrous part)

internal auditory meatus

jugular foramen

semicircular canals

hypo-glossal canal

groove for sigmoid sinus

foramen magnum

occipital b.

internal aspect of base of skull

zygomatic process

articular tubercle

mandibular fossa

external auditory meatus

mastoid process

mastoid notch

inferior aspect

opening of bony auditory tube

carotid canal

temporal b. **A** (petrous part)

cochlear canaliculus (external orifice)

mastoid canaliculus

jugular fossa

stylomastoid foramen

occipital groove

2nd

3rd

4th

5th

metacarpal b.'s

1st

capitate b.

B **trapezium**

scaphoid b.

facet for 2nd metacarpal b.

dorsal surface

C **trapezoid b.**

dorsal surface

facet for scaphoid b.

facet for scaphoid b.

facet for trapezoid b.

facet for capitate b.

tubercle

medial aspect

medial aspect

© MELLONI

	BONE	LOCATION	DESCRIPTION	ARTICULATION	MUSCLE/TENDON ATTACHMENTS
A	**os triquetrum** *triquetral bone* *pyramidal bone* *triangular bone*	wrist; proximal row of carpal bones; 2nd from ulnar side	small pyramidal bone; has oval articular facet on its palmar surface; four SURFACES (palmar, hamate, lunate, and mediodorsal)	palmar surface: with dorsal surface of pisiform bone hamate surface: with hamate bone lunate surface: with lunate bone	none
B	**os zygomaticum** *zygomatic bone*	side of face	quadrangular cheek bone; composed of: three SURFACES (lateral, temporal, orbital) and two PROCESSES (frontal, temporal)	frontal process: with zygomatic process of frontal bone, greater wing of sphenoid temporal process: with zygomatic process of temporal bone anteroinferior border: with maxilla	zygomaticus (major and minor), levator labii superioris, masseter
C	**patella** *patella*	front of knee	large, flat, triangular sesamoid bone; consists of: ANTERIOR SURFACE, POSTERIOR SURFACE (with articular facets and ridge), BASE (superiorly) and APEX (inferiorly)	femur	anterior surface: tendon quadratus femoris (joint tendon of rectus femoris and vastus lateralis, medialis, and intermedius)
D	**pelvis** *pelvis*	between femoral heads and 5th lumbar vertebra	bony girdle composed of: ilium, ischium, and pubis on either side and sacrum posteriorly; has: GREATER PELVIS (with superior pelvic aperture and pelvic brim); LESSER PELVIS (with inferior pelvic aperture) OBTURATOR FORAMINA, and ACETABULAR	base of sacrum: with 5th lumbar vertebra apex of sacrum: with base of coccyx	see individual bones

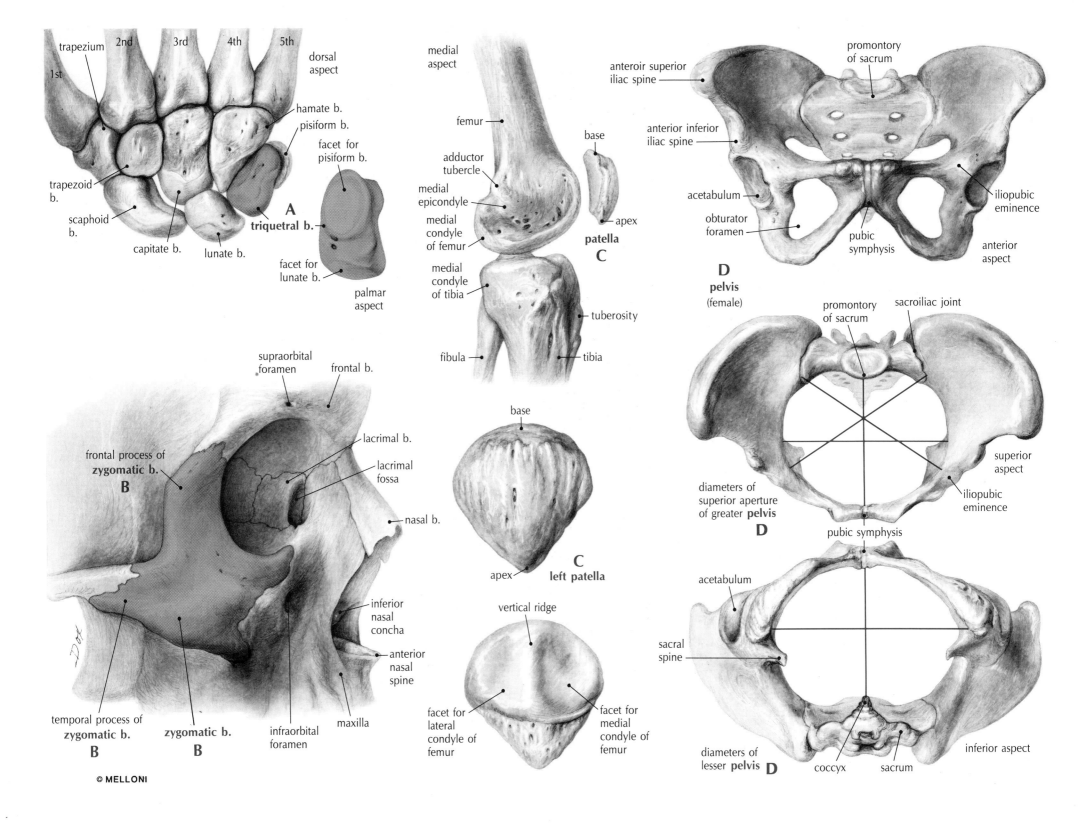

A

1st
trapezium
2nd
3rd
4th
5th
dorsal aspect
hamate b.
pisiform b.
facet for pisiform b.
trapezoid b.
scaphoid b.
capitate b.
lunate b.
triquetral b.
facet for lunate b.
palmar aspect

B

supraorbital foramen
frontal b.
lacrimal b.
lacrimal fossa
frontal process of **zygomatic b.**
B
nasal b.
inferior nasal concha
anterior nasal spine
temporal process of **zygomatic b.**
B
zygomatic b.
B
infraorbital foramen
maxilla

© MELLONI

C

medial aspect
femur
base
adductor tubercle
medial epicondyle
apex
patella
C
medial condyle of femur
medial condyle of tibia
tuberosity
fibula
tibia

base
apex
C
left patella

vertical ridge
facet for lateral condyle of femur
facet for medial condyle of femur

D

promontory of sacrum
anteroir superior iliac spine
anterior inferior iliac spine
acetabulum
obturator foramen
pubic symphysis
iliopubic eminence
anterior aspect
D
pelvis (female)

promontory of sacrum
sacroiliac joint
diameters of superior aperture of greater **pelvis**
D
superior aspect
iliopubic eminence
pubic symphysis

acetabulum
sacral spine
diameters of lesser **pelvis** **D**
coccyx
sacrum
inferior aspect

	BONE	LOCATION	DESCRIPTION	ARTICULATION	MUSCLE/TENDON ATTACHMENTS

A	**radius**
	radius
		lateral aspect of forearm, between elbow and wrist	shortest of two bones of forearm; consists of: small PROXIMAL END at elbow (with head, fovea, articular circumference, and neck); SHAFT with tuberosity, 3 surfaces (anterior, posterior, lateral) and 3 borders (interosseous, anterior, posterior); and broad DISTAL END at wrist (with styloid process, dorsal tubercle, carpal articular surface, and ulnar notch)	PROXIMAL END
				  head: with radial notch of ulna and capitulum of humerus
				DISTAL END
				  carpal articular surface: with lunate and scaphoid bones
				  ulnar notch: with head of ulna
					tuberosity: biceps brachii
					anterior border of shaft: flexor digitorum superficialis
					anterior surface of shaft: flexor pollicis longus, pronator quadratus
					lateral surface of shaft: pronator teres, supinator
					posterior surface of shaft: abductor pollicis longus, extensor pollicis brevis
					styloid process: brachioradialis

B	**scapula** *scapula*	superior and lateral part of back	flat, triangular bone forming posterior part of pectoral girdle; composed of: two SURFACES (costal [with subscapular fossa] and posterior [with spine of scapula, supraspinous fossa, and infraspinous fossa]), ACROMION (with articular surface), three BORDERS (lateral, medial, and superior [with suprascapular notch]), CORACOID PROCESS, three ANGLES (superior, lateral, and inferior), GLENOID CAVITY, and two TUBERCLES (supraglenoid and infraglenoid)	acromion: with clavicle glenoid cavity: with head of humerus	costal surface: subscapular, serratus anterior dorsal surface: supraspinatus, infraspinatus, teres (major, minor) superior border: omohyoid (inferior belly) medial border: levator scapulae rhomboideus (major, minor) . inferior angle: latissimus dorsi infraglenoid tubercle: triceps brachii (long head) scapular spine: trapezius, deltoid (posterior fibers) acromion: deltoid (middle fibers), trapezius (horizontal fibers) coracoid process: coracobrachialis, biceps brachii (short head), pectoralis minor
C	**stapes** *stapes*	middle ear, between incus and oval window (medial wall of middle-ear chamber)	stirrup-shaped and smallest ear ossicle; composed of: HEAD (with articular surface), NECK, anterior and posterior LIMBS (crura), and BASE	head: lentiform process of incus base: margins of oval window	neck: stapedius
D	**sternum** *sternum*	anterior wall of thorax	elongated, flat bone with two SURFACES (anterior and posterior); composed of: manubrium (with jugular notch, clavicular notch); BODY (with four sternebrae); and XIPHOID PROCESS	on both sides, manubrium: with clavicle, cartilage of 1st rib and part of 2nd rib body: with part of cartilage of 2nd rib, cartilages of 3rd, 4th, 5th, 6th, and part of 7th ribs xiphoid process: with part of cartilage of 7th rib	on both sides, manubrium: pectoralis major, sternocleidomastoid, sternothyroid, sternohyoid body: pectoralis major, transversus thoracic (sternocostalis) xiphoid process: rectus abdominis, diaphragm, and (through their aponeuroses) internal oblique, external oblique, transversus abdominis

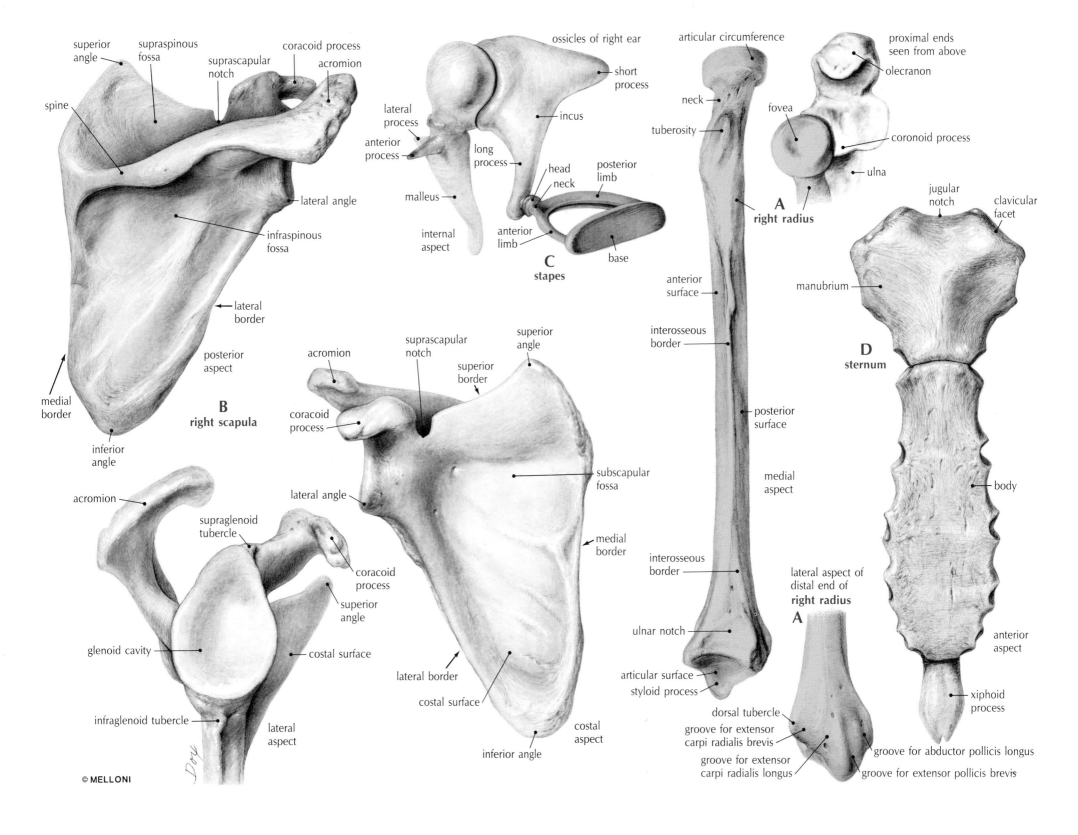

superior angle

supraspinous fossa

suprascapular notch

coracoid process

acromion

spine

lateral angle

infraspinous fossa

lateral border

posterior aspect

medial border

inferior angle

B
right scapula

acromion

supraglenoid tubercle

coracoid process

superior angle

glenoid cavity

costal surface

infraglenoid tubercle

lateral aspect

© MELLONI

ossicles of right ear

short process

lateral process

incus

anterior process

long process

malleus

head

neck

posterior limb

internal aspect

anterior limb

base

C
stapes

acromion

suprascapular notch

superior angle

superior border

coracoid process

lateral angle

subscapular fossa

medial border

lateral border

costal surface

costal aspect

inferior angle

articular circumference

proximal ends seen from above

olecranon

neck

fovea

tuberosity

coronoid process

anterior surface

ulna

A
right radius

interosseous border

jugular notch

clavicular facet

manubrium

posterior surface

D
sternum

medial aspect

body

interosseous border

lateral aspect of distal end of **right radius**

ulnar notch

A

articular surface

styloid process

dorsal tubercle

groove for extensor carpi radialis brevis

anterior aspect

groove for abductor pollicis longus

groove for extensor carpi radialis longus

groove for extensor pollicis brevis

xiphoid process

	BONE	LOCATION	DESCRIPTION	ARTICULATION	MUSCLE/TENDON ATTACHMENTS
A	**talus** *talus*	tarsus at ankle	second largest bone of tarsus connecting the foot to the leg; composed of: HEAD, NECK with sulcus for tendon of flexor hallucis longus muscle; BODY with two processes (lateral and posterior), two tubercles (lateral and medial), and trochlea; seven ARTICULAR SURFACES (navicular trochlear, medial, lateral, and three plantar)	navicular surface: with navicular bone trochlear surface: with tibia medial surface: with medial malleolus (tibia) lateral surface: with lateral malleolus (fibula) plantar surfaces (anterior, middle, posterior): with calcaneus	none
B	**tarsalia** *tarsus*	foot	the seven bones of the posterior half of the foot; arranged in two rows: PROXIMAL ROW (with talus and calcaneus) and DISTAL ROW (with medial cuneiform, intermediate cuneiform, lateral cuneiform, and cuboid bones)	proximal row (talus): with tibia distal row: with metatarsal bones	see individual bones
C	**tibia** *tibia*	medial aspect of leg between knee and ankle	largest of two bones of the leg; consists of: large PROXIMAL END at the knee with two condyles (lateral, medial), two intercondylar areas (anterior, posterior), two intercondylar tubercles (medial, lateral), intercondylar eminence, superior articular surface, and fibular facet; SHAFT with tibial tuberosity, three surfaces (lateral, medial, posterior), three borders (anterior medial, interosseous), and soleal line; and DISTAL END at the ankle (with medial malleolus, malleolar articular facet, malleolar groove, fibular notch, and inferior articular surface)	PROXIMAL END superior articular surface: with condyles of femur fibular facet: with head of fibula DISTAL END inferior articular surface: with body of talus (trochlear surface) malleolar articular surface: with body of talus (medial surface)	lateral condyle: biceps femoris medial surface of shaft: semimembranosus, sartorius, gracilis, semitendinosus lateral surface of shaft: tibialis anterior posterior surface of shaft: popliteus, soleus, flexor digitorum longus, tibialis posterior

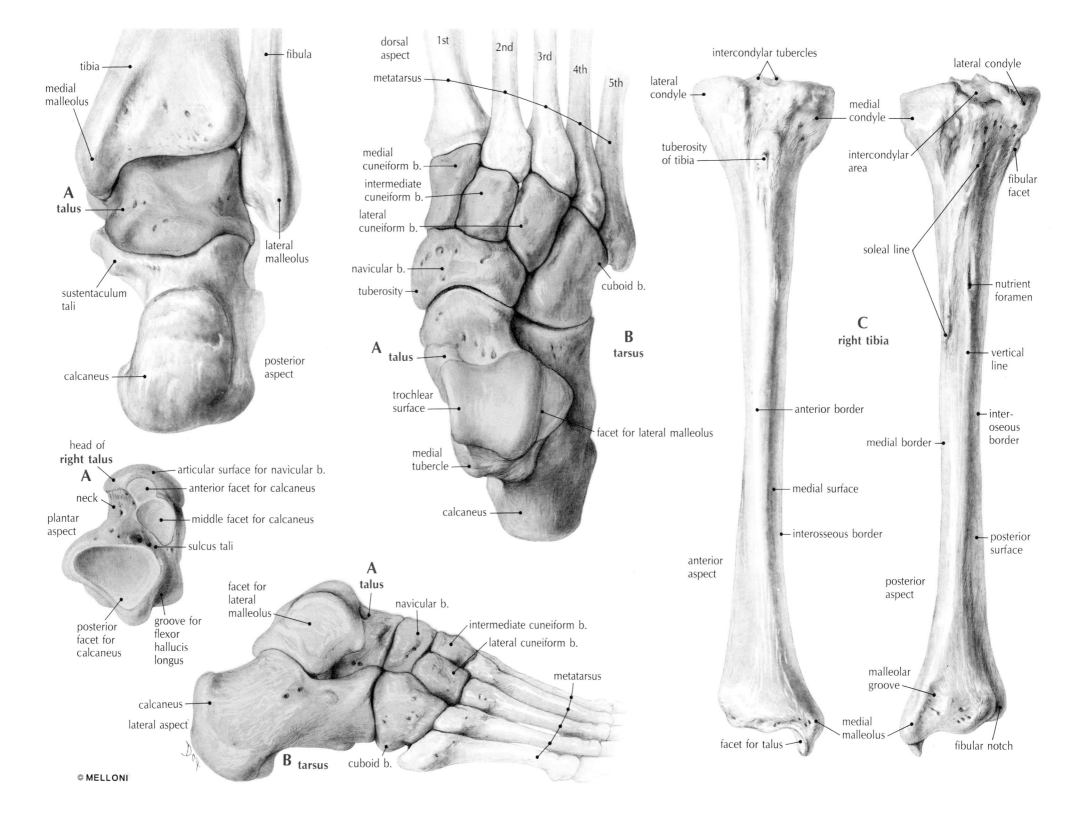

tibia

medial
malleolus

fibula

A **talus**

sustentaculum
tali

lateral
malleolus

calcaneus

posterior
aspect

head of
right talus

A

neck

plantar
aspect

posterior
facet for
calcaneus

articular surface for navicular b.

anterior facet for calcaneus

middle facet for calcaneus

sulcus tali

groove for
flexor
hallucis
longus

dorsal
aspect

metatarsus

1st 2nd 3rd 4th 5th

medial
cuneiform b.

intermediate
cuneiform b.

lateral
cuneiform b.

navicular b.

tuberosity

cuboid b.

A **talus**

B **tarsus**

trochlear
surface

facet for lateral malleolus

medial
tubercle

calcaneus

facet for
lateral
malleolus

A **talus**

navicular b.

intermediate cuneiform b.

lateral cuneiform b.

metatarsus

calcaneus

lateral aspect

B **tarsus**

cuboid b.

© MELLONI

intercondylar tubercles

lateral
condyle

tuberosity
of tibia

lateral condyle

medial
condyle

intercondylar
area

fibular
facet

soleal line

nutrient
foramen

C **right tibia**

vertical
line

anterior border

inter-
osseous
border

medial border

medial surface

posterior
surface

interosseous border

anterior
aspect

posterior
aspect

malleolar
groove

medial
malleolus

fibular notch

facet for talus

BONE	LOCATION	DESCRIPTION	ARTICULATION	MUSCLE/TENDON ATTACHMENTS
ulna *ulna*	forearm, medial aspect	longest of two bones of forearm; composed of: hook-like PROXIMAL END at elbow (with olecranon, coronoid process, tuberosity, radial notch, and trochlear notch); SHAFT with three surfaces (anterior, medial, posterior), three margins (interosseous, anterior, posterior), and supinator crest; DISTAL END at wrist (with head, styloid process, and articular circumference)	PROXIMAL END trochlear notch: with trochlea of humerus radial notch: with head of radius DISTAL END head: with ulnar notch of radius	olecranon: triceps brachii, flexor carpi ulnaris, flexor digitorum profundus, anconeus coronoid process: brachialis, flexor digitorum superficialis, pronator teres, flexor pollicis longus (occasionally), flexor digitorum profundus anterior surface of shaft: flexor digitorum profundus, pronator quadratus anterior border of shaft: flexor digitorum profundus medial surface of shaft: flexor digitorum profundus posterior surface of shaft: anconeus, abductor pollicis longus, extensor pollicis longus, extensor indicis, extensor carpi ulnaris posterior border of shaft: extensor carpi ulnaris, flexor carpi ulnaris
vertebrae *vertebrae*	back, from skull to pelvis	32 to 34 bones that form vertebral column; grouped as follows: 7 cervical, 12 thoracic, 5 lumbar, 5 sacral, 3 to 5 coccygeal. For individual descriptions see atlas (1st cervical), axis (2nd cervical), sacrum (5 fused sacral), and coccyx (fused 3 to 5 coccygeal)	all vertebrae: with contiguous vertebrae atlas: with skull (occipital condyles) thoracic: with heads of ribs, tubercles of ribs (except 11th and 12th) sacrum: with auricular surface of ilium	at different levels of vertebral column (except atlas, axis, sacrum and coccyx): longus coli, longus capitis, scalenus (anterior, medius, posterior), splenius (capitis, cervicis), erector spinae, semispinalis (thoracic, cervicis, capitis), multifidi (cervicis, thoracic, lumborum), rotatores (thoracis, cervicis, lumborum), interspinales, intertransversarii, levatores costarum, serratus posterior superior, serratus posterior inferior, diaphragm, latissimus dorsi, trapezius, rhomboideus (major, minor), levator scapulae, transversus abdominus, quadratus lumborum, psoas (major, minor)
vomer *vomer*	nasal cavity	unpaired flat, thin bone forming posteroinferior part of nasal cavity framework; has two ALA and four BORDERS: anterior, superior (with furrow)	alae: with sphenoidal conchae, palatine bones inferior border: with maxillae, palatine bones anterior border (upper half): with ethmoid bone	none

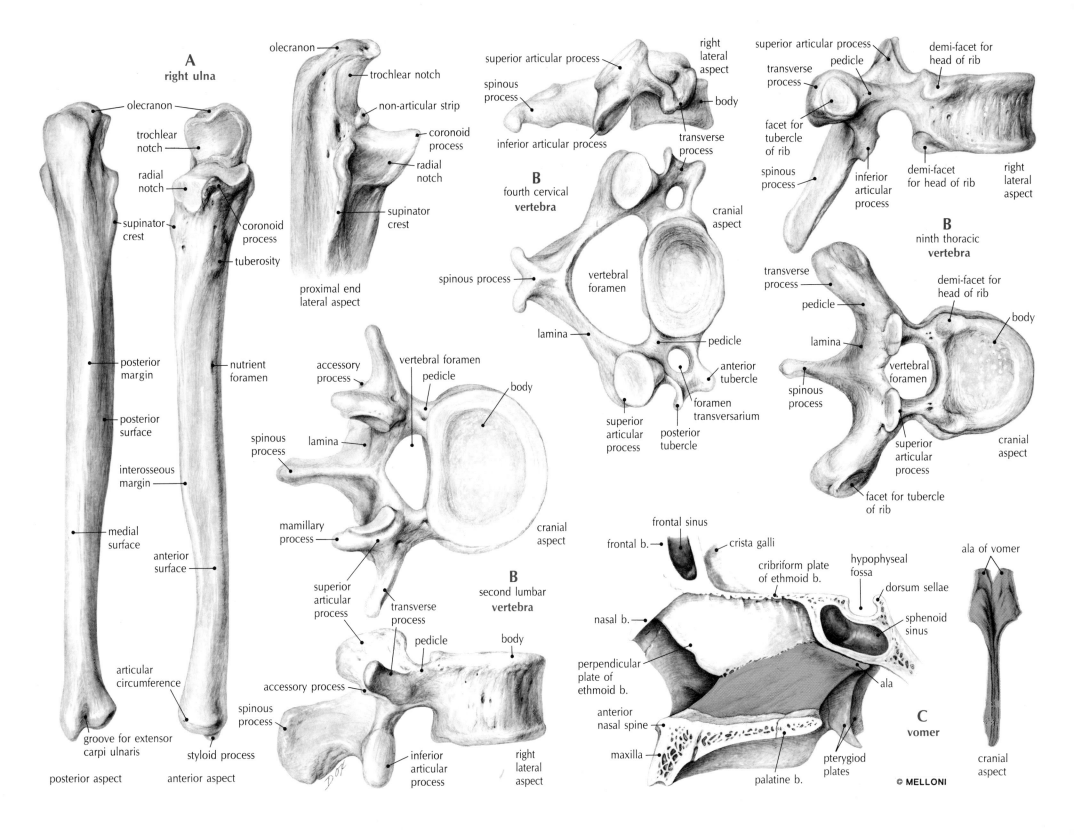

A
right ulna

olecranon
trochlear notch
non-articular strip
coronoid process
radial notch
supinator crest

proximal end lateral aspect

olecranon
trochlear notch
radial notch
supinator crest
coronoid process
tuberosity
nutrient foramen
posterior margin
posterior surface
interosseous margin
medial surface
anterior surface
articular circumference
groove for extensor carpi ulnaris
styloid process

posterior aspect   anterior aspect

B
fourth cervical vertebra

superior articular process
spinous process
inferior articular process
right lateral aspect
body
transverse process

spinous process
vertebral foramen
lamina
cranial aspect
superior articular process
pedicle
anterior tubercle
foramen transversarium
posterior tubercle

B
second lumbar vertebra

accessory process
vertebral foramen
pedicle
body
spinous process
lamina
mamillary process
cranial aspect
superior articular process
transverse process

accessory process
spinous process
pedicle
body
transverse process
inferior articular process
right lateral aspect

superior articular process
transverse process
pedicle
demi-facet for head of rib
facet for tubercle of rib
inferior articular process
spinous process
demi-facet for head of rib
right lateral aspect

B
ninth thoracic vertebra

transverse process
pedicle
lamina
spinous process
superior articular process
demi-facet for head of rib
body
vertebral foramen
cranial aspect
facet for tubercle of rib

frontal sinus
frontal b.
crista galli
cribriform plate of ethmoid b.
hypophyseal fossa
dorsum sellae
nasal b.
sphenoid sinus
perpendicular plate of ethmoid b.
ala
anterior nasal spine
maxilla
pterygoid plates
palatine b.
C
vomer

ala of vomer
cranial aspect

© MELLONI

MUSCLES

	MUSCLE	ORIGIN	INSERTION	INNERVATION	ACTION
A	**m. abductor digiti minimi manus** *abductor m. of little finger*	pisiform bone; tendon of m. flexor carpi ulnaris	base of proximal phalanx of 5th finger	deep branch of ulnar nerve	abducts little finger
B	**m. abductor digiti minimi pedis** *abductor m. of little toe*	lateral and medial tubercles of calcaneus; plantar aponeurosis	lateral surface of base of proximal phalanx of little toe	lateral plantar nerve (S2, S3)	abducts and flexes little toe
C	**m. abductor hallucis** *abductor m. of big toe*	calcanean tuberosity; flexor retinaculum; plantar aponeurosis	inner side of base of proximal phalanx of big toe (in common with tendon of m. flexor hallucis brevis	medial plantar nerve (S2, S3)	abducts and aids in flexion of big toe
D	**m. abductor pollicis brevis** *short abductor m. of thumb*	flexor retinaculum; scaphoid bone; trapezium	proximal phalanx of thumb	lateral terminal branch of median nerve (8th cranial nerve and T1)	abducts thumb; aids in flexion of thumb
E	**m. abductor pollicis longus** *long abductor m. of thumb*	posterior surface of ulna; middle third of radius; interosseous membrane	base of 1st metacarpal bone; trapezium	posterior interosseous nerve (7th and 8th cranial nerves)	abducts and extends thumb
F	**m. adductor brevis** *short adductor m.*	body and inferior ramus of pubis	upper part of shaft of femur	obturator nerve (L2, L3, L4)	adducts, flexes, and rotates thigh laterally
G	**m. adductor hallucis** *adductor m. of big toe*	oblique head: bases of middle three metatarsal bones; sheath of m. peroneus longus	oblique head: outer side of the base of the proximal phalanx of the big toe; lateral sesamoid bone	lateral plantar nerve (S2, S3)	oblique head: adducts and flexes big toe
		transverse head: plantar metatarsophalangeal ligaments of lateral three toes	transverse head: proximal phalanx of big toe (joined by m. flexor hallucis longus); lateral sesamoid bone		transverse head: supports transverse arch; adducts great toe
H	**m. adductor longus** *long adductor m.*	front of pubis, below pubic crest	linea aspera femoris	anterior division of obturator nerve (L2, L3, L4)	adducts, flexes, and rotates thigh medially
I	**m. adductor magnus** *great adductor m.*	deep (adductor) part: inferior ramus of pubis; ramus of ischium	deep (adductor) part: linea aspera femoris	obturator nerve and tibial division of sciatic nerve (L2, L3, L4)	adducts, flexes, and rotates thigh medially
		superficial (extensor) part: ischial tuberosity	superficial (extensor) part: adductor tubercle of femur		

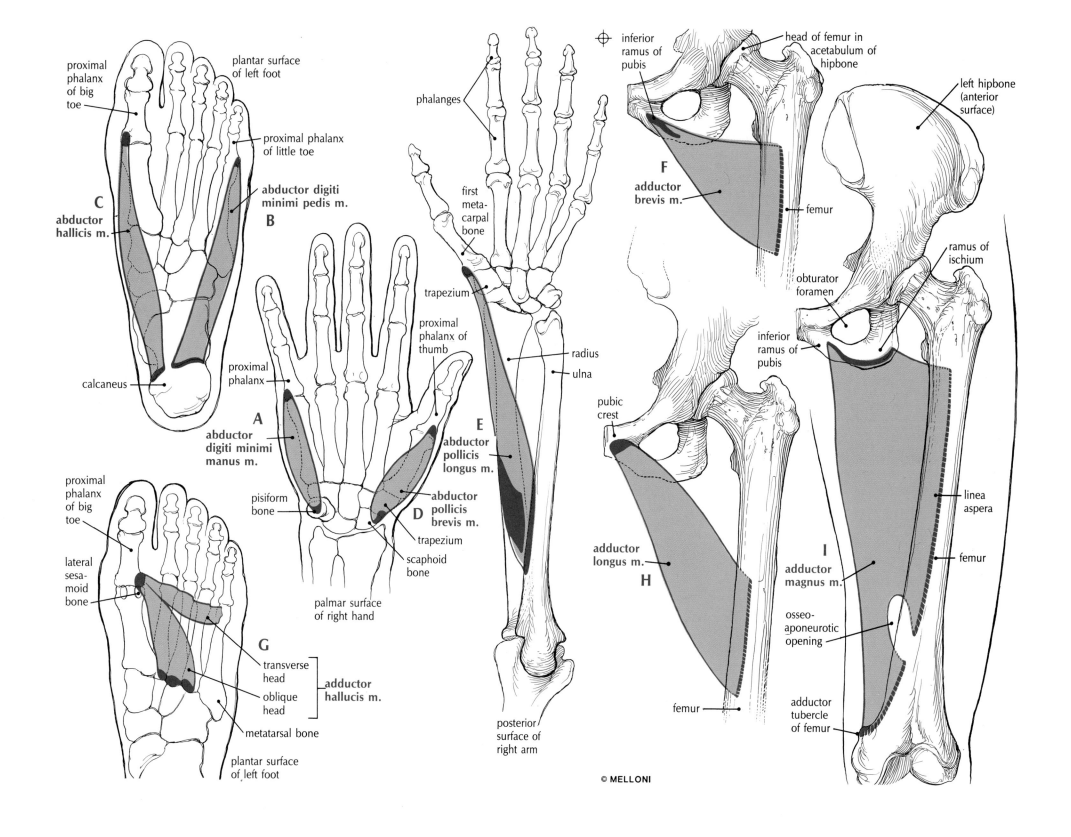

proximal phalanx of big toe

plantar surface of left foot

proximal phalanx of little toe

abductor digiti minimi pedis m.

B

C

abductor hallicis m.

calcaneus

proximal phalanx

A

abductor digiti minimi manus m.

pisiform bone

palmar surface of right hand

proximal phalanx of thumb

D

abductor pollicis brevis m.

trapezium

scaphoid bone

phalanges

first meta-carpal bone

trapezium

radius

ulna

E

abductor pollicis longus m.

posterior surface of right arm

proximal phalanx of big toe

lateral sesa-moid bone

G

transverse head

oblique head

adductor hallicis m.

metatarsal bone

plantar surface of left foot

inferior ramus of pubis

F

adductor brevis m.

head of femur in acetabulum of hipbone

left hipbone (anterior surface)

femur

obturator foramen

inferior ramus of pubis

ramus of ischium

pubic crest

adductor longus m.

H

femur

I

adductor magnus m.

osseo-aponeurotic opening

adductor tubercle of femur

linea aspera

femur

© MELLONI

	MUSCLE	ORIGIN	INSERTION	INNERVATION	ACTION
A	**m. adductor minimus** *smallest adductor m.*	the proximal portion of m. adductor magnus when it forms a distinct muscle			adducts, flexes, and rotates thigh medially
B	**m. adductor pollicis** *adductor m. of thumb*	oblique head: capitate, 2nd, and 3rd metacarpal bones; radial carpal ligament transverse head: 3rd metacarpal bone	proximal phalanx of thumb; medial sesamoid bone	deep branch of ulnar nerve (8th cranial nerve and T1)	adducts thumb; assists in apposition
C	**m. anconeus** *anconeus m.*	posterior surface of lateral epicondyle of humerus	lateral surface of olecranon process; posterior surface of shaft of ulna	radial nerve (7th and 8th cranial nerves and T1)	extends forearm; abducts ulna in pronation of wrist
D	**m. antitragicus** *antitragus m.*	outer surface of antitragus of ear	tail of helix and antihelix	posterior auricular and temporal branches of facial nerve (7th cranial nerve)	thought to be vestigial
E	**mm. arrectores pilorum** *arrector muscles of hair*	superficial layer of dermis (corium)	outer layer of hair follicle	sympathetic nerves	elevates hairs of skin (goose flesh); aids in discharging sebum
F	**m. articularis cubiti** *articular m. of elbow; subanconeus m.*	deep surface of lower part of m. triceps brachii	posterior aspects of fibrous capsule of elbow joint	radial nerve (6th, 7th, and 8th cranial nerves)	elevates capsule in extension of elbow joint
G	**m. articularis genus** *articular m. of knee*	lower part of anterior surface of femur	upper part of synovial membrane of knee joint	femoral nerve (L2, L3, L4)	elevates capsule of knee joint during extension of leg
H	**m. aryepiglotticus** *aryepiglottic m.*	apex of arytenoid cartilage	lateral margin of epiglottis	recurrent nerve and internal laryngeal branch of superior laryngeal nerve of vagus nerve (10th cranial nerve)	narrows inlet of larynx by lowering epiglottis
I	**m. arytenoideus obliquus** *oblique arytenoid m.*	muscular process of arytenoid cartilage	apex of opposite arytenoid cartilage; prolonged as aryepiglottic muscle	recurrent nerve and internal laryngeal branch of superior laryngeal nerve of vagus nerve (10th cranial nerve)	helps to close the inlet of larynx by approximating arytenoid cartilages
J	**m. arytenoideus transversus** *transverse arytenoid m.*	posterior surface of arytenoid cartilage	posterior surface of arytenoid cartilage on opposite side	recurrent nerve of vagus nerve (10th cranial nerve)	helps to close the glottis by approximating the arytenoid cartilages

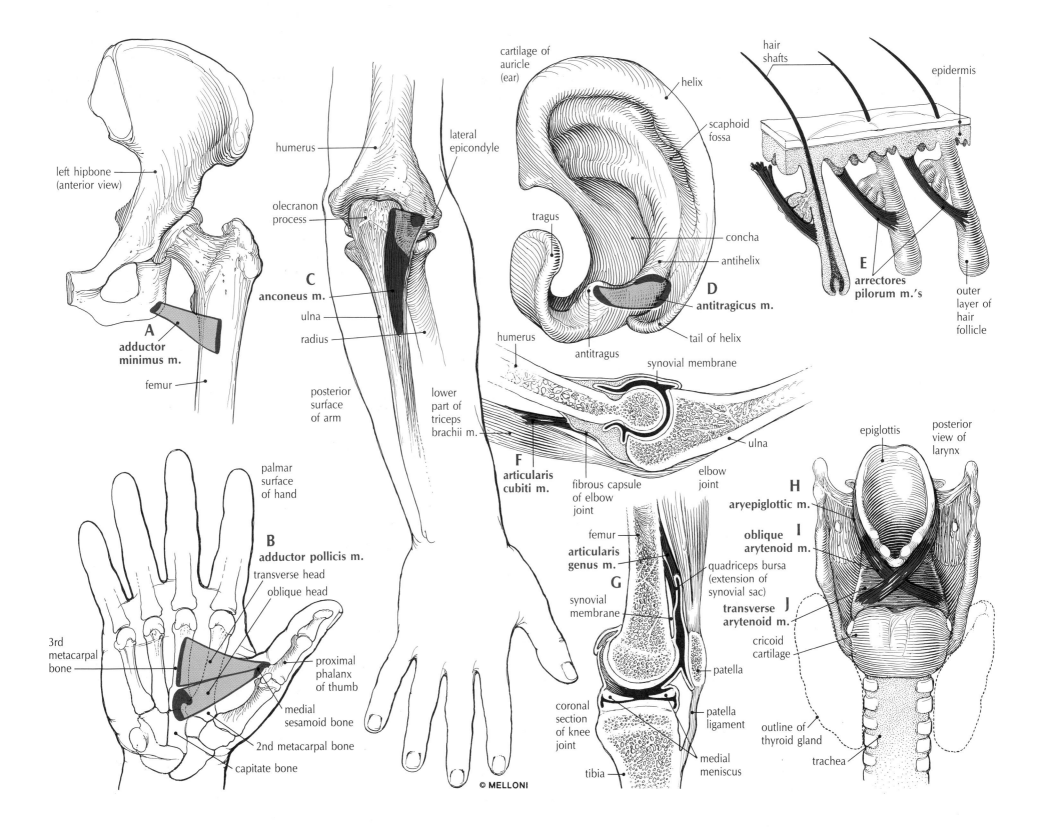

left hipbone
(anterior view)

A

**adductor
minimus m.**

femur

palmar
surface
of hand

B

adductor pollicis m.

transverse head

oblique head

3rd
metacarpal
bone

proximal
phalanx
of thumb

medial
sesamoid bone

2nd metacarpal bone

capitate bone

humerus

olecranon
process

C

anconeus m.

ulna

radius

posterior
surface
of arm

lateral
epicondyle

lower
part of
triceps
brachii m.

cartilage
of auricle
(ear)

tragus

D

antitragicus m.

antitragus

tail of helix

helix

scaphoid
fossa

concha

antihelix

hair
shafts

epidermis

E

**arrectores
pilorum m.'s**

outer
layer of
hair
follicle

humerus

F

**articularis
cubiti m.**

synovial membrane

fibrous capsule
of elbow
joint

ulna

elbow
joint

femur

**articularis
genus m.**

synovial
membrane

G

coronal
section
of knee
joint

tibia

quadriceps bursa
(extension of
synovial sac)

patella

patella
ligament

medial
meniscus

epiglottis

posterior
view of larynx

H

aryepiglottic m.

I

**oblique
arytenoid m.**

J

**transverse
arytenoid m.**

cricoid
cartilage

outline of
thyroid gland

trachea

© MELLONI

	MUSCLE	ORIGIN	INSERTION	INNERVATION	ACTION
A	**m. auricularis anterior** *anterior auricular m.*	superficial temporal fascia	anterior part of medial surface of cartilaginous helix of ear	temporal branches of facial nerve (7th cranial nerve)	feeble forward movement of auricle
B	**m. auricularis posterior** *posterior auricular m.*	mastoid process of temporal bone	medial surface of cartilage of ear	posterior auricular branch of facial nerve (7th cranial nerve)	feeble backward movement of auricle
C	**m. auricularis superior** *superior auricular m.*	epicranial aponeurosis	upper part of medial surface of cartilage of ear	temporal branches of facial nerve (7th cranial nerve)	feeble elevation of auricle
D	**m. biceps brachii** *biceps m. of arm*	long head: supraglenoid tubercle of scapula (within shoulder joint) short head: apex of coracoid process (in common with m. coracobrachialis)	tuberosity of radius; posterior border of ulna through bicipital aponeurosis	musculocutaneous nerve (5th and 6th cranial nerves)	flexes forearm; supinates hand
E	**m. biceps femoris** *biceps m. of thigh*	long head: ischial tuberosity (in common with m. semi-tendinosus) short head: middle of linea aspera femoris; 2nd supracondylar ridge of femur	head of fibula; lateral condyle of tibia	long head: tibial part of sciatic nerve short head: common peroneal portion of sciatic nerve (L5, S1, S2)	flexes leg and rotates it laterally; extends thigh
F	**m. brachialis** *brachial m.*	anterior surface of distal two thirds of humerus	coronoid process of ulna	musculocutaneous nerve (5th and 6th cranial nerves); radial nerve (7th cranial nerve)	flexes forearm
G	**m. brachioradialis** *brachioradial m.*	intermuscular septum; lateral supracondylar ridge of humerus	lower end of radius	radial nerve (5th, 6th, and 7th cranial nerves)	flexes forearm
H	**m. bronchoesophageus** *bronchoesophageal m.*	left primary bronchus	musculature at middle of esophagus	small branch of vagus nerve (10th cranial nerve)	reinforces esophagus
I	**m. buccinator** *buccinator m.*	pterygomandibular raphe; surrounding portions of alveolar processes of jaws	m. orbicularis oris at angle of mouth	lower buccal branch of facial nerve (7th cranial nerve)	retracts angle of mouth; compresses cheek against teeth; aids in mastication

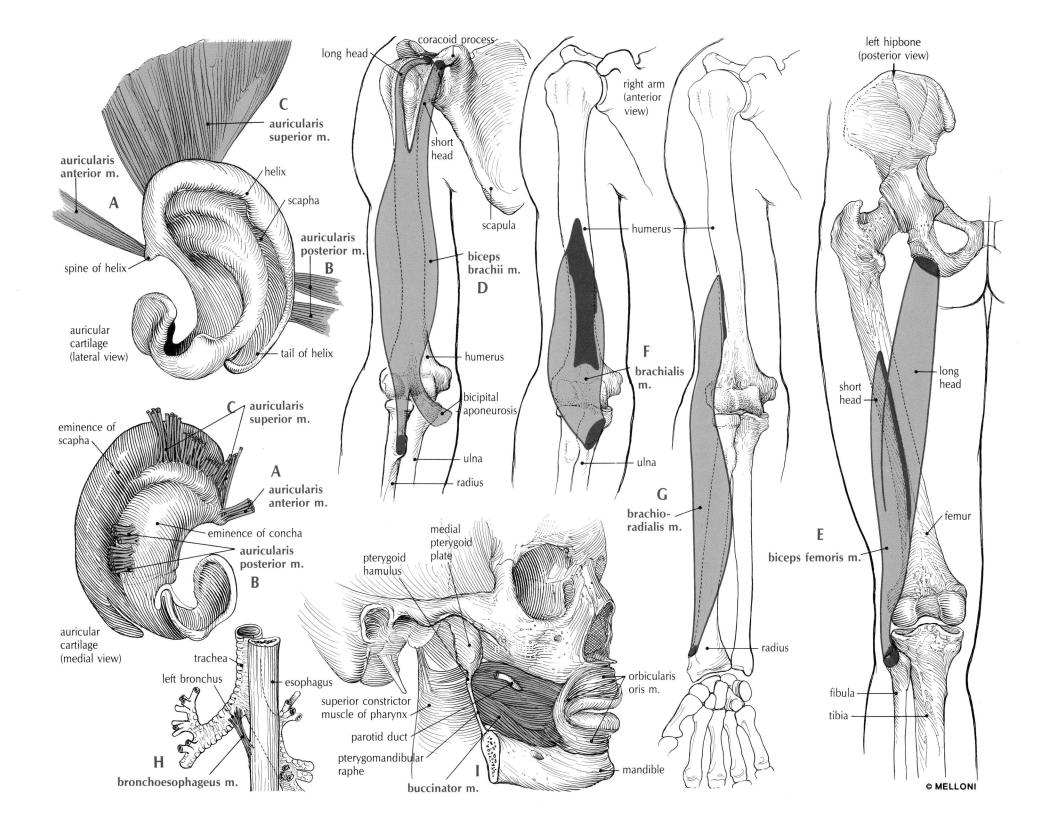

**auricularis
anterior m.**

C **auricularis
superior m.**

helix

scapha

**auricularis
posterior m.**

B

A

spine of helix

auricular
cartilage
(lateral view)

tail of helix

C **auricularis
superior m.**

eminence of
scapha

A **auricularis
anterior m.**

eminence of concha

**auricularis
posterior m.**

B

auricular
cartilage
(medial view)

trachea

left bronchus

esophagus

H

bronchoesophageus m.

coracoid process

long head

short
head

scapula

**biceps
brachii m.**

D

humerus

bicipital
aponeurosis

ulna

radius

right arm
(anterior
view)

humerus

F brachialis
m.

ulna

G

**brachio-
radialis m.**

radius

medial
pterygoid
plate

pterygoid
hamulus

superior constrictor
muscle of pharynx

parotid duct

pterygomandibular
raphe

I

buccinator m.

orbicularis
oris m.

mandible

left hipbone
(posterior view)

short
head

long
head

E

biceps femoris m.

femur

fibula

tibia

© MELLONI

	MUSCLE	ORIGIN	INSERTION	INNERVATION	ACTION
A	**m. bulbospongiosus** *bulbocavernous m.*	female: perineal body (central tendon of perineum); inferior fascia of urogenital diaphragm male: perineal body (central tendon of perineum); median raphe over bulb of penis	female: dorsum of clitoris male: deep layer of fascia encircling corpus spongiosum; inferior fascia of urogenital diaphragm	perineal branch of pudendal nerve (S2, S3, S4)	female: compresses vaginal orifice; contributes to erection of clitoris; protects vestibular bulb male: compresses bulb of penis and urethra; contributes to erection of penis; assists in ejaculation
B	**m. ceratocricoideus** *ceratocricoid m.*	lower margin of cricoid cartilage	inferior horn (cornu) of thyroid cartilage	laryngeal branch of vagus nerve (10th cranial nerve)	aids m. cricoarytenoideus posterior separate vocal cords
C	**m. chondroglossus** *chondroglossus m.*	lesser horn (cornu) and body of hyoid bone	side of tongue	hypoglossal nerve (12th cranial nerve)	depresses tongue
D	**m. ciliaris** *ciliary m.*	meridional, radial, and circular parts attached to the scleral spur	ciliary process	oculomotor nerve (3rd cranial nerve)	makes lens more convex in accommodation for near vision
E	**m. coccygeus** *(part of pelvic diaphragm)* *coccygeus m.*	spine of ischium; sacrospinous ligament	coccyx; lateral border of 5th sacral vertebra	branch frcom spinal nerves (S4, S5)	draws coccyx forward; forms part of pelvic floor
F	**m. compressor naris** *(transverse part of m. nasalis)* *compressor m. of nose*	maxilla, lateral to nasal notch, just above area of cuspid root	aponeurosis on nasal cartilage and bridge of nose	upper buccal branches of facial nerve (7th cranial nerve)	compresses nostril
G	**m. constrictor pharyngis inferior** *inferior constrictor m. of pharynx*	cricopharyngeal part: side of cricoid cartilage thyropharyngeal part: inferior cornu and oblique line of thyroid cartilage	median raphe of posterior wall of pharynx	pharyngeal plexus; recurrent and external laryngeal branches of vagus nerve (10th cranial nerve)	narrows lower part of pharynx in swallowing
H	**m. constrictor pharyngis medius** *middle constrictor m. of pharynx*	chondropharyngeal part: lesser cornu of hyoid bone; lower portion of stylohyoid ligament ceratopharyngeal part: greater cornu of hyoid bone	median raphe of posterior wall of pharynx	pharyngeal plexus of vagus nerve (10th cranial nerve)	narrows pharynx in swallowing

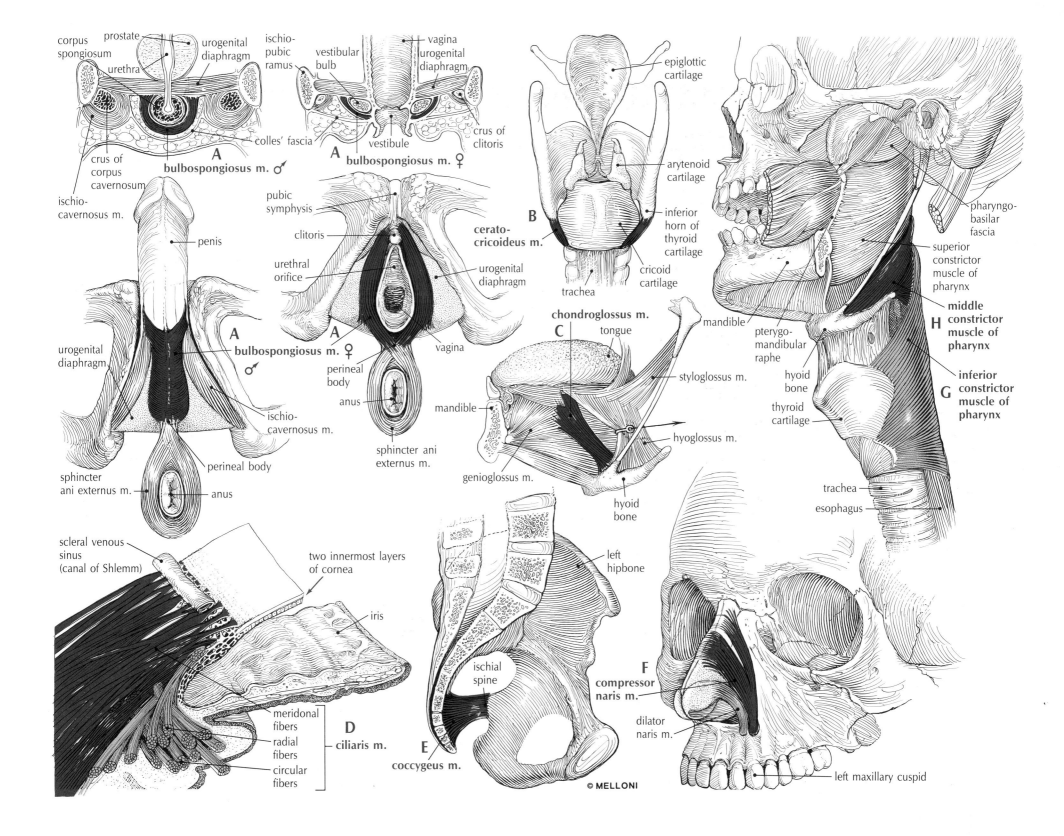

corpus spongiosum

prostate

urethra

urogenital diaphragm

crus of corpus cavernosum

ischio-cavernosus m.

colles' fascia

bulbospongiosus m. ♂

A

ischio-pubic ramus

vestibular bulb

vagina

urogenital diaphragm

crus of clitoris

vestibule

bulbospongiosus m. ♀

A

epiglottic cartilage

arytenoid cartilage

inferior horn of thyroid cartilage

cricoid cartilage

trachea

B

pharyngo-basilar fascia

superior constrictor muscle of pharynx

H

middle constrictor muscle of pharynx

G

inferior constrictor muscle of pharynx

penis

pubic symphysis

clitoris

urethral orifice

urogenital diaphragm

urogenital diaphragm

cerato-cricoideus m.

vagina

ischio-cavernosus m.

bulbospongiosus m. ♀

A

perineal body

anus

sphincter ani externus m.

sphincter ani externus m.

perineal body

anus

pterygo-mandibular raphe

hyoid bone

thyroid cartilage

mandible

chondroglossus m.

tongue

C

styloglossus m.

hyoglossus m.

mandible

genioglossus m.

hyoid bone

trachea

esophagus

scleral venous sinus (canal of Shlemm)

two innermost layers of cornea

iris

meridonal fibers

radial fibers

circular fibers

ciliaris m.

D

left hipbone

ischial spine

E

coccygeus m.

compressor naris m.

F

dilator naris m.

left maxillary cuspid

© MELLONI

MUSCLE	ORIGIN	INSERTION	INNERVATION	ACTION
m. constrictor pharyngis superior *superior constrictor m. of pharynx*	pterygopharyngeal part: pterygoid hamulus; medial pterygoid plate buccopharyngeal part: pterygomandibular raphe mylopharyngeal part: inner part of mandible glossopharyngeal part: side of tongue	median raphe; pharyngeal tubercle of occipital bone	pharyngeal plexus of vagus nerve (10th cranial nerve)	narrows pharynx in swallowing
m. coracobrachialis *coracobrachial m.*	coracoid process of scapula (in common with tendon of short head of m. biceps brachii)	midway along inner side of shaft of humerus	musculocutaneous nerve (5th, 6th, and 7th cranial nerves)	flexes and assists in adduction of arm
m. corrugator cutis ani *corrugator cutis ani m.*	fine strands of involuntary muscle derived from the conjoint longitudinal coat of the anal canal and attached to the dermis of the perianal skin		fibers from the inferior rectal branch of pudendal nerve (S2, S3)	aids in corrugating perianal skin
m. corrugator supercilii *superciliary corrugator m.* *corrugator m.*	medial portion of supraorbital margin	skin over middle of eyebrow	temporal branches of facial nerve (7th cranial nerve)	draws eyebrow medially and downward; furrows eyebrow
m. cremaster *cremaster m.*	lateral part: inguinal ligament; inferior margin of m. obliquus internus (often from m. transversus abdominis) medial part: pubic tubercle; inferior margin of m. transversus abdominis	lateral part: saclike cremastic fascia over anterior and lateral surfaces of spermatic cord; superior part of tunica vaginalis medial part: saclike cremastic fascia over posterior and medial surfaces of spermatic cord	genital branch of genitofemoral nerve (L1, L2)	male: elevates testis toward superficial inguinal ring (female: encircles part of the round ligament of the uterus)
m. cricoarytenoideus lateralis *lateral cricoarytenoid m.*	upper margin of arch of cricoid cartilage	muscular process of arytenoid cartilage	recurrent nerve of vagus nerve (10th cranial nerve)	the paired muscles rotate the arytenoid cartilages thereby closing the glottis and approximating the vocal cords for phonation
m. cricoarytenoideus posterior *posterior cricoarytenoid m.*	posterior surface of lamina of cricoid cartilage	muscular process of arytenoid cartilage	recurrent nerve of vagus nerve (10th cranial nerve)	the paired muscles rotate the arytenoid cartilages thereby opening the glottis and separating the vocal cords

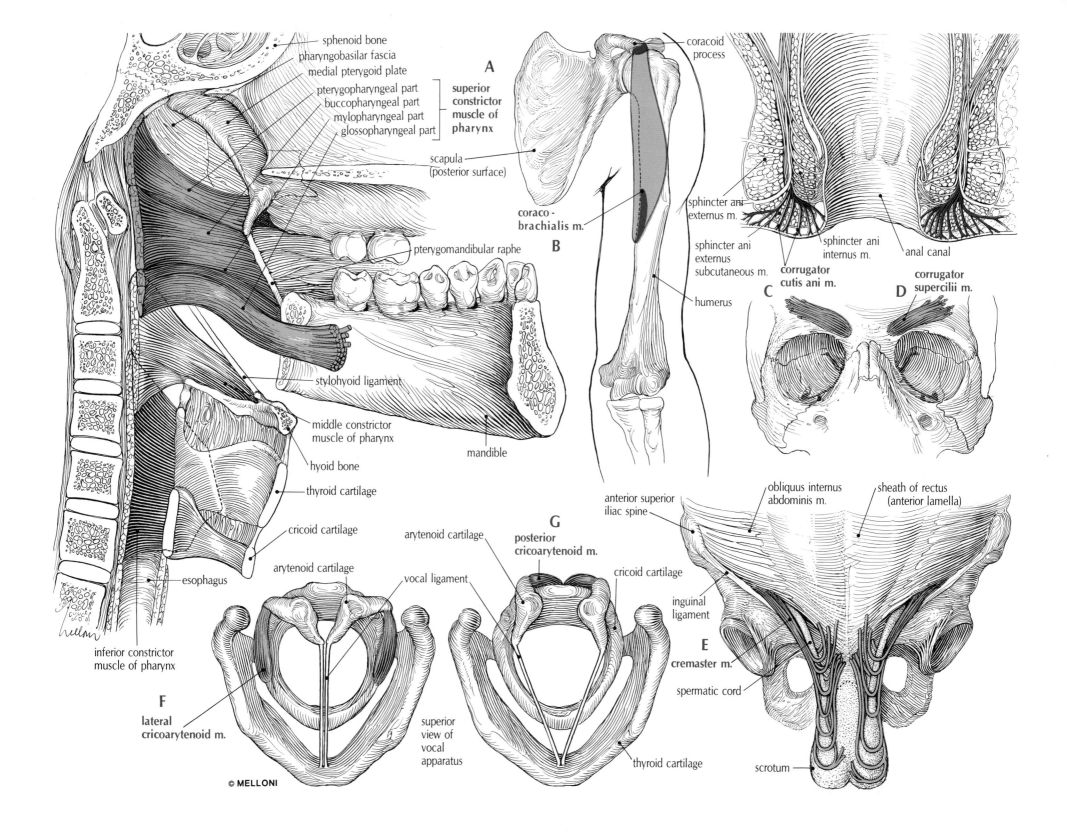

sphenoid bone
pharyngobasilar fascia
medial pterygoid plate
pterygopharyngeal part
buccopharyngeal part
mylopharyngeal part
glossopharyngeal part
superior constrictor muscle of pharynx
scapula (posterior surface)

A

coracoid process

coraco-brachialis m.

B

humerus

pterygomandibular raphe

stylohyoid ligament

middle constrictor muscle of pharynx

hyoid bone

thyroid cartilage

cricoid cartilage

esophagus

inferior constrictor muscle of pharynx

mandible

sphincter ani externus m.
sphincter ani externus subcutaneous m.
sphincter ani internus m.
anal canal

corrugator cutis ani m.

C

corrugator supercilii m.

D

obliquus internus abdominis m.
sheath of rectus (anterior lamella)

anterior superior iliac spine

inguinal ligament

E

cremaster m.

spermatic cord

scrotum

arytenoid cartilage
vocal ligament

F

lateral cricoarytenoid m.

superior view of vocal apparatus

arytenoid cartilage

posterior cricoarytenoid m.

cricoid cartilage

G

thyroid cartilage

© MELLONI

	MUSCLE	ORIGIN	INSERTION	INNERVATION	ACTION
A	**m. cricothyroideus** *cricothyroid m.*	anterolateral surface of cricoid thyroid cartilage	straight part: lower margin of lamina of thyroid cartilage oblique part: inferior horn of thyroid cartilage	superior laryngeal branch of vagus nerve (10th cranial nerve)	lengthens, stretches and tenses vocal cord (main tensor of vocal cord)
B	**m. deltoideus** *deltoid m.*	lateral third of clavicle; acromion; spine of scapula	deltoid tuberosity of shaft of humerus	axillary nerve	main abductor of arm; aids in flexion, extension, and lateral rotation of arm
C	**m. depressor anguli oris** *depressor m. of angle of mouth* *triangular m*	anterolateral part of mandible (oblique line)	angle of mouth	mandibular marginal branch of facial nerve (7th cranial nerve)	pulls down angle of mouth
D	**m. depressor labii inferioris** *depressor m. of lower lip* *quadrate m. of lower lip*	mandible adjacent to mental foramen; m. platysma	skin of lower lip	mandibular marginal branch facial nerve (7th cranial nerve)	draws lower lip downward and somewhat laterally
E	**m. depressor septi nasi** *depressor m. of nasal septum*	incisive fossa of maxilla (over roots of incisor teeth)	back part of cartilaginous ala and adjacent part of nasal septum	upper buccal branch of facial nerve (7th cranial nerve)	widens nostril in deep inspiration
F	**m. depressor supercilii** *(one of three parts of m. orbicularis oculi)* *superciliary depressor m.*	frontal process of maxilla; nasal part of frontal bone; medial palpebral ligament	skin of eyebrow	temporal and zygomatic branches of facial nerve (7th cranial nerve)	pulls eyebrow downward
G	**m. detrusor vesicae** *detrusor m. of urinary bladder*	the muscular coat of the bladder, consisting of three layers of nonstriated muscular fibers; an external longitudinal layer, a middle circular layer, and an internal longitudinal layer		vesicular plexus, primarily parasympathetic component (S2, S3, S4); to a lesser degree, a sympathetic component (T11, T12, L2)	empties urinary bladder
H	**m. diaphragma** *diaphragm*	costal part: internal surfaces of lower six ribs and costal cartilages sternal part: internal surface of xiphoid process lumbar part: via a tendinous crus on the anterolateral surfaces of vertebral bodies L1, L2, L3 (left side) and L1, L2 (right side); arcuate ligament	central tendon of diaphragm	phrenic nerve; lower six intercostal nerves	major muscle of inspiration

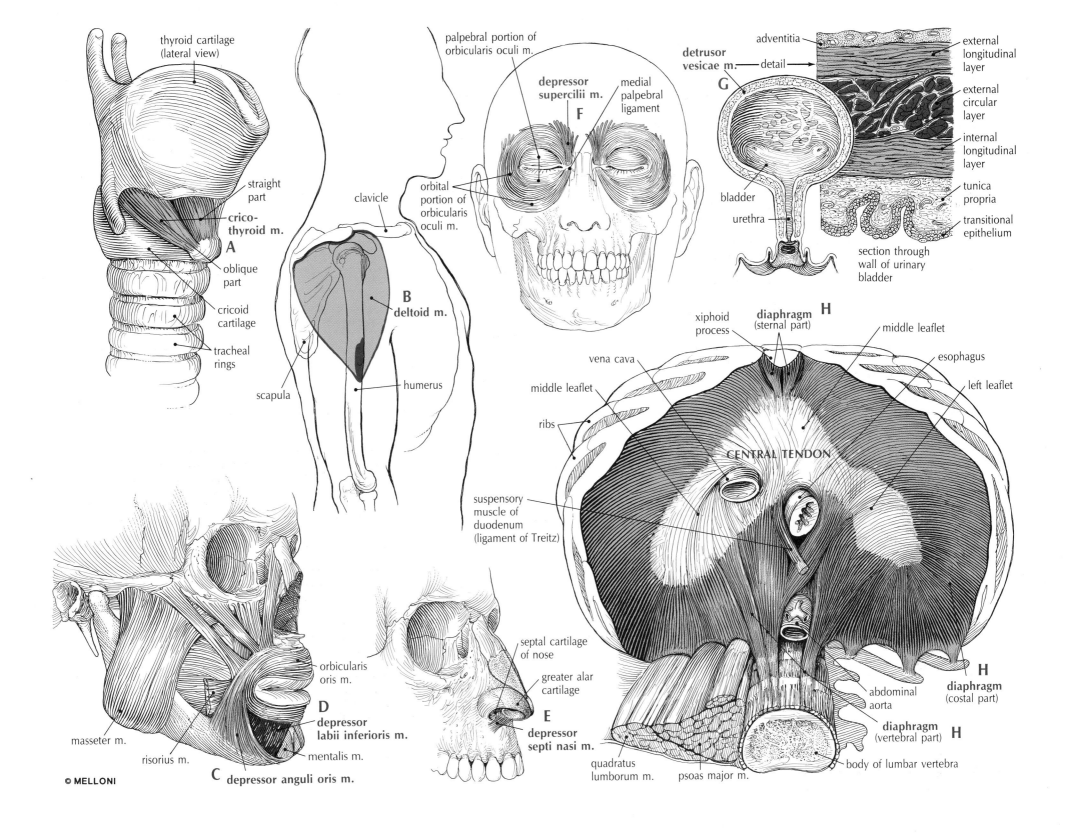

thyroid cartilage (lateral view)

straight part

crico-thyroid m.

A

oblique part

cricoid cartilage

tracheal rings

clavicle

B **deltoid m.**

scapula

humerus

palpebral portion of orbicularis oculi m.

depressor supercilii m.

medial palpebral ligament

F

orbital portion of orbicularis oculi m.

adventitia

detrusor vesicae m.

detail

G

bladder

urethra

external longitudinal layer

external circular layer

internal longitudinal layer

tunica propria

transitional epithelium

section through wall of urinary bladder

orbicularis oris m.

masseter m.

risorius m.

C **depressor anguli oris m.**

mentalis m.

D **depressor labii inferioris m.**

septal cartilage of nose

greater alar cartilage

E **depressor septi nasi m.**

diaphragm (sternal part) **H**

xiphoid process

middle leaflet

esophagus

left leaflet

vena cava

middle leaflet

ribs

CENTRAL TENDON

suspensory muscle of duodenum (ligament of Treitz)

H

diaphragm (costal part)

abdominal aorta

diaphragm (vertebral part) **H**

quadratus lumborum m.

psoas major m.

body of lumbar vertebra

© MELLONI

	MUSCLE	ORIGIN	INSERTION	INNERVATION	ACTION
A	**diaphragma pelvis** *pelvic diaphragm*	a funnel-shaped musculotendinous structure composed of the paired m. levator ani and m. coccygeus and sheathed in a superior and inferior layer of fascia			forms the partition between the pelvic cavity and the perineum; it supports the pelvic viscera
B	**diaphragma urogenitale** *urogenital diaphragm*	a musculotendinous structure composed of the m. transversus perinei profundus, m. transversus perinei superficialis (inconstant), and m. sphincter urethrae and sheathed in a superior and inferior layer of fascia			forms partition across the anterior half of the pelvic outlet between the ischiopubic rami
C	**m. digastricus** *digastric m.*	anterior belly: digastric fossa on base of mandible near median plane posterior belly: mastoid notch of temporal bone	anterior belly: intermediate tendon bound to hyoid bone by loop of fascia posterior belly: intermediate tendon bound to hyoid bone by loop of fascia	anterior belly: mylohyoid branch of inferior alveolar nerve posterior belly: facial nerve (7th cranial nerve)	lowers mandible; raises hyoid bone
D	**m. dilator naris** *(the ala part of m. nasalis)* *dilator m. of nose*	nasal notch of maxilla	ala cartilage of nose	upper buccal branches of facial nerve (7th cranial nerve)	widens nostril
E	**m. dilator pupillae** *dilator m. of pupil*	ciliary margin of iris	near margin of pupil	sympathetic nerves derived from the superior cervical ganglion	dilates pupil
F	**m. epicranius** *epicranial m.*	the muscular and tendinous layer of the scalp composed of the m. occipitofrontalis and m. temporoparietalis connected by an extensive epicranial aponeurosis (galea aponeurotica)			elevates eyebrows; draws scalp forward and backward; tightens scalp
G	**m. erector spinae** *erector m. of spine* *sacrospinal m.*	deep muscle arising from the broad and thick tendon attached to the middle and lateral sacral crest, spinous processes of vertebrae (L1, L2, L3, L4, L5, T11, T12), supraspinous ligament, and back part of iliac crest; it splits in the upper lumbar region into three columns: m. iliocostalis (lateral division), m. longissimus (intermediate division), and m. spinalis (medial division)			extends vertebral column and bends trunk to one side
H	**m. extensor carpi radialis brevis** *short radial extensor m. of wrist*	lateral epicondyle of humerus; radial collateral ligament of elbow joint	base of 3rd metacarpal bone	posterior interosseous nerve of radial nerve (7th and 8th cranial nerves)	extends wrist; abducts hand
I	**m. extensor carpi radialis longus** *long radial extensor m. of wrist*	lateral supracondylar ridge of humerus	dorsal surface of 2nd metacarpal bone	radial nerve (6th and 7th cranial nerves)	extends wrist; abducts hand
J	**m. extensor carpi ulnaris** *ulnar extensor m. of wrist*	humeral head: lateral epicondyle of humerus ulnar head: posterior border of ulna	base of 5th metacarpal bone	posterior interosseous nerve of deep radial nerve (7th and 8th cranial nerves)	extends wrist; adducts hand

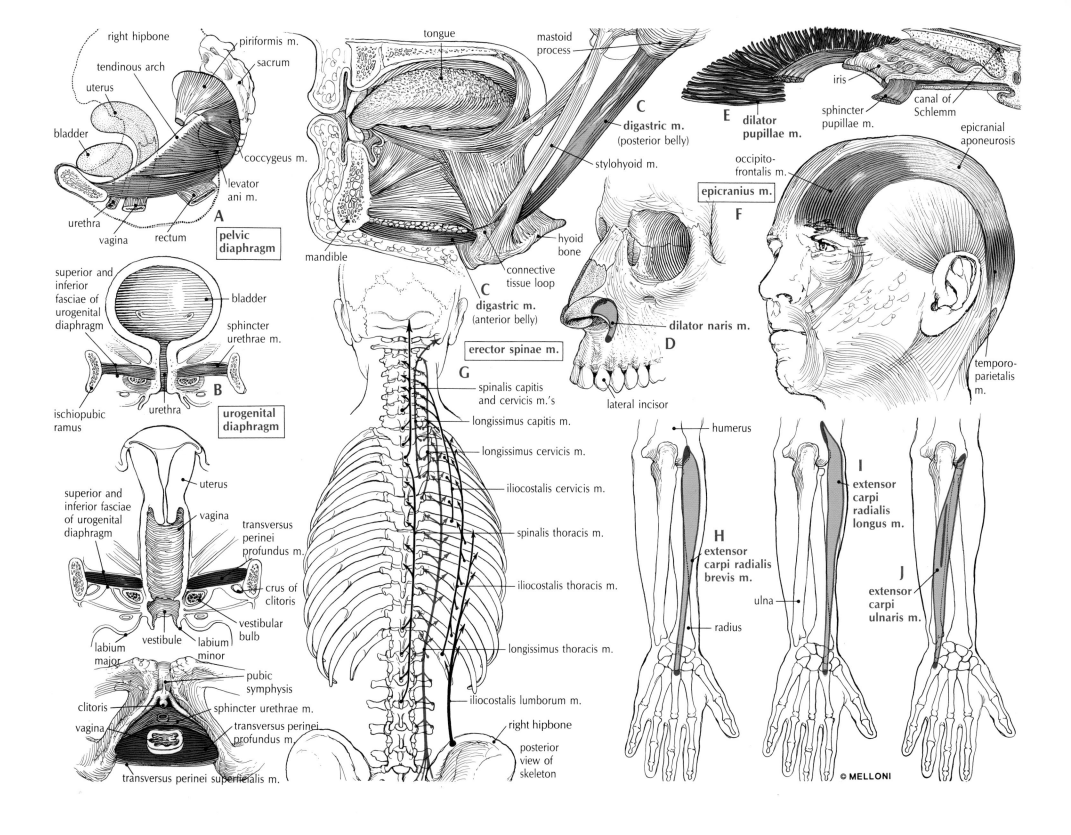

right hipbone

piriformis m.

tendinous arch

sacrum

uterus

bladder

coccygeus m.

urethra

levator ani m.

vagina

rectum

A

pelvic diaphragm

superior and inferior fasciae of urogenital diaphragm

bladder

sphincter urethrae m.

ischiopubic ramus

urethra

B

urogenital diaphragm

superior and inferior fasciae of urogenital diaphragm

uterus

vagina

transversus perinei profundus m.

crus of clitoris

vestibular bulb

labium major

labium minor

vestibule

pubic symphysis

clitoris

sphincter urethrae m.

vagina

transversus perinei profundus m.

transversus perinei superficialis m.

tongue

mastoid process

digastric m. (posterior belly)

stylohyoid m.

C

mandible

hyoid bone

connective tissue loop

C digastric m. (anterior belly)

erector spinae m.

G

spinalis capitis and cervicis m.'s

longissimus capitis m.

longissimus cervicis m.

iliocostalis cervicis m.

spinalis thoracis m.

iliocostalis thoracis m.

longissimus thoracis m.

iliocostalis lumborum m.

right hipbone

posterior view of skeleton

iris

dilator pupillae m.

E

sphincter pupillae m.

canal of Schlemm

epicranial aponeurosis

occipito-frontalis m.

epicranius m.

F

dilator naris m.

D

lateral incisor

temporo-parietalis m.

humerus

I

extensor carpi radialis longus m.

H extensor carpi radialis brevis m.

ulna

radius

J extensor carpi ulnaris m.

© MELLONI

	MUSCLE	ORIGIN	INSERTION	INNERVATION	ACTION
A	**m. extensor digiti minimi** *extensor m. of little finger*	lateral epicondyle of humerus	dorsal aponeurosis of little finger	posterior interosseous nerve of deep radial nerve (7th and 8th cranial nerves)	extends little finger
B	**m. extensor digitorum** *extensor m. of fingers*	lateral epicondyle of humerus	common extensor tendon on dorsum of each finger	posterior interosseous nerve of deep radial nerve (7th and 8th cranial nerves)	extends fingers and wrist
C	**m. extensor digitorum brevis** *short extensor m. of toes*	dorsolateral surface of calcaneus	dorsal aponeurosis of proximal phalanx of big toe; extensor tendons of 2nd, 3rd, and 4th toes	lateral terminal branch of deep peroneal nerve (S1, S2)	extends toes
D	**m. extensor digitorum longus** *long extensor m. of toes*	lateral condyle of tibia; medial surface of upper three fourths of fibula; interosseous membrane	dorsal aponeurosis of middle and distal phalanges of lateral four toes	deep peroneal nerve (L5, S1)	extends toes; dorsiflexes foot
E	**m. extensor hallucis brevis** *(medial part of m. extensor digitorum brevis)* *short extensor m. of big toe*	dorsal surface of calcaneus; interosseous talocalcaneal ligament	dorsal surface of base of proximal phalanx of big toe	deep peroneal nerve (S1, S2)	dorsiflexes big toe
F	**m. extensor hallucis longus** *long extensor m. of big toe*	middle of fibula; interosseous membrane	dorsal surface of distal phalanx of big toe	deep peroneal nerve (L5, S1)	extends big toe; dorsiflexes foot
G	**m. extensor indicis** *extensor m. of index finger*	posterior surface of ulna; interosseous membrane	dorsal aponeurosis of index finger (joins tendon of m. extensor digitorum)	posterior interosseous nerve of deep radial nerve (7th and 8th cranial nerves)	extends index finger; aids in extending hand
H	**m. extensor pollicis brevis** *short extensor m. of thumb*	dorsal surface of middle third of radius; interosseous membrane	dorsal surface of proximal phalanx of thumb	posterior interosseous nerve of deep radial nerve (7th and 8th cranial nerves)	extends and abducts thumb
I	**m. extensor pollicis longus** *long extensor m. of thumb*	middle third of ulna; interosseous membrane	base of distal phalanx of thumb	posterior interosseous nerve of deep radial nerve (7th and 8th cranial nerves)	extends distal phalanx of thumb; abducts thumb
J	**m. flexor carpi radialis** *radial flexor m. of wrist*	medial epicondyle of humerus; antebrachial fascia	bases of 2nd and 3rd metacarpal bones	median nerve (6th and 7th cranial nerves)	flexes wrist; abducts hand
K	**m. flexor carpi ulnaris** *ulnar flexor m. of wrist*	humeral head: medial epicondyle of humerus ulnar head: medial side of olecranon; upper two thirds of posterior border of ulna	pisiform, hamate, and 5th metacarpal bones; flexor retinaculum	ulnar nerve (7th and 8th cranial nerves)	flexes wrist; adducts hand

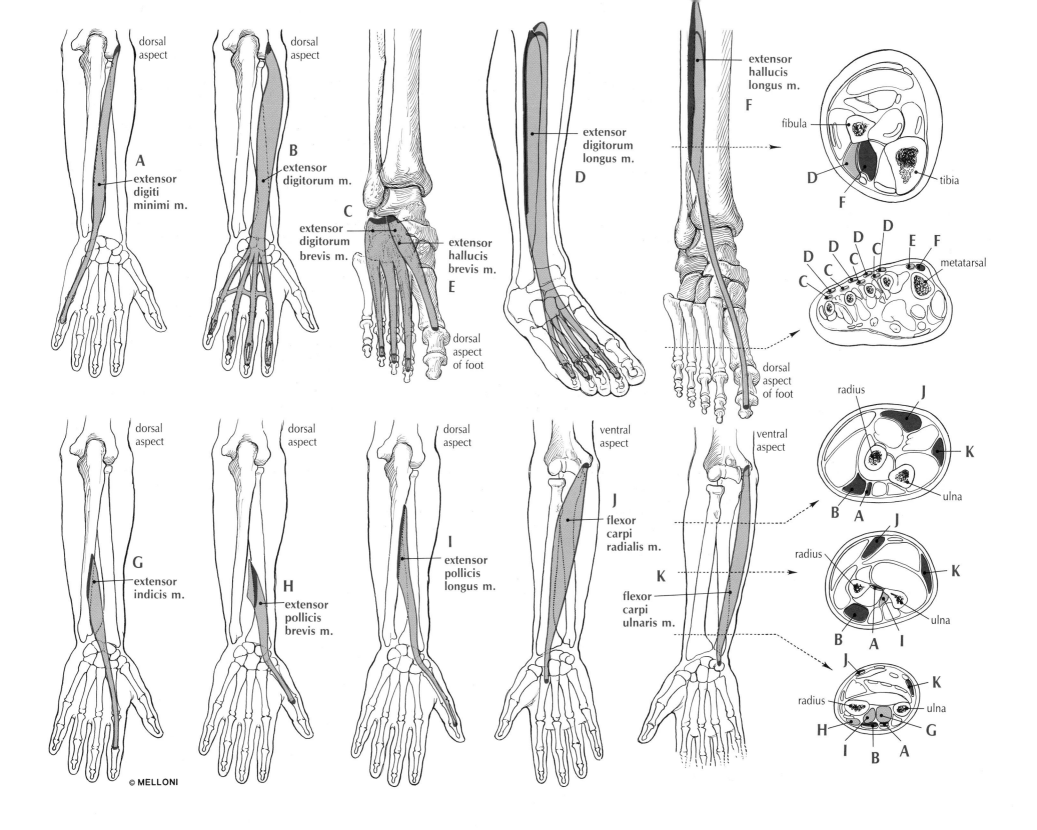

A extensor digiti minimi m.

dorsal aspect

B extensor digitorum m.

dorsal aspect

C extensor digitorum brevis m.

E extensor hallucis brevis m.

dorsal aspect of foot

D extensor digitorum longus m.

dorsal aspect of foot

F extensor hallucis longus m.

fibula

D

F

tibia

D D D
D D C C
C C C
E F

metatarsal

G extensor indicis m.

dorsal aspect

H extensor pollicis brevis m.

dorsal aspect

I extensor pollicis longus m.

dorsal aspect

J flexor carpi radialis m.

ventral aspect

K flexor carpi ulnaris m.

ventral aspect

radius

J

K

ulna

B A

radius

J

K

ulna

B A I

J

radius

K

ulna

H

I B A

G

© MELLONI

	MUSCLE	ORIGIN	INSERTION	INNERVATION	ACTION
A	**m. flexor digiti minimi brevis manus** *short flexor m. of little finger*	hook of hamate bone; flexor retinaculum	base of proximal phalanx of little finger	deep branch of ulnar nerve (8th cranial nerve and T1)	flexes proximal phalanx of little finger
B	**m. flexor digiti minimi brevis pedis** *short flexor m. of little toe*	base of 5th metatarsal bone; sheath of m. peroneous longus	proximal phalanx of little toe	superficial branch of lateral plantar nerve (S2, S3)	flexes little toe
C	**m. flexor digitorum brevis** *short flexor m. of toes*	medial surface of tuberosity of calcaneus; long plantar ligament	middle phalanges of lateral four toes	lateral plantar nerve (S2, S3)	flexes lateral four toes
D	**m. flexor digitorum longus** *long flexor m. of toes*	posterior surface of middle half of tibia	distal phalanges of lateral four toes	tibial nerve (S2, S3)	flexes 2nd to 5th toes; plantarflexes foot
E	**m. flexor digitorum profundus** *deep flexor m. of fingers*	upper three fourths of ulna; adjacent interosseous membrane	distal phalanges of fingers	ulnar nerve; anterior interosseous branch of median nerve (8th cranial nerve and T1)	flexes terminal phalanges of lateral four digits; aids in flexing wrist
F	**m. flexor digitorum superficialis** *superficial flexor m. of fingers*	humeroulnar head: medial epicondyle of humerus; coronoid process of ulna radial head: anterior border of radius	middle phalanges of 2nd to 5th fingers	median nerve (7th and 8th cranial nerves and T1)	flexes phalanges and wrist
G	**m. flexor hallucis brevis** *short flexor m. of big toe*	underside of cuboid bone; lateral cuneiform bone	both sides of proximal phalanx of big toe	medial plantar nerve (S2, S3)	flexes big toe
H	**m. flexor hallucis longus** *long flexor m. of big toe*	lower two thirds of posterior surface of fibula; inter-muscular septum; interosseous membrane	plantar aspect of distal phalanx of big toe	tibial nerve (S2, S3)	flexes big toe; plantarflexes foot
I	**m. flexor pollicis brevis** *short flexor m. of thumb*	superficial part: distal border of flexor retinaculum; tubercle of trapezium deep part: trapezoid and capitate bones of wrist; palmar ligament	superficial part: base of proximal phalanx of thumb deep part: base of proximal phalanx of thumb	superficial part: lateral branch of median nerve deep part: deep branch of ulnar nerve	flexes thumb
J	**m. flexor pollicis longus** *long flexor m. of thumb*	anterior surface of radius; adjacent interosseous membrane; coronoid process of ulna	distal phalanx of thumb	anterior interosseous branch of median nerve (8th cranial nerve and T1)	flexes thumb

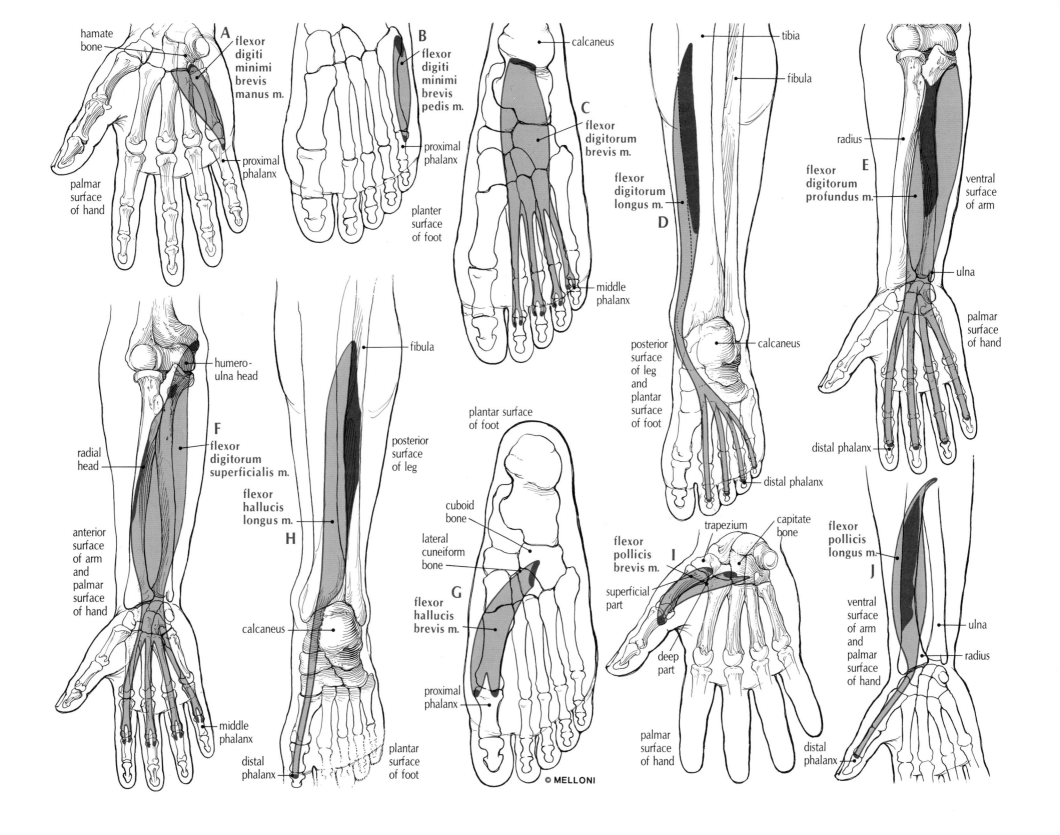

hamate bone

A flexor digiti minimi brevis manus m.

proximal phalanx

palmar surface of hand

B flexor digiti minimi brevis pedis m.

proximal phalanx

planter surface of foot

calcaneus

C flexor digitorum brevis m.

middle phalanx

tibia

fibula

flexor digitorum longus m.

D

posterior surface of leg and plantar surface of foot

calcaneus

distal phalanx

radius

flexor digitorum profundus m.

E

ventral surface of arm

ulna

palmar surface of hand

distal phalanx

humero-ulna head

radial head

F flexor digitorum superficialis m.

anterior surface of arm and palmar surface of hand

middle phalanx

distal phalanx

fibula

posterior surface of leg

flexor hallucis longus m.

H

calcaneus

plantar surface of foot

plantar surface of foot

cuboid bone

lateral cuneiform bone

G flexor hallucis brevis m.

proximal phalanx

trapezium

capitate bone

flexor pollicis brevis m.

I

superficial part

deep part

palmar surface of hand

distal phalanx

flexor pollicis longus m.

J

ventral surface of arm and palmar surface of hand

ulna

radius

distal phalanx

© MELLONI

	MUSCLE	ORIGIN	INSERTION	INNERVATION	ACTION
A	**m. gastrocnemius** *gastrocnemius m.*	medial head: popliteal surface of femur; upper part of medial condyle of femur; capsule of knee joint lateral head: lateral condyle of femur; lower part of supracondylar line; capsule of knee joint	calcaneus via calcaneal tendon (in common with m. soleus)	tibial nerve (S1, S2)	plantarflexes foot; flexes knee
B	**m. gemellus inferior** *inferior gemellus m.*	upper part of ischial tuberosity	medial side of greater trochanter of femur via the internal obturator tendon	nerve to quadratus femoris (L5, S1)	rotates thigh laterally
C	**m. gemellus superior** *superior gemellus m.*	spine of ischium	medial side of greater trochanter of femur via internal obturator tendon	obturator internus nerve (L5, S1)	rotates and extends thigh laterally; abducts flexed thigh
D	**m. genioglossus** *genioglossus m.*	upper genial tubercle on inner surface of mandibular symphysis	entire ventral surface of tongue; hyoid bone; middle constrictor muscle of pharynx	muscular branches of hypoglossal nerve (12th cranial nerve)	protrudes and depresses tongue
E	**m. geniohyoideus** *geniohyoid m.*	lower genial tubercle on inner surface of mandibular symphysis	anterior surface of body of hyoid bone	1st cervical spine nerve through hypoglossal nerve (12th cranial nerve)	elevates hyoid bone and draws it forward
F	**m. gluteus maximus** *greatest gluteal m.*	upper portion of outer surface of ilium, sacrum and coccyx; sacrotuberous ligament; gluteal aponeurosis	iliotibial tract of fascia lata; gluteal tuberosity of femur	inferior gluteal nerve (L5, S1, S2)	rotates thigh laterally and extends and abducts it
G	**m. gluteus medius** *middle gluteal m.*	midportion of outer surface of ilium	lateral surface of greater trochanter of femur	superior gluteal nerve (L5, S1)	abducts and rotates thigh medially; tilts pelvis to raise opposite foot from floor
H	**m. gluteus minimus** *least gluteal m.*	lower portion of outer surface of ilium between the anterior and inferior gluteal lines	anterior surface of greater trochanter of femur; fibrous capsule of hip joint	superior gluteal nerve (L5, S1)	abducts and rotates thigh medially
I	**m. gracilis** *gracilis m.*	lower half of pubis	medial side of upper part of tibia	obturator nerve (L2, L3)	flexes and rotates leg medially; adducts thigh

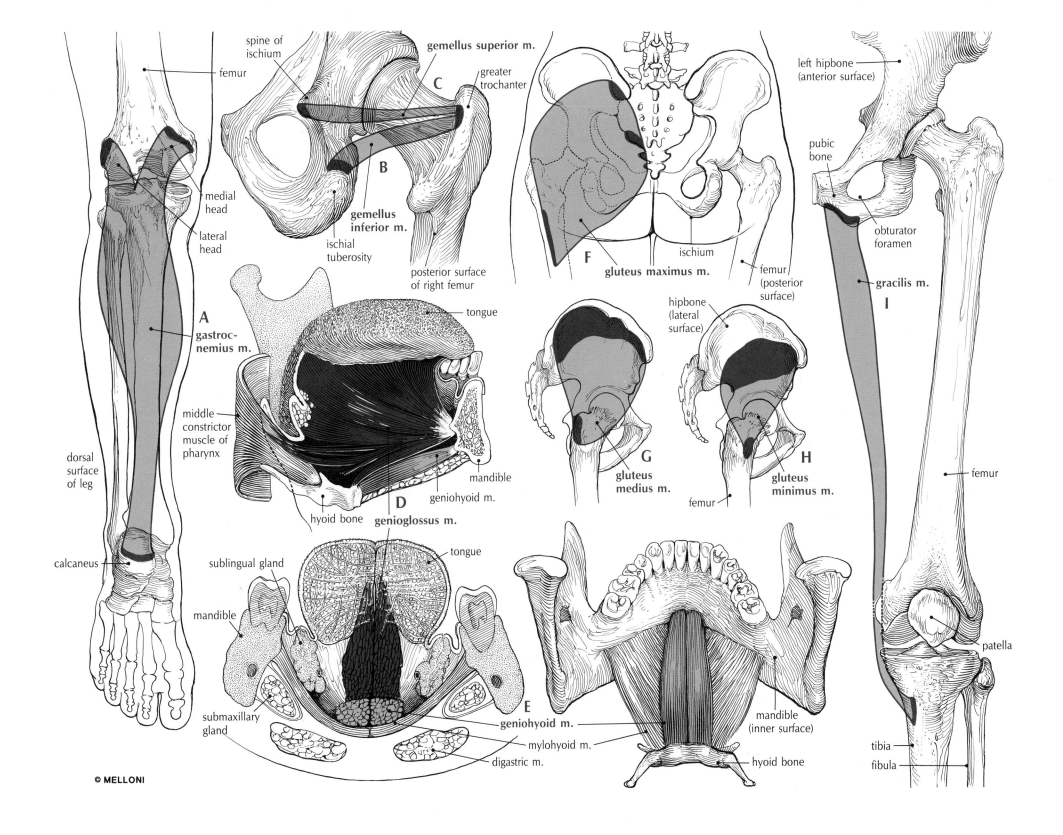

femur

medial head

lateral head

A
**gastroc-
nemius m.**

dorsal surface of leg

calcaneus

spine of ischium

gemellus superior m.

greater trochanter

C

B

gemellus inferior m.

ischial tuberosity

posterior surface of right femur

tongue

middle constrictor muscle of pharynx

mandible

geniohyoid m.

hyoid bone

D
genioglossus m.

sublingual gland

mandible

tongue

submaxillary gland

E

geniohyoid m.

mylohyoid m.

digastric m.

mandible (inner surface)

hyoid bone

left hipbone (anterior surface)

pubic bone

obturator foramen

gracilis m.

I

femur

patella

tibia

fibula

ischium

F
gluteus maximus m.

femur (posterior surface)

hipbone (lateral surface)

G
gluteus medius m.

femur

H
gluteus minimus m.

© MELLONI

	MUSCLE	ORIGIN	INSERTION	INNERVATION	ACTION
A	**m. helicis major** *larger m. of helix*	spine of helix	anterior border of helix	posterior auricular branch of facial nerve (7th cranial nerve)	thought to be vestigial
B	**m. helicis minor** *smaller m. of helix*	anterior rim of helix	crux of helix	temporal branch of facial nerve (7th cranial nerve)	thought to be vestigial
C	**m. hyoglossus** *hyoglossus m.*	body and greater horn of hyoid bone	side of tongue	muscular branch of hypoglossal nerve (12th cranial nerve)	retracts and depresses tongue
D	**m. iliacus** *iliac m.*	iliac fossa (inner surface of iliac bone); lateral aspect of sacrum	greater psoas tendon; lesser trochanter of femur	branches of femoral nerve (L2, L3)	flexes thigh
E	**m. iliococcygeus** *(part of m. levator ani)* *iliococcygeal m.*	ischial spine; tendinous arch of pelvic fascia	coccyx; medial raphe between the tip of coccyx and anal canal	branch from S4; branch from inferior rectal nerve	supports pelvic viscera
F	**m. iliocostalis** *iliocostal m.*	the lateral portion of m. erector spinae (sacrospinalis) composed of three parts: m. iliocostalis cervicis, m. iliocostalis thoracis, m. iliocostalis lumborum			extends vertebral column; assists in lateral movement of trunk
G	**m. iliocostalis cervicis** *iliocostal m. of neck*	angles of 3rd, 4th, 5th, and 6th ribs	transverse processes of 4th, 5th, and 6th cervical vertebrae	dorsal branches of lower cervical spinal nerves	extends cervical vertebral column and flexes it laterally
H	**m. iliocostalis lumborum** *iliocostal m. of loins* *sacrolumbalis m.*	iliac crest; thoracolumbar fascia	transverse processes of lumbar vertebrae; inferior border of angles of lower seven ribs	dorsal branches of thoracic and upper lumbar spinal nerves	extends lumbar vertebral column and flexes it laterally
I	**m. iliocostalis thoracis** *iliocostal m. of thorax* *iliocostal m. of back*	upper borders of lower six ribs, medial to angles	angles of upper six ribs; transverse process of 7th cervical vertebra	dorsal branches of thoracic spinal nerves	extends thoracic vertebral column and flexes it laterally
J	**m. iliopsoas** *iliopsoas m.*	a compound muscle consisting of the m. iliacus and m. psoas major, which inserts by a common tendon to the lesser trochanter of femur			flexes thigh upon pelvis; raises trunk from supine to sitting position
K	**m. incisurae helicis** *m. of incisure of helix*	muscular slips occasionally seen on the medial surface of the cartilage of the ear as a caudal continuation of m. transversus auriculae		posterior auricular branch of facial nerve (7th cranial nerve)	retracts helix feebly
L	**m. incisivus labii inferioris** *incisive muscle of lower lip*	mandible adjacent to m. mentalis	angle of mouth	mandibular marginal branch of facial nerve (7th cranial nerve)	make vestibule of mouth shallow; aid in articulation and mastication

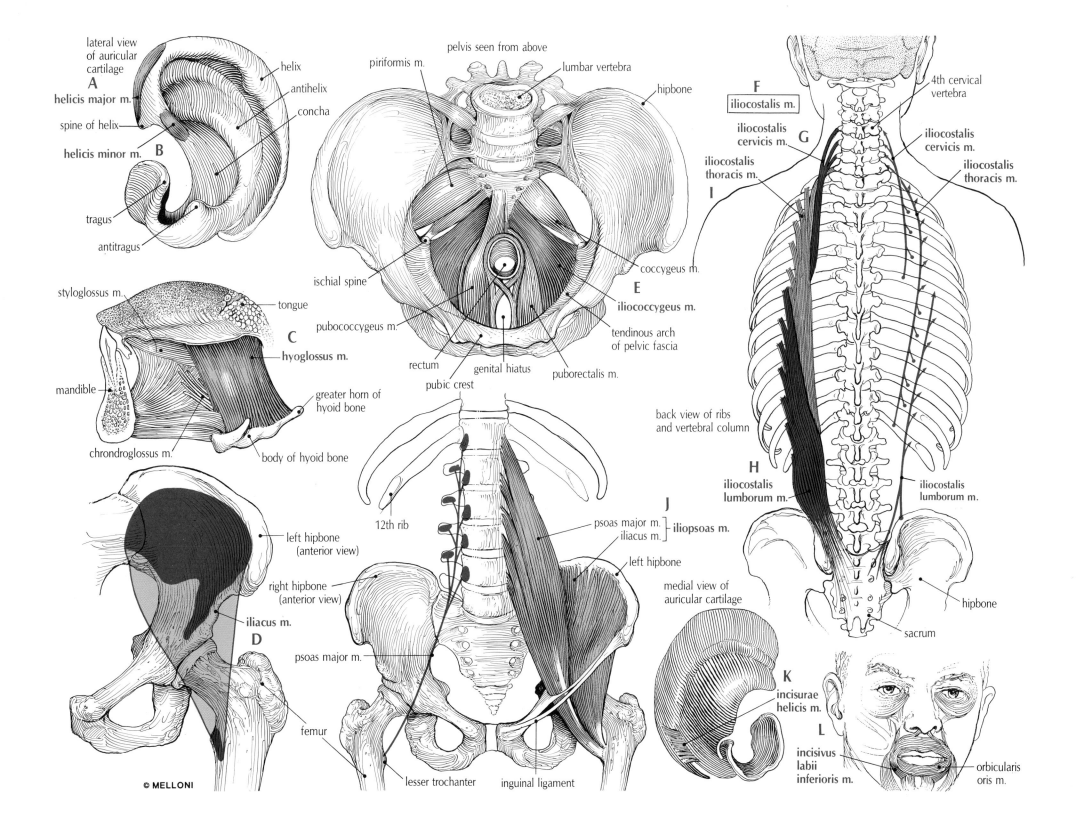

A lateral view of auricular cartilage

helicis major m.

spine of helix

helicis minor m.   **B**

helix

antihelix

concha

tragus

antitragus

C

styloglossus m.

tongue

mandible

hyoglossus m.

chrondroglossus m.

greater horn of hyoid bone

body of hyoid bone

D

left hipbone (anterior view)

iliacus m.

femur

pelvis seen from above

piriformis m.

lumbar vertebra

hipbone

ischial spine

pubococcygeus m.

rectum

pubic crest

genital hiatus

coccygeus m.

iliococcygeus m.   **E**

tendinous arch of pelvic fascia

puborectalis m.

right hipbone (anterior view)

psoas major m.

12th rib

psoas major m.
iliacus m. } **iliopsoas m.**

left hipbone

lesser trochanter

inguinal ligament

F   iliocostalis m.

iliocostalis cervicis m.   **G**

iliocostalis thoracis m.

I

4th cervical vertebra

iliocostalis cervicis m.

iliocostalis thoracis m.

back view of ribs and vertebral column

H

iliocostalis lumborum m.

iliocostalis lumborum m.

hipbone

sacrum

J

medial view of auricular cartilage

K

incisurae helicis m.

L

incisivus labii inferioris m.

orbicularis oris m.

© MELLONI

	MUSCLE	ORIGIN	INSERTION	INNERVATION	ACTION
A	**m. incisivus labii superioris** *incisive muscle of upper lip*	maxilla near root of lateral incisor tooth	angle of mouth	lower buccal branch of facial nerve (7th cranial nerve)	make vestibule of mouth shallow; aid in articulation and mastication
B	**mm. infrahyoidei** *infrahyoid muscles*	ribbonlike muscles below the hyoid bone including the m. omohyoideus, m. sternohyoideus, m. sternothyroideus, and the m. thyrohyoideus			stabilize the hyoid bone to the sternum, clavicle, and scapula and as a group are antagonists to the suprahyoid group
C	**m. infraspinatus** *infraspinous m.*	medial two thirds of infraspinous fossa; infraspinous fascia	posterior surface of greater tubercle of humerus	suprascapular nerve (4th, 5th, and 6th cranial nerves)	rotates arm laterally
D	**mm. intercostales externi** *external intercostal muscles*	lower border of rib	upper border of rib below	intercostal nerves	draw ribs together
E	**mm. intercostales interni** *internal intercostal muscles*	lower border of rib; costal cartilage	upper border of rib and costal cartilage below	intercostal nerves	draw ribs together
F	**mm. intercostales intimi** *innermost intercostal muscles*	internal surface of superior border of rib	internal surface of inferior border of rib below	intercostal nerves	draw ribs together
G	**mm. interossei dorsales manus** *(four in number)* *dorsal interosseous muscles of hand*	adjacent sides of metatarsal bones	proximal phalanges of 2nd, 3rd, and 4th fingers and their dorsal digital expansions	deep branch of ulnar nerve (8th cranial nerve and T1)	abduct fingers 2, 3, 4; aid in flexion of proximal phalanges; spread fingers
H	**mm. interossei dorsales pedis** *(four in number)* *dorsal interosseous muscles of foot*	adjacent sides of metatarsal bones	proximal phalanges of both sides of 2nd toe, lateral side of 3rd and 4th toes, and their dorsal digital expansions	lateral plantar nerve (S2, S3)	abduct lateral toes, move 2nd toe from side to side; flex proximal phalanges
I	**mm. interossei palmares manus** *(three in number)* *palmar interosseous muscles of hand*	medial side of 2nd and lateral side of 4th and 5th metacarpal bones	proximal phalanges of 2nd, 4th, and 5th fingers and their dorsal digital expansion	deep branch of ulnar nerve (8th cranial nerve and T1)	adduct fingers 2, 4, 5; aid in flexing proximal phalanges; close fingers
J	**mm. interossei plantares pedis** *(three in number)* *plantar interosseous muscles of foot*	base and medial side of 3rd, 4th, and 5th metatarsal bones	medial side of proximal phalanges of 3rd, 4th, and 5th toes and their dorsal digital expansions	lateral plantar nerve (S2, S3)	adduct three lateral toes; flex toes

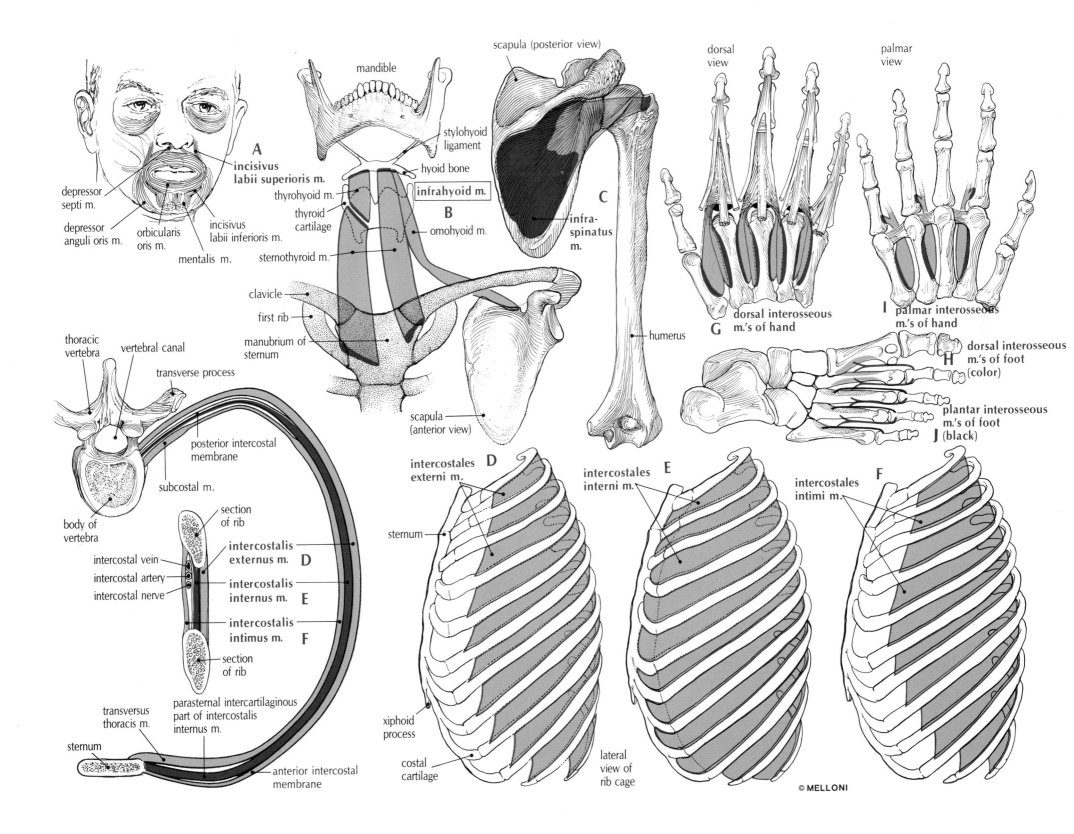

A

incisivus labii superioris m.

depressor septi m.

depressor anguli oris m.

orbicularis oris m.

incisivus labii inferioris m.

mentalis m.

mandible

stylohyoid ligament

hyoid bone

thyrohyoid m.

thyroid cartilage

infrahyoid m.

B

omohyoid m.

sternothyroid m.

clavicle

first rib

manubrium of sternum

scapula (anterior view)

scapula (posterior view)

C

infra-spinatus m.

humerus

dorsal view

palmar view

G dorsal interosseous m.'s of hand

I palmar interosseous m.'s of hand

H dorsal interosseous m.'s of foot (color)

J plantar interosseous m.'s of foot (black)

thoracic vertebra

vertebral canal

transverse process

posterior intercostal membrane

subcostal m.

body of vertebra

section of rib

intercostal vein

intercostal artery

intercostal nerve

intercostalis externus m. **D**

intercostalis internus m. **E**

intercostalis intimus m. **F**

section of rib

transversus thoracis m.

sternum

parasternal intercartilaginous part of intercostalis internus m.

anterior intercostal membrane

intercostales externi m. **D**

sternum

xiphoid process

costal cartilage

lateral view of rib cage

intercostales interni m. **E**

intercostales intimi m. **F**

© MELLONI

	MUSCLE	ORIGIN	INSERTION	INNERVATION	ACTION
A	**mm. interspinales** *interspinal muscles*	short muscles between the spinous processes of contiguous vertebrae on either side of the interspinous ligament, including the mm. interspinales cervicis, mm. interspinales thoracis, and mm. interspinales lumborum			extend vertebral column
B	**mm. interspinales cervicis** *interspinal muscles of neck*	superior surface of spinous process of vertebrae C3, C4, C5, C6, C7, and T1	inferior surface of spinous process of vertebra above vertebra of origin	dorsal branches of spinal nerves	aid in extending the vertebral column
C	**mm. interspinales lumborum** *interspinal muscles of loins*	superior surface of spinous process of vertebrae L2, L3, L4, and L5	inferior surface of spinous process of vertebra above vertebra of origin	dorsal branches of spinal nerves	aid in extending the vertebral column
D	**mm. interspinales thoracis** *interspinal muscles of thorax*	superior surface of spinous process of vertebrae T2, T3, and T12	inferior surface of spinous process of vertebra above vertebra of origin	dorsal branches of spinal nerves	aid in extending the vertebral column
E	**mm. intertransversarii** *intertransverse muscles*	small paired muscles between the transverse processes of contiguous vertebrae, including: mm. intertransversarii anteriores cervicis, mm. intertransversarii posteriorea cervicis, mm. intertransversarii mediales lumborum, mm. intertransversarii laterales lumborum, mm. intertransversarii thoracis			aid in maintaining erect posture by extension, lateral flexion, and rotation of the body
F	**mm. intertransversarii anteriores cervicis** *anterior intertransverse muscles of neck*	superior surface of anterior tubercles of vertebrae C3, C4, C5, C6, C7, T1	inferior surface of anterior tubercles of vertebrae C2, C3, C4, C5, C6, C7	ventral branches of spinal nerves (C2–C6)	aid in bending vertebral column laterally
G	**mm. intertransversarii laterales lumborum** *lateral intertransverse lumbar muscles*	ventral part: superior surface of costal processes of vertebrae L2, L3, L4, L5, S1 dorsal part: superior surface of accessory processes of vertebrae L2, L3, L4, L5, S1	ventral part: inferior surface of costal processes of vertebrae above vertebra of origin dorsal part: inferior surface of transverse processes of vertebrae above vertebra of origin	ventral branches of spinal nerves (L1–L4)	aid in bending vertebral column laterally
H	**mm. intertransversarii mediales lumborum** *medial intertransverse lumbar muscles*	accessory processes of vertebrae L2, L3, L4, L5, S1	mamillary processes of vertebrae above vertebra of origin	dorsal branches of spinal nerves (L1–L4)	aid in bending vertebral column laterally

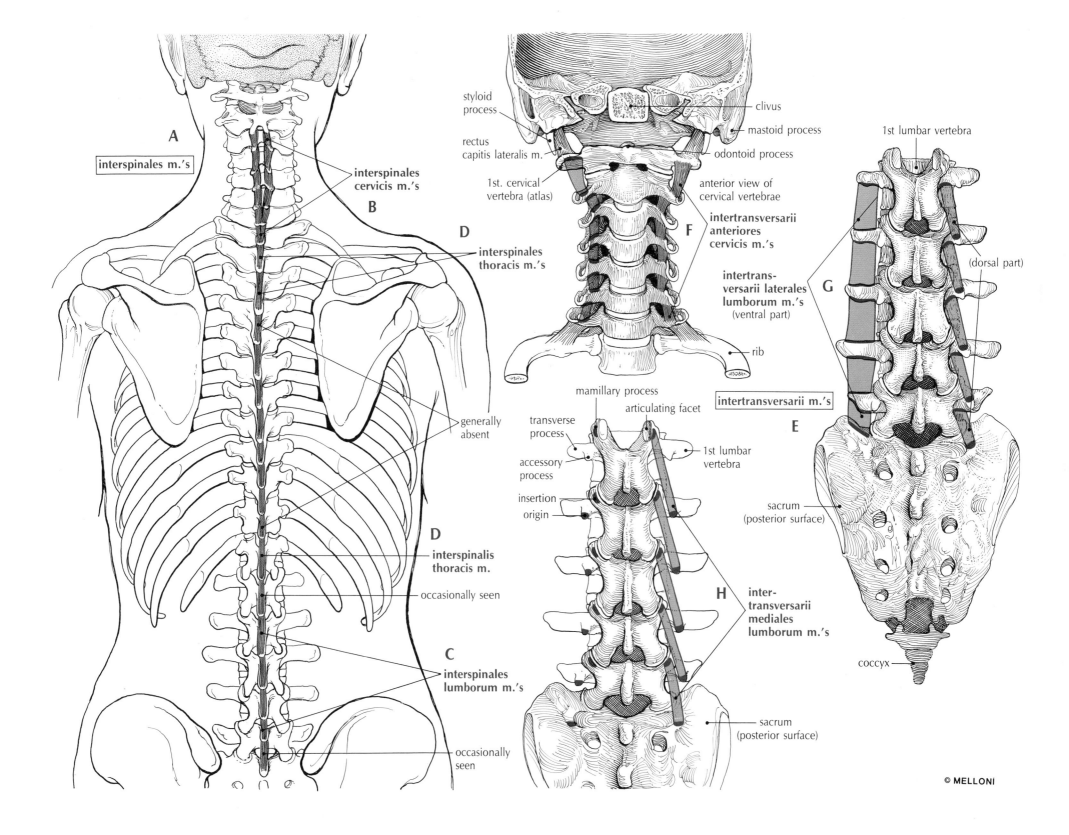

interspinales m.'s

A

interspinales cervicis m.'s

B

D

interspinales thoracis m.'s

generally absent

D

interspinalis thoracis m.

occasionally seen

C

interspinales lumborum m.'s

occasionally seen

styloid process

clivus

rectus capitis lateralis m.

mastoid process

odontoid process

1st. cervical vertebra (atlas)

anterior view of cervical vertebrae

intertransversarii anteriores cervicis m.'s

F

intertransversarii laterales lumborum m.'s (ventral part)

rib

mamillary process

articulating facet

transverse process

intertransversarii m.'s

E

accessory process

1st lumbar vertebra

insertion

origin

H

intertransversarii mediales lumborum m.'s

sacrum (posterior surface)

1st lumbar vertebra

(dorsal part)

G

sacrum (posterior surface)

coccyx

© MELLONI

	MUSCLE	ORIGIN	INSERTION	INNERVATION	ACTION
A	**mm. intertransversarii posteriores cervicis** *(inconstant muscles)* *posterior intertransverse muscles of neck*	medial part: superior surface of posterior tubercles of vertebrae C2, C3, C4, C5, C6, C7, T1 lateral part: superior surface of transverse processes of vertebrae C2, C3, C4, C5, C6, C7, T1	medial part: inferior surface of posterior tubercles of vertebrae C1, C2, C3, C4, C5, C6, C7 lateral part: inferior surface of transverse processes of vertebrae C1, C2, C3, C4, C5, C6, C7	medial part: ventral branches of spinal nerves (C1–C6) lateral part: dorsal branches of spinal nerves (C1–C6)	aid in bending vertebral column laterally
B	**mm. intertransversarii thoracis** *(inconstant muscle)* *intertransverse muscles of thorax*	superior surface of transverse process of vertebrae T11 to L1	inferior surface of transverse process of vertebrae T10 to T12	dorsal branches of spinal nerves	aid in bending vertebral column laterally
C	**m. ischiocavernosus** *ischiocavernosus m.* male: erector m. of penis female: erector m. of clitoris	ramus of ischium adjacent to crus of penis or clitoris	tunica albuginea of crus of penis or clitoris	perineal branch of the pudendal nerve (S2, S3, S4)	male: maintains erection of penis female: maintains erection of clitoris
D	**m. latissimus dorsi** *latissimus dorsi m.*	spinous processes of vertebrae T7 to S3; thoracolumbar fascia; iliac crest; lower four ribs; inferior angle of scapula	floor of intertubercular (bicipital) groove of humerus	thoracodorsal nerve from the posterior cord of the brachial plexus (6th, 7th, and 8th cranial nerves)	adducts, extends and rotates arm medially
E	**m. levator anguli oris** *levator m. of angle of mouth* *canine m.*	cuspid fossa of maxilla just below infraorbital foramen	angle of mouth	buccal branches of facial nerve (7th cranial nerve)	raises angle of mouth
F	**m. levator ani** *(part of pelvic diaphragm)* *levator ani m.*	the main muscle of the pelvic floor within the lesser pelvis; comprised of the m. pubococcygeus, m. iliococcygeus, m. puborectalis, and m. levator prostatae			supports pelvic viscera and separates it from the perineum
G	**mm. levatores costarum** *levator muscles of ribs*	16 small muscles on either side that arise from the transverse processes of vertebrae and pass to a rib below; consist of m. levator costarum brevis and m. levator costarum longus		corresponding spinal nerves	elevate ribs, extend vertebral column and bend it laterally
H	**mm. levatores costarum breves** *(12 in number)* *short levator muscles of ribs*	transverse processes of vertebrae C7, T1 to T11	upper margin of dorsal side of rib below, between angle and tubercle	dorsal branches of C8 and thoracic spinal nerves	elevate ribs, extend spinal column and bend it laterally
I	**mm. levatores costarum longi** *(4 in number)* *long levator muscles of ribs*	transverse processes of vertebrae T7 to T10	upper margin of dorsal side of second rib below, near the angle	dorsal branches of lower thoracic spinal nerves	elevate ribs; extend spinal column and bend it laterally

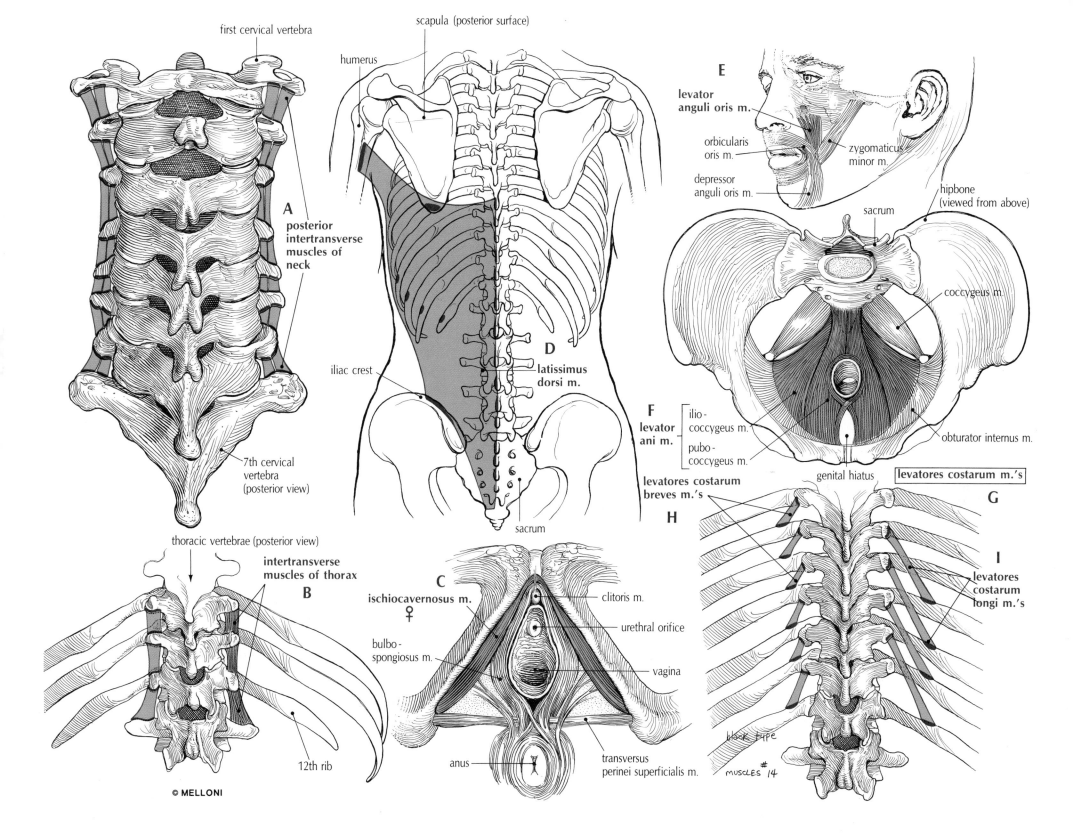

first cervical vertebra

A
posterior intertransverse muscles of neck

7th cervical vertebra (posterior view)

thoracic vertebrae (posterior view)

intertransverse muscles of thorax

B

12th rib

© MELLONI

scapula (posterior surface)

humerus

iliac crest

D
latissimus dorsi m.

sacrum

E
levator anguli oris m.

orbicularis oris m.

depressor anguli oris m.

zygomaticus minor m.

hipbone (viewed from above)

sacrum

coccygeus m

F
levator ani m.
ilio-coccygeus m.
pubo-coccygeus m.

obturator internus m.

genital hiatus

levatores costarum breves m.'s

H

C
ischiocavernosus m.
♀

bulbo-spongiosus m.

clitoris m.

urethral orifice

vagina

anus

transversus perinei superficialis m.

levatores costarum m.'s

G

I
levatores costarum longi m.'s

block type

muscles #14

	MUSCLE	ORIGIN	INSERTION	INNERVATION	ACTION
A	**m. levator glandulae thyroideae** *(inconstant muscle)* *levator m. of thyroid gland*	isthmus or pyramidal lobe of thyroid gland	body of hyoid bone	branch of hypoglossal nerve (12th cranial nerve) containing fibers of C1	stabilizes thyroid gland
B	**m. levator labii superioris** *levator m. of upper lip*	zygomatic bone and maxilla above the infraorbital foramen	muscular substance of upper lip and margin of nostril	buccal branches of facial nerve (7th cranial nerve)	raises upper lip; dilates nostril
C	**m. levator labii superioris alaeque nasi** *levator m. of upper lip and ala of nose*	frontal process of maxilla	skin of upper lip; ala of nose	buccal branches of facial nerve (7th cranial nerve)	raises upper lip; dilates nostril
D	**m. levator palpebrae superioris** *levator m. of upper eyelid*	roof of orbital cavity above optic canal	skin and tarsal plate of upper eyelid and superior conjunctical fornix	oculomotor nerve (3rd cranial nerve)	raises upper eyelid
E	**m. levator prostatae** *(part of m. pubococcygeus)* *levator m. of prostate*	in the male, the most anterior fibers of the m. pubococcygeus (part of m. levator ani), which pass back from the pubis, around the prostate, and insert into the perineal body (central tendon of perineum)		branch from inferior rectal nerve or pudendal nerve	elevates and compresses the prostate; aids in controlling micturition
F	**m. levator scapulae** *levator m. of scapula*	transverse processes of upper four cervical vertebrae	medial border of scapula	C3, C4	raises scapula; aids in rotating the neck
G	**m. levator vaginae** *(part of m. pubococcygeus)* *levator m. of vagina*	in the female, the most anterior fibers of the m. pubococcygeus (part of m. levator ani), which pass back from the pubis, around the vagina, and insert into the perineal body (central tendon of perineum)		branch from inferior rectal nerve or pudendal nerve	elevates and compresses the vagina; aids in controlling micturition
H	**m. levator veli palatini** *levator m. of soft palate*	undersurface of petrous part of temporal bone; undersurface of cartilagenous part of auditory tube	aponeurosis of soft palate	pharyngeal plexus of vagus nerve (10th cranial nerve)	raises soft palate in swallowing; aids in opening orifice of auditory tube
I	**m. longissimus** *longissimus m.*	the largest and intermediate part of the m. erector spinae; it consists of m. longissimus capitis, m. longissimus cervicis, and m. longissimus thoracis		dorsal branches of spinal nerves from lower cervical to lower lumbar	bends vertebral column backward and laterally; extends and rotates head
J	**m. longissimus capitis** *longissimus m. of head*	transverse and articular processes of vertebrae C3 to C7; transverse processes of vertebrae T1 to T4	back of mastoid process of temporal bone	dorsal branch of middle and lower cervical spinal nerves	extends head; rotates head to same side

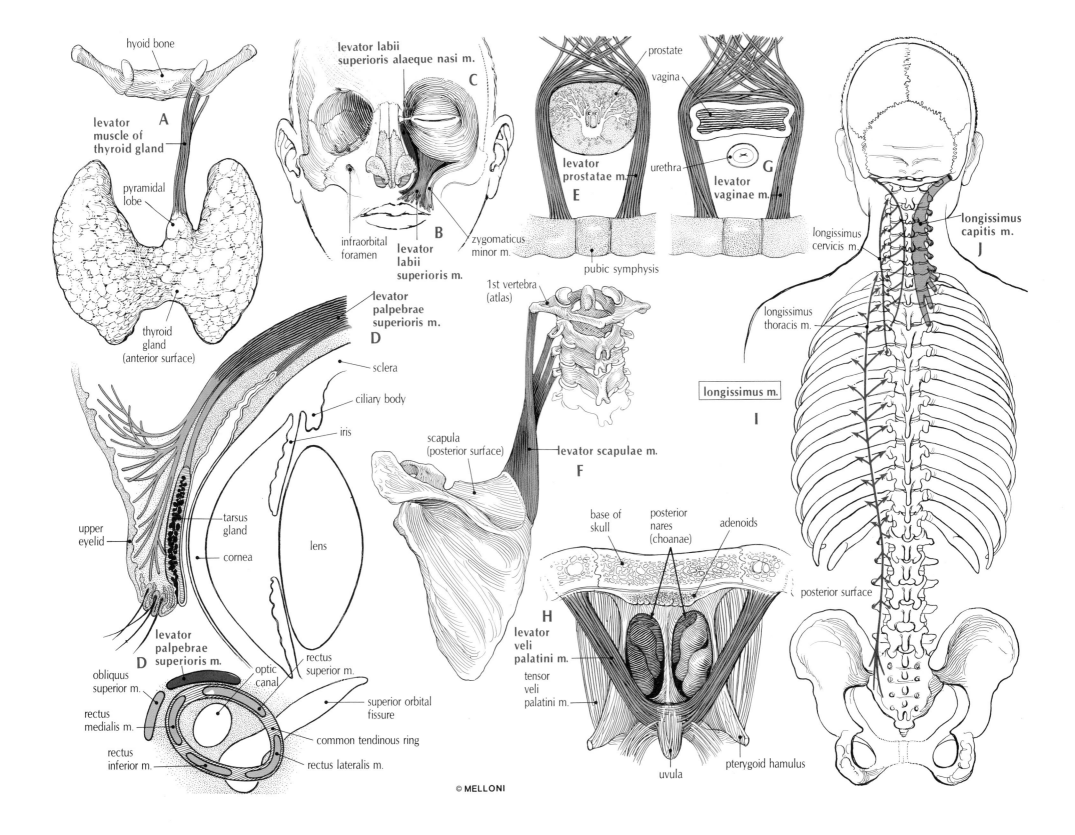

hyoid bone

levator muscle of thyroid gland

pyramidal lobe

thyroid gland (anterior surface)

A

levator labii superioris alaeque nasi m.

C

infraorbital foramen

levator labii superioris m.

B

zygomaticus minor m.

prostate

levator prostatae m.

E

pubic symphysis

vagina

urethra

levator vaginae m.

G

longissimus capitis m.

J

longissimus cervicis m.

longissimus thoracis m.

longissimus m.

I

posterior surface

levator palpebrae superioris m.

D

sclera

ciliary body

iris

lens

upper eyelid

tarsus gland

cornea

rectus superior m.

levator palpebrae superioris m.

D

obliquus superior m.

rectus medialis m.

rectus inferior m.

optic canal

superior orbital fissure

common tendinous ring

rectus lateralis m.

1st vertebra (atlas)

scapula (posterior surface)

levator scapulae m.

F

base of skull

posterior nares (choanae)

adenoids

levator veli palatini m.

tensor veli palatini m.

uvula

pterygoid hamulus

© MELLONI

	MUSCLE	ORIGIN	INSERTION	INNERVATION	ACTION
A	**m. longissimus cervicis** *longissimus m. of neck*	transverse processes of vertebrae T1 to T5	transverse processes of vertebrae C2 to C6	dorsal branches of cervical and upper thoracic spinal nerves	bends vertebral column backward and laterally
B	**m. longissimus thoracis** *longissimus m. of thorax* *longissimus m. of back*	transverse and accessory processes of lumbar vertebrae; thoracolumbar fascia	transverse processes of vertebrae T1 to T12; angles of lower 10 ribs	dorsal branch of thoracic and lumbar spinal nerves	extends vertebral column and bends it to one side
C	**m. longitudinalis inferior linguae** *inferior longitudinal m. of tongue*	undersurface of tongue at base	tip of tongue	hypoglossal nerve (12th cranial nerve)	acts to alter shape of tongue
D	**m. longitudinalis superior linguae** *superior longitudinal m. of tongue*	submucosa and median septum of tongue	margins of tongue	hypoglossal nerve (12th cranial nerve)	acts to alter shape of tongue
E	**m. longus capitis** *long m. of head*	transverse processes of 3rd to 6th cervical vertebrae	basal part of occipital bone	ventral branches of spinal nerves (1st, 2nd, and 3rd cranial nerves)	flexes head
F	**m. longus colli** *long m. of neck*	superior oblique part: anterior tubercles of the transverse processes of vertebrae C3, C4, C5 vertical part: front of bodies of vertebrae C5, C6, C7, T1, T2, T3 inferior oblique part: front of bodies of vertebrae T1, T2, T3	superior oblique part: by a narrow tendon to the anterior tubercle of 1st vertebra (atlas) vertical part: front of the bodies of vertebrae C2, C3, C4 inferior oblique part: anterior tubercles of the transverse processes of vertebrae C5, C6	ventral branches of C2 to C6	bends neck forward; slightly rotates the cervical portion of vertebral column
G	**mm. lumbricales manus** *(four in number)* *lumbrical muscles of hand*	tendons of m. flexor digitorum profundus	extensor tendons of the 2nd through 5th fingers	1st and 2nd lumbricals: branches of median nerve (8th cranial nerve and T1) 3rd and 4th lumbricals: branches of ulnar nerve (8th cranial nerve and T1)	aid in flexion of digits at metacarpophalangeal joints and extension of the interphalangeal joints
H	**mm. lumbricales pedis** *(four in number)* *lumbrical muscles of foot*	tendons of m. flexor digitorum longus	medial side of proximal phalanges and extensor tendons of the 2nd through 5th toes	1st lumbrical: medial plantar nerve 2nd, 3rd, and 4th lumbricals: deep branch of lateral plantar nerve (S2, S3)	aid in flexion of digits at metatarsophalangeal joints

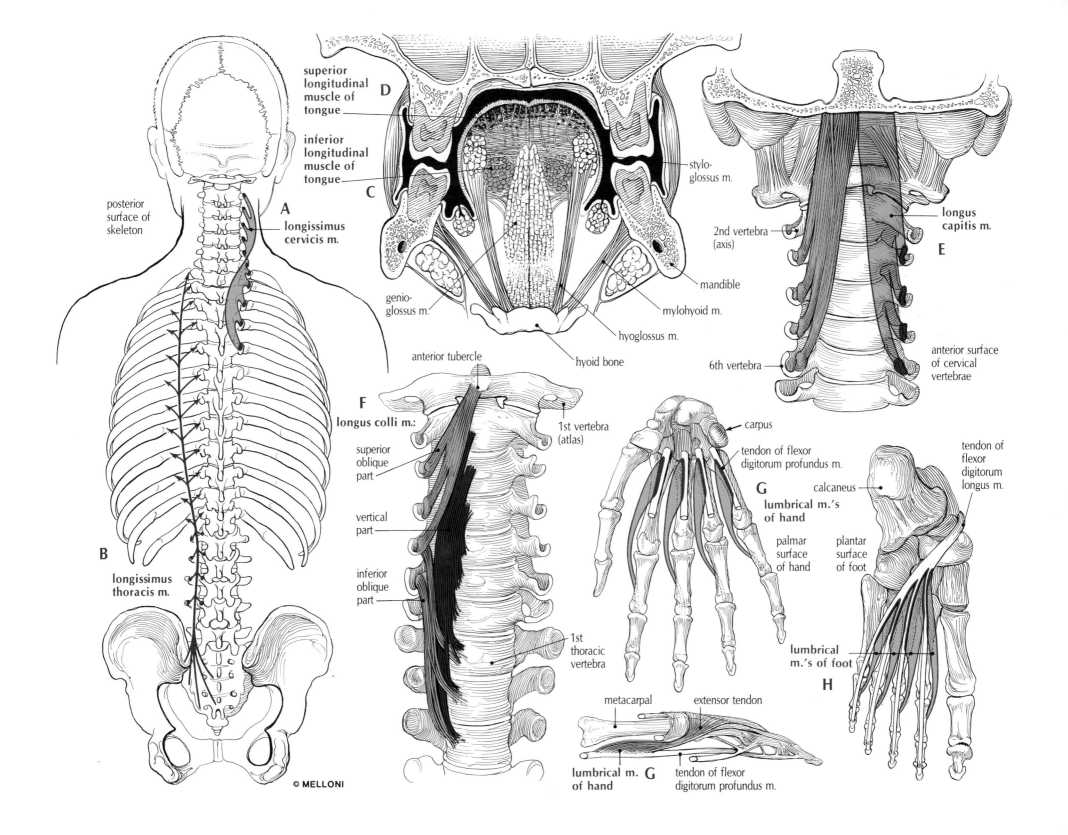

superior longitudinal muscle of tongue

inferior longitudinal muscle of tongue

D

C

posterior surface of skeleton

longissimus cervicis m.

A

stylo-glossus m.

2nd vertebra (axis)

longus capitis m.

E

genio-glossus m.

mandible

mylohyoid m.

hyoglossus m.

hyoid bone

6th vertebra

anterior surface of cervical vertebrae

B

longissimus thoracis m.

anterior tubercle

F

longus colli m.:

superior oblique part

1st vertebra (atlas)

carpus

tendon of flexor digitorum profundus m.

G

lumbrical m.'s of hand

vertical part

palmar surface of hand

plantar surface of foot

tendon of flexor digitorum longus m.

calcaneus

inferior oblique part

1st thoracic vertebra

metacarpal

extensor tendon

lumbrical m.'s of foot

H

lumbrical m. G of hand

tendon of flexor digitorum profundus m.

© MELLONI

	MUSCLE	ORIGIN	INSERTION	INNERVATION	ACTION
A	**m. masseter** *masseter m.*	superficial part: zygomatic process of maxilla; anterior two thirds of lower border of zygomatic arch deep part: medial surface of zygomatic arch; lower border of zygomatic arch	superficial part: angle of mandible; lateral surface of lower half of ramus of mandible deep part: lateral surface of upper half of ramus of mandible; lateral surface of coronoid process	masseteric nerve of mandibular division of trigeminal nerve (5th cranial nerve)	elevates mandible and closes jaws
B	**m. mentalis** *mentalis m.* *chin m.*	incisive fossa of mandible	skin of chin	mandibular marginal branch of facial nerve (7th cranial nerve)	raises and protrudes lower lip
C	**mm. multifidi** *multifidus muscles*	cervical area: articular processes of vertebrae C4, C5, C6, and C7 thoracic area: transverse processes of thoracic vertebrae lumbar area: mamillary processes of lumbar vertebrae sacral area: posterior surface of sacrum, origin aponeurosis of m. erector spinae, posterior iliac spine, sacroiliac ligament	deep fibers: entire length of spines of contiguous vertebrae above middle fibers: entire length of spines of 2nd and 3rd vertebrae above superficial fibers: entire length of spine of 3rd and 4th vertebrae above superficial fibers: entire length of spine of 3rd and 4th vertebrae above	dorsal branches of spinal nerves	maintain posture; slightly rotate and extend vertebral column
D	**m. mylohyoideus** *mylohyoid m.* *m. of floor of mouth*	entire mylohyoid line of mandible	superior surface of body of hyoid bone; mylohyoid raphe (stretches from symphysis menti of mandible to hyoid bone)	mylohyoid branch of inferior alveolar nerve (mandibular division of trigeminal nerve)	supports floor of mouth; elevates hyoid bone and larynx upward and forward; lowers mandible
E	**m. nasalis** *nasal m.*	transverse part: maxilla, lateral to nasal notch alar part: nasal notch of maxilla	transverse part: aponeurosis on nasal cartilage and bridge of nose alar part: ala cartilage of nose	upper buccal branches of facial nerve (7th cranial nerve)	transverse part: compresses nostril alar part: widens nostril
F	**m. obliquus auriculae** *oblique m. of auricle*	eminence of concha on medial surface of auricular cartilage	eminence of triangular fossa on medial surface of auricular cartilage	posterior auricular branch of facial nerve (7th cranial nerve)	thought to be vestigal

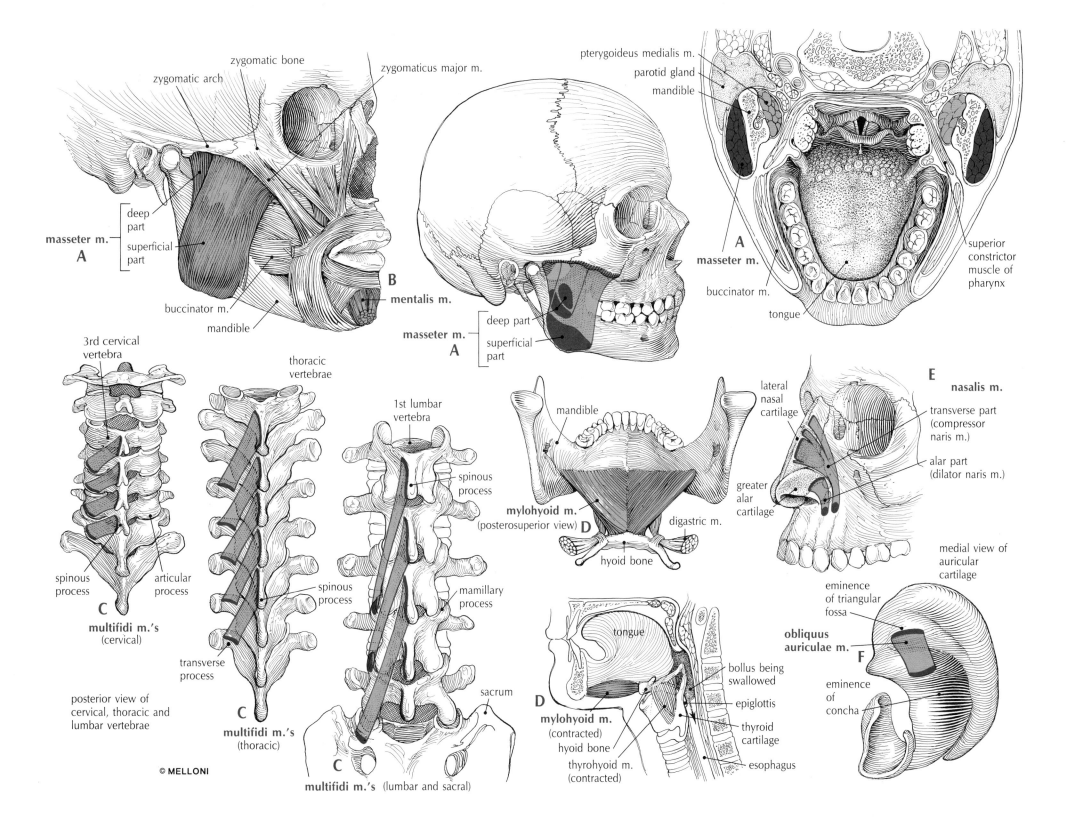

zygomatic arch

zygomatic bone

zygomaticus major m.

pterygoideus medialis m.

parotid gland

mandible

deep part
superficial part
masseter m.
A

buccinator m.

mandible

B

mentalis m.

deep part
superficial part
masseter m.
A

A

masseter m.

buccinator m.

tongue

superior constrictor muscle of pharynx

3rd cervical vertebra

thoracic vertebrae

1st lumbar vertebra

spinous process

mandible

lateral nasal cartilage

nasalis m.
E

transverse part (compressor naris m.)

alar part (dilator naris m.)

greater alar cartilage

medial view of auricular cartilage

spinous process

mamillary process

spinous process

articular process

mylohyoid m.
(posterosuperior view) **D**

digastric m.

hyoid bone

eminence of triangular fossa

obliquus auriculae m.
F

eminence of concha

C

multifidi m.'s
(cervical)

transverse process

C

multifidi m.'s
(thoracic)

sacrum

posterior view of cervical, thoracic and lumbar vertebrae

© MELLONI

C

multifidi m.'s (lumbar and sacral)

tongue

bollus being swallowed

epiglottis

thyroid cartilage

D

mylohyoid m.
(contracted)

hyoid bone

thyrohyoid m.
(contracted)

esophagus

	MUSCLE	ORIGIN	INSERTION	INNERVATION	ACTION
A	**m. obliquus capitis inferior** *inferior oblique m. of head*	spinous process of 2nd vertebra (axis)	transverse process of 1st vertebra (atlas)	dorsal branch of 1st spinal nerve	turns the face toward the same side; rotates head laterally
B	**m. obliquus capitis superior** *superior oblique m. of head*	transverse process of 1st vertebra (atlas)	occipital bone between the superior and inferior nuchal lines	dorsal branch of 1st spinal nerve	rotates head laterally; bends head backward
C	**m. obliquus externus abdominis** *external oblique m. of abdomen*	inferior borders of lower eight ribs	anterior half of iliac crest; outer layer of rectus sheath and linea alba; inguinal ligament	ventral branches of lower six thoracic spinal nerves	tenses abdominal wall and supports abdominal contents; aids in micturition and defecation; flexes and rotates vertebral column
D	**m. obliquus inferior bulbi** *inferior oblique m. of eyeball*	anterior margin of orbital plate of maxilla, lateral to nasolacrimal groove	lateral surface of eyeball behind the equator	oculomotor nerve (3rd cranial nerve)	rotates the eyeball upward and laterally
E	**m. obliquus internus abdominis** *internal oblique m. of abdomen*	lateral two thirds of inguinal ligament; anterior two thirds of iliac crest; thoracolumbar fascia	inferior border of ribs 10, 11, and 12; rectus sheath and linea alba; conjoined tendon to pubis (formed along with aponeurosis of m. transversus abdominis); cartilages of ribs 7, 8, and 9	ventral branches of lower six thoracic and 1st lumbar spinal nerves	tenses abdominal wall and supports abdominal contents; rotates vertebral column; lowers ribs
F	**m. obliquus superior bulbi** *superior oblique m. of eyeball*	body of sphenoid medial to and slightly above the optic canal	lateral surface of eyeball behind the equator	trochlear nerve (4th cranial nerve)	rotates eyeball downward and laterally
G	**m. obturatorius externus** *external obturator m.*	external medial margin of obturator foramen; obturator membrane	trochanteric fossa of femur	posterior branch of obturator nerve (L3, L4)	rotates thigh laterally
H	**m. obturatorius internus** *internal obturator m.* *obturator internus m.*	internal margin of obturator foramen; obturator membrane; tendinous arch of obturator canal	upper medial surface of greater trochanter of femur	nerve to obturator internus (L5, S1, S2)	abducts and rotates thigh laterally
I	**m. occipitofrontalis** *occipitofrontal m.*	frontal part: epicranial aponeurosis occipital part: highest nuchal line of occipital bone; mastoid process	frontal part: skin of eyebrows; root of nose occipital part: epicranial aponeurosis	frontal part: temporal branch of facial nerve (7th cranial nerve) occipital part: posterior auricular branch of facial nerve (7th cranial nerve)	frontal part: elevates eyebrows; draws scalp forward wrinkling forehead occipital part: draws scalp backward

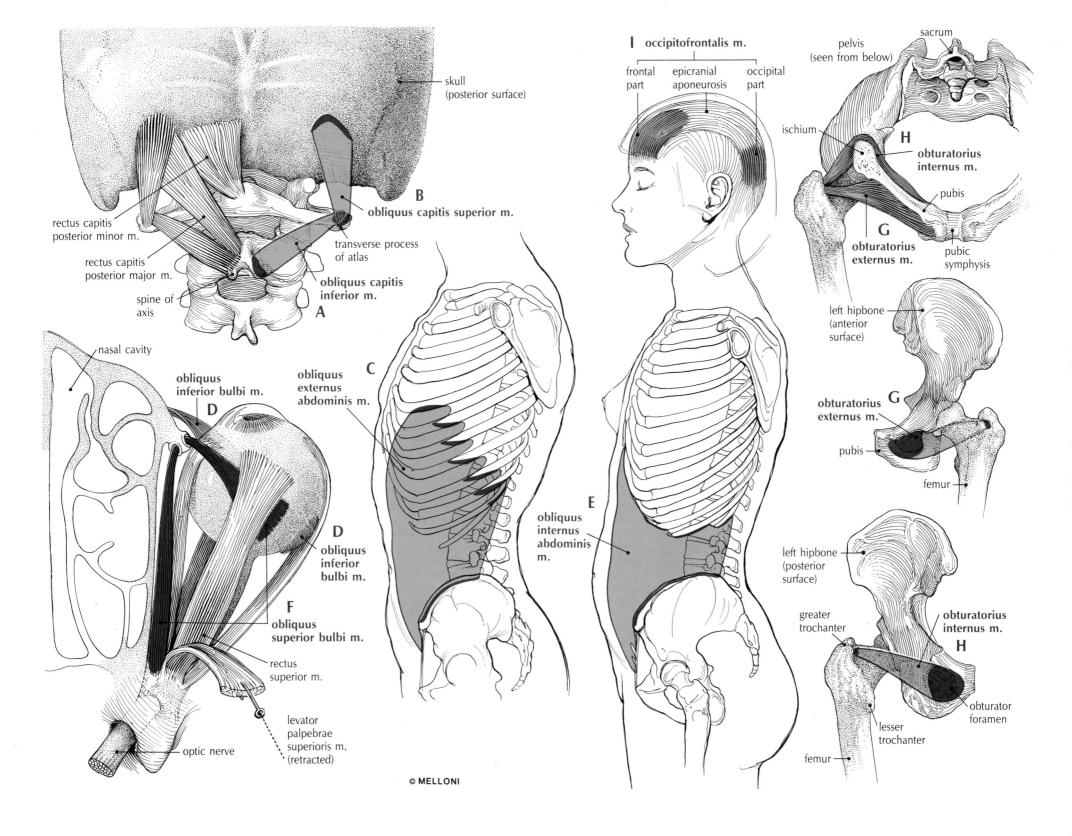

skull (posterior surface)

rectus capitis posterior minor m.

rectus capitis posterior major m.

spine of axis

B **obliquus capitis superior m.**

transverse process of atlas

obliquus capitis inferior m.

A

nasal cavity

obliquus inferior bulbi m.

D

obliquus externus abdominis m.

C

D **obliquus inferior bulbi m.**

F **obliquus superior bulbi m.**

rectus superior m.

levator palpebrae superioris m. (retracted)

optic nerve

E obliquus internus abdominis m.

I occipitofrontalis m.

frontal part | epicranial aponeurosis | occipital part

pelvis (seen from below)

sacrum

ischium

H **obturatorius internus m.**

G **obturatorius externus m.**

pubis

pubic symphysis

left hipbone (anterior surface)

G **obturatorius externus m.**

pubis

femur

left hipbone (posterior surface)

greater trochanter

obturatorius internus m.

H

obturator foramen

lesser trochanter

femur

© MELLONI

	MUSCLE	ORIGIN	INSERTION	INNERVATION	ACTION
A	**m. omohyoideus** *omohyoid m.*	medial border of suprascapular notch on upper surface of scapula	lower margin of body of hyoid bone	superior belly: branch from upper root of ansa cervicalis inferior belly: branch from lower root of ansa cervicalis	lowers hyoid bone after it has been elevated
B	**m. opponens digiti minimi** *opposing m. of little finger*	hook of hamate bone; flexor retinaculum	5th metacarpal bone	deep branch of ulnar nerve (8th cranial nerve and T1)	draws 5th metacarpal bone forward toward the center of palm (in opposition with thumb); rotates bone laterally
C	**m. opponens pollicis** *opposing m. of thumb*	tubercle of trapezium; flexor retinaculum	lateral border of 1st metacarpal bone	branch of median nerve (8th cranial nerve and T1)	draws 1st metacarpal bone toward center of palm
D	**m. orbicularis oculi** *orbicularis oculi m.* *orbicular m. of eye*	orbital part: medial palpebral ligament, adjacent bones palpebral part: medial palpebral ligament, adjacent bones lacrimal part: posterior lacrimal crest, lacrimal fascia, lateral surface of lacrimal bone	orbital part: near origin after encircling orbit palpebral part: lateral palpebral raphe lacrimal part: superior and inferior tarsi, medial to puncta lacrimalia	temporal and zygomatic branches of facial nerve (7th cranial nerve)	closes eyelids; tightens skin of forehead; compresses lacrimal sac
E	**m. orbicularis oris** *orbicularis oris m.* *orbicular m. of mouth*	marginal part: peripheral fibers blending with adjacent facial muscles (m. buccinator, m. levator anguli oris, m. depressor anguli oris, m. levator labii superioris, m. depressor labii inferioris, m. zygomaticus minor, and m. zygomaticus major) labial part: central fibers restricted to lips	muscles interlace to encircle orifice of mouth	mandibular marginal and lower buccal branches of facial nerve (7th cranial nerve)	protrudes lips forward and brings them together
F	**m. orbitalis** *orbital m.*	orbital periosteum	fascia of inferior orbital fissure	sympathetic nerves derived from pterygopalatine ganglion	thought to be rudimentary; may feebly protrude the eyeball

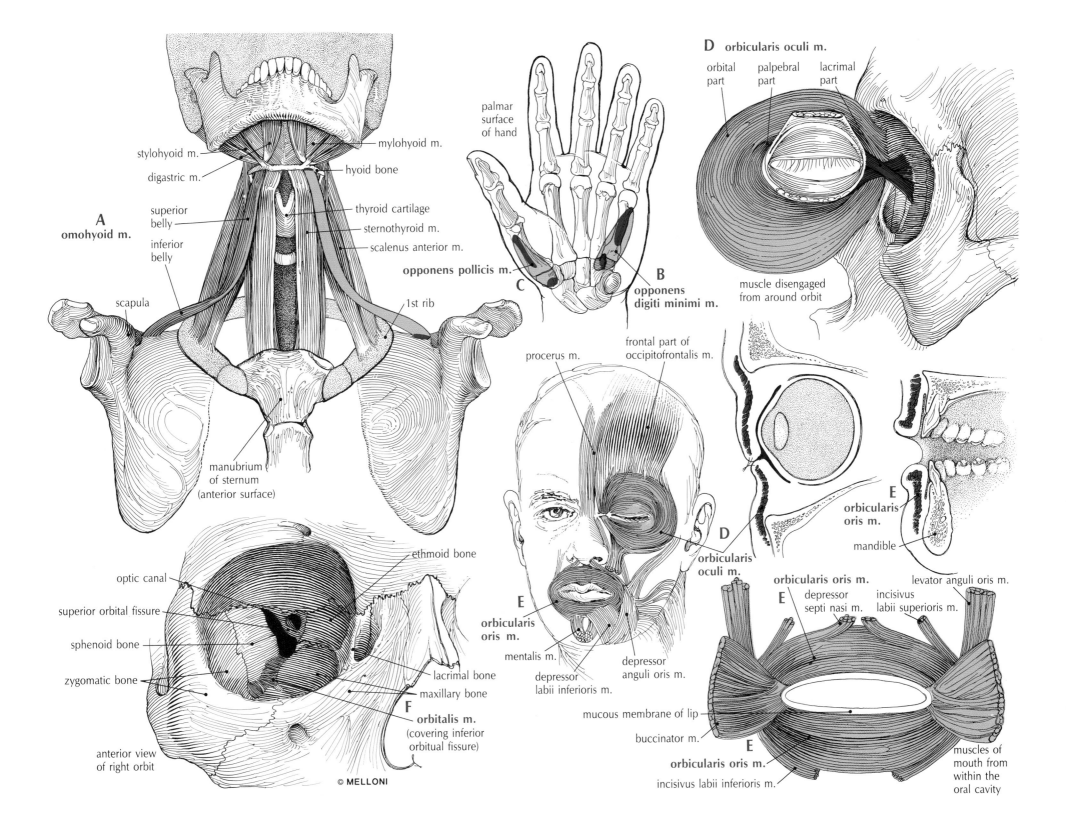

A
omohyoid m.

stylohyoid m.
digastric m.
superior belly
inferior belly
scapula
mylohyoid m.
hyoid bone
thyroid cartilage
sternothyroid m.
scalenus anterior m.
1st rib
manubrium of sternum (anterior surface)

palmar surface of hand

opponens pollicis m.
C
B
opponens digiti minimi m.

D orbicularis oculi m.
orbital part
palpebral part
lacrimal part

muscle disengaged from around orbit

procerus m.
frontal part of occipitofrontalis m.

D
orbicularis oculi m.

E
orbicularis oris m.

mandible

E
orbicularis oris m.

mentalis m.
depressor labii inferioris m.
depressor anguli oris m.

optic canal
superior orbital fissure
sphenoid bone
zygomatic bone
ethmoid bone
lacrimal bone
maxillary bone
F
orbitalis m. (covering inferior orbital fissure)

anterior view of right orbit

© MELLONI

orbicularis oris m.
E
depressor septi nasi m.
incisivus labii superioris m.
levator anguli oris m.

mucous membrane of lip
buccinator m.
E
orbicularis oris m.
incisivus labii inferioris m.

muscles of mouth from within the oral cavity

	MUSCLE	ORIGIN	INSERTION	INNERVATION	ACTION
A	**m. palatoglossus** *palatoglossus m.*	undersurface of soft palate	side and dorsum of tongue	pharyngeal plexus of vagus nerve (10th cranial nerve)	elevates back of tongue; narrows fauces
B	**m. palatopharyngeus** *palatopharyngeal m.*	back of hard palate; soft palate	posterior wall of thyroid cartilage; wall of pharynx	pharyngeal plexus of vagus nerve (10th cranial nerve)	elevates pharynx and shortens it during act of swallowing; narrows fauces
C	**m. palmaris brevis** *short palmar m.*	flexor retinaculum; medial side of palmar aponeurosis	skin over hypothenar eminence	superficial branch of ulnar nerve (8th cranial nerve and T1)	wrinkles skin on ulnar side of palm of hand
D	**m. palmaris longus** *long palmar m.*	medial epicondyle of humerus	anterior surface of flexor retinaculum; palmar aponeurosis	median nerve (7th and 8th cranial nerves)	flexes hand
E	**mm. papillares** *papillary muscles*	conical muscles projecting from the walls of the ventricles into the cavity of the heart, attached to the right and left atrioventricular valves by the chordae tendinae (tendinous cords)			aid atrioventricular valves of the heart to function properly
F	**m. papillaris anterior ventriculi dextri** *anterior papillary m. of right ventricle*	moderate band (septomarginal trabeculae) of right ventricle	chordae tendinae attached to anterior and posterior cusps of right atrioventricular valve	cardiac plexus	aids right atrioventricular valve to function properly
G	**m. papillaris anterior ventriculi sinistri** *anterior papillary m. of left ventricle*	wall of left ventricle	chordae tendinae attached to anterior and posterior cusps of atrioventricular valve	cardiac plexus	aids left atrioventricular valve to function properly
H	**m. papillaris posterior ventriculi dextri** *posterior papillary m. of right ventricle*	posterior wall of right ventricle of heart	chordae tendinae attached to posterior and septal cusps of right atrioventricular valve	cardiac plexus	aids right atrioventricular valve to function properly
I	**m. papillaris posterior ventriculi sinistri** *posterior papillary m. of left ventricle*	wall of left ventricle	chordae tendinae attached to anterior and posterior cusps of atrioventricular valve	cardiac plexus	aids left atrioventricular valve to function properly
J	**m. papillaris septalis ventriculi dextri** *septal papillary m. of right ventricle*	interventricular septum	chordae tendinae attached to anterior and septal (medial) cusps of right atrioventricular valve	cardiac plexus	aids right atrioventricular valve to function properly
K	**mm. pectinati** *pectinate muscles*	a number of muscular ridges in the wall of the right atrium, right auricle, and left auricle of the heart		branches from the cardiac plexus	contract the atria during systole

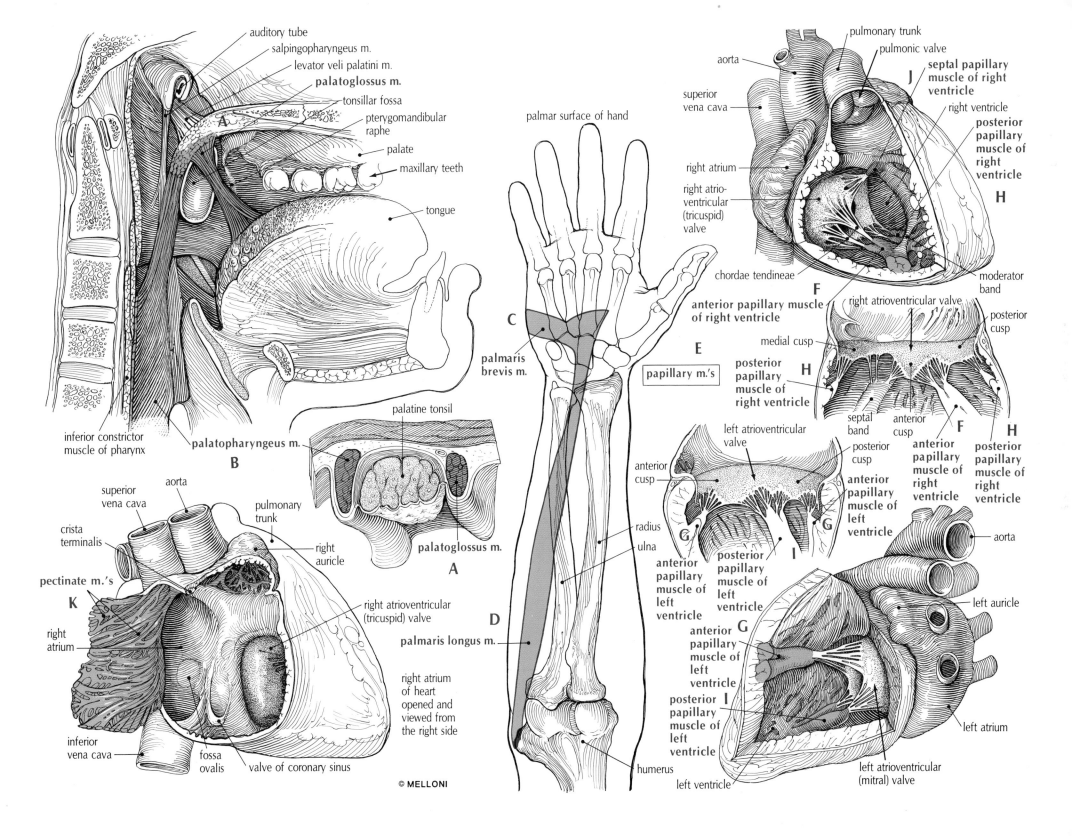

auditory tube

salpingopharyngeus m.

levator veli palatini m.

palatoglossus m.

tonsillar fossa

pterygomandibular raphe

palate

maxillary teeth

tongue

A

inferior constrictor muscle of pharynx

palatopharyngeus m.

B

palatine tonsil

palatoglossus m.

A

aorta

superior vena cava

pulmonary trunk

crista terminalis

right auricle

pectinate m.'s

K

right atrium

right atrioventricular (tricuspid) valve

inferior vena cava

fossa ovalis

valve of coronary sinus

© MELLONI

palmar surface of hand

C

palmaris brevis m.

E

papillary m.'s

radius

ulna

D

palmaris longus m.

right atrium of heart opened and viewed from the right side

humerus

pulmonary trunk

aorta

superior vena cava

right atrium

right atrioventricular (tricuspid) valve

chordae tendineae

F

septal papillary muscle of right ventricle

right ventricle

posterior papillary muscle of right ventricle

H

moderator band

anterior papillary muscle of right ventricle

right atrioventricular valve

medial cusp

posterior cusp

posterior papillary muscle of right ventricle

H

septal band

anterior cusp

F

anterior papillary muscle of right ventricle

H

posterior papillary muscle of right ventricle

left atrioventricular valve

anterior cusp

posterior cusp

G

G

anterior papillary muscle of left ventricle

I

anterior papillary muscle of left ventricle

posterior papillary muscle of left ventricle

aorta

left auricle

anterior papillary muscle of left ventricle

G

posterior papillary muscle of left ventricle

I

left atrium

left ventricle

left atrioventricular (mitral) valve

	MUSCLE	ORIGIN	INSERTION	INNERVATION	ACTION
A	**m. pectineus** *pectineal m.*	pectineal line of pubis	pectineal line of femur from lesser trochanter to linea aspera	branches of obturator and femoral nerves (L2, L3, L4)	flexes and adducts thigh
B	**m. pectoralis major** *greater pectoral m.*	medial half of clavicle, sternum, and costal cartilages of 4th to 6th ribs; aponeurosis of m. obliquus externus abdominis; often at anterior extremity of 6th rib	lateral lip of intertubercular groove of humerus	lateral and medial pectoral nerves derived from the 5th through 8th cranial nerves and T1	adduction and medial rotation of arm; draws arm forward
C	**m. pectoralis minor** *smaller pectoral m.*	anterior surface of ribs 3, 4, 5, near the costal cartilages; upper part of coracoid process of scapula	upper part of coracoid process	lateral and medial pectoral nerves (6th, 7th, and 8th cranial nerves)	draws shoulder forward and downward; raises rib cage
D	**m. peroneus brevis** *short peroneal m.* *short fibular m.*	lateral side of lower two thirds of fibula; crural septum	lateral side of 5th metatarsal bone	superficial peroneal nerve (L5, S1, S2)	everts foot; aids in plantar flexion; aids in preventing over-inversion of foot
E	**m. peroneus longus** *long peroneal m.* *long fibular m.*	lateral side of upper two thirds of fibula; crural septum	medial cuneiform; base of first metatarsal bone	superficial peroneal nerve (L5, S1, S2)	helps maintain transverse arch of foot; everts foot; aids in plantar flexion
F	**m. peroneus tertius** *(part of m. extensor digitorum longus)* *third peroneal m.* *third fibular m.*	medial side of distal third of fibula; crural fascia	dorsal surface of base of 5th metatarsal bone	deep peroneal nerve (L5, S1)	dorsiflexes foot
G	**m. piriformis** *piriform m.*	anterior surface of middle three sacral vertebrae; ilium near posterior iliac spine	upper part of greater trochanter of femur	spinal nerves (L5, S1, S2)	rotates thigh laterally
H	**m. plantaris** *plantar m.*	supracondylar line just above lateral condyle of femur; oblique popliteal ligament	posterior part of calcaneus (along with calcaneal tendon)	tibial nerve (S1, S2)	plantar flexes foot
I	**m. platysma** *platysma m.*	superficial fascia of upper chest	skin of lower portion of face	cervical branch of facial nerve (7th cranial nerve)	depresses lower jaw; forms ridges in skin of neck; draws down angle of mouth

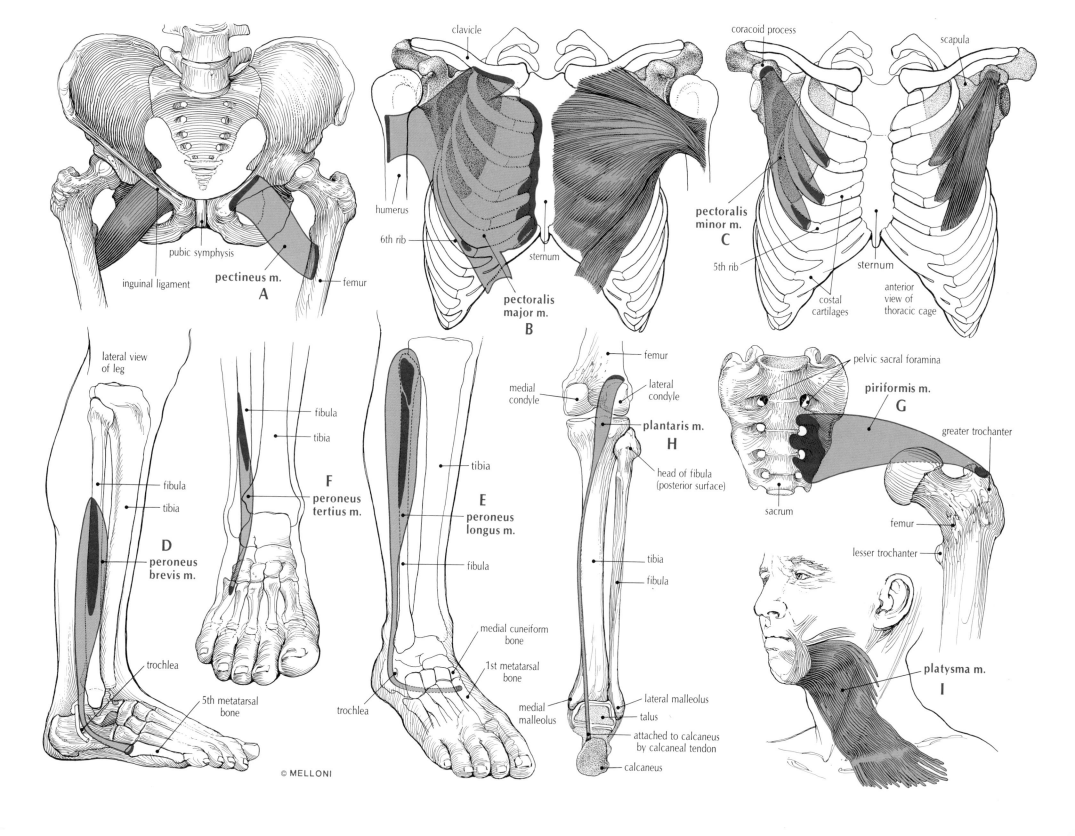

pubic symphysis

inguinal ligament

pectineus m.

A

femur

clavicle

coracoid process

scapula

humerus

6th rib

sternum

pectoralis major m.

B

pectoralis minor m.

C

5th rib

sternum

costal cartilages

anterior view of thoracic cage

lateral view of leg

fibula

tibia

fibula

tibia

D
peroneus brevis m.

trochlea

5th metatarsal bone

fibula

tibia

F
peroneus tertius m.

trochlea

tibia

fibula

medial cuneiform bone

1st metatarsal bone

medial malleolus

E
peroneus longus m.

femur

medial condyle

lateral condyle

plantaris m.

H

head of fibula (posterior surface)

tibia

fibula

lateral malleolus

talus

attached to calcaneus by calcaneal tendon

calcaneus

pelvic sacral foramina

piriformis m.

G

greater trochanter

sacrum

femur

lesser trochanter

platysma m.

I

© MELLONI

	MUSCLE	ORIGIN	INSERTION	INNERVATION	ACTION
A	**m. pleuroesophageus** *pleuroesophageal m.*	left mediastinal pleura	musculature of middle of esophague just below insertion of m. bronchoesophageus	small branch of vagus nerve (10th cranial nerve)	reinforces esophagus
B	**m. popliteus** *popliteal m.*	popliteal groove of lateral condyle of femur; arcuate popliteal ligament; back of lateral meniscus	upper part of posterior surface of tibia	tibial nerve (L4, L5, S1)	rotates tibia medially; helps to flex knee
C	**m. procerus** *procerus m.*	fascia covering bridge of nose	skin above nose between eyebrows	upper buccal branches of facial nerve (7th cranial nerve)	wrinkles skin over bridge of nose; draws down medial angle of eyebrow
D	**m. pronator quadratus** *quadrate pronator m.*	lower fourth of ulnar	lower fourth of radius	anterior interosseous branch of median nerve (8th cranial nerve and T1)	pronates forearm
E	**m. pronator teres** *round pronator m.*	humeral part: medial epicondyle of humerus ulnar part: coronoid process of ulna	lateral side of midshaft of radius at point of maximum convexity	median nerve (6th and 7th cranial nerves)	pronates (medial rotation of radius on ulna) forearm and hand
F	**m. psoas major** *greater psoas m.*	body of 12th thoracic vertebra; transverse processes and bodies of first four lumbar vertebrae	lesser trochanter of femur	ventral branches of lumbar nerves (L1, L2, L3)	flexes thigh
G	**m. psoas minor** *smaller psoas m.*	bodies of last thoracic and 1st lumbar vertebrae	iliac fascia; iliopubic (iliopectineal) eminence; pecten pubis	L1	flexes trunk
H	**m. pterygoideus lateralis** *lateral pterygoid m.* *external pterygoid m.*	upper part: lower surface of greater wing of sphenoid bone lower part: lateral surface of lateral pterygoid plate	pterygoid fovea of condyle of mandible; capsule and disk of temporomandibular joint	branch of mandibular division of trigeminal nerve (5th cranial nerve)	opens mouth; assists in protruding mandible
I	**m. pterygoideus medialis** *(functions synergistically with m. temporalis and m. masseter)* *medial pterygoid m.* *internal pterygoid m.*	medial surface of lateral pterygoid plate; tubercle of palatine bone; tuberosity of maxilla	medial surface of ramus and angle of mandible	branch of mandibular division of trigeminal nerve (5th cranial nerve)	closes mouth; assists in protruding mandible and moving it side-to-side
J	**m. pubococcygeus** *(part of m. levator ani)* *pubococcygeal m.*	back of pubis; obturator fascia	side of coccyx; median fibrous raphe	branch of inferior rectal nerve; branch of sacral nerve (S4)	supports pelvic viscera

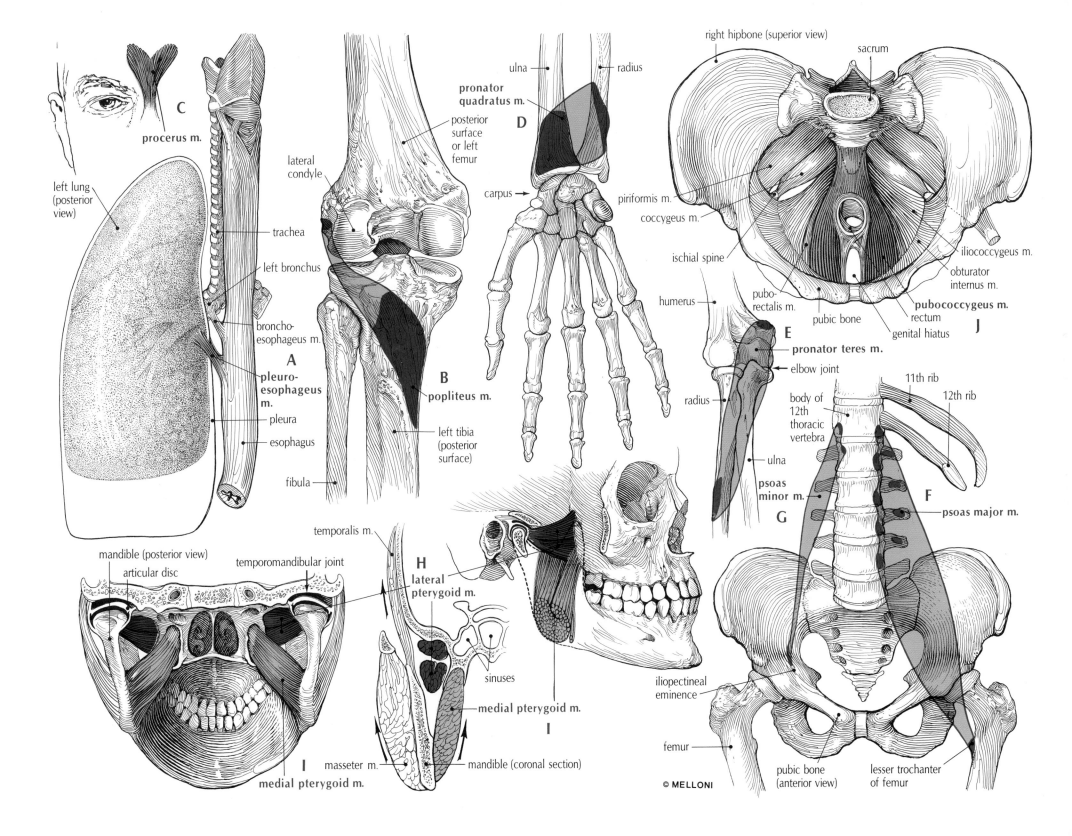

procerus m. **C**

left lung (posterior view)

trachea

left bronchus

broncho-esophageus m.

A

pleuro-esophageus m.

pleura

esophagus

lateral condyle

B

popliteus m.

left tibia (posterior surface)

fibula

pronator quadratus m.

posterior surface or left femur

carpus →

ulna

radius

D

right hipbone (superior view)

sacrum

piriformis m.

coccygeus m.

ischial spine

humerus

pubo-rectalis m.

pubic bone

radius

ulna

psoas minor m.

G

iliococcygeus m.

obturator internus m.

pubococcygeus m.

rectum

genital hiatus

J

pronator teres m.

elbow joint

E

11th rib

body of 12th thoracic vertebra

12th rib

F

psoas major m.

mandible (posterior view)

articular disc

temporomandibular joint

temporalis m.

H

lateral pterygoid m.

sinuses

medial pterygoid m.

I

masseter m.

mandible (coronal section)

medial pterygoid m.

I

iliopectineal eminence

femur

pubic bone (anterior view)

lesser trochanter of femur

© MELLONI

	MUSCLE	ORIGIN	INSERTION	INNERVATION	ACTION
A	**m. puboprostaticus** *(part of m. pubococcygeus)* *puboprostatic m.*	lower part of pubic symphysis in male	prostate	branches from vesical plexus	secures prostate and base of bladder
B	**m. puborectalis** *(part of m. pubococcygeus)* *puborectal m.*	back of pubis	interdigitates to form a sling that passes posteriorly around the rectum at the junction with the anal canal	branch of inferior rectal nerve; branch of sacral nerve (S4)	holds anal canal at right angle to rectum
C	**m. pubovaginalis** *(part of m. pubococcygeus)* *pubovaginal m.*	fibers of m. pubococcygeus passing into musculature of vagina and urethra		perineal division of pudendal nerve; branch of sacral nerve (S4)	sphincter for vagina
D	**m. pubovesicalis** *pubovesical m.* *pubovesical ligament*	posterior surface of lower part of pubis in female	neck of urinary bladder	sympathetic and parasympathetic branches from vesical plexus	secures base of bladder
E	**m. pyramidalis** *pyramidal m.*	pubic bone and pubic symphysis	linea alba	ventral ramus of T12 (subcostal nerve)	tenses linea alba of abdominal wall
F	**m. pyramidalis auriculae** *pyramidal m. of auricle*	a slip of muscle fibers extending vertically from m. tragicus to spine of helix		temporal branch of facial nerve (7th cranial nerve)	feebly alters shape of ear
G	**m. quadratus femoris** *quadrate m. of thigh*	upper part of lateral border of ischial tuberosity	upper part of trochanteric crest of femur	nerve to quadratus femoris (L5, S1)	rotates thigh laterally
H	**m. quadratus lumborum** *quadrate m. of loins*	iliac crest; iliolumbar ligament	12th rib; transverse processes of upper 4 lumbar vertebrae	ventral rami of T12, L1, L2, L3	draws rib cage downward; bends vertebral column laterally
I	**m. quadratus plantae** *quadrate m. of sole* *accessory flexor m.*	medial head: medial surface of calcaneus lateral head: lateral surface of calcaneus	lateral margins of tendon of m. flexor digitorum longus	branch of lateral plantar nerve (S1, S2)	aids in flexing all toes except the big one
J	**m. quadriceps femoris** *quadriceps m. of thigh*	the large four-headed muscle mass that covers the front and sides of the femur, consisting of the m. rectus femoris, m. vastus lateralis, m. vastus medialis, and m. vastus intermedius			great extensor of leg (m. rectus femoris also flexes thigh)
K	**m. rectococcygeus** *rectococcygeal m.*	band of muscle fibers connecting the anterior surface of coccygeal vertebrae 2 and 3 with the posterior wall of rectum		branches from inferior hypogastric plexus	secures rectum
L	**m. rectourethralis** *rectourethral m.*	band of muscle fibers connecting the membranous part of the urethra with the rectum		inferior rectal branch of pudendal nerve (S2, S3)	secures urethra

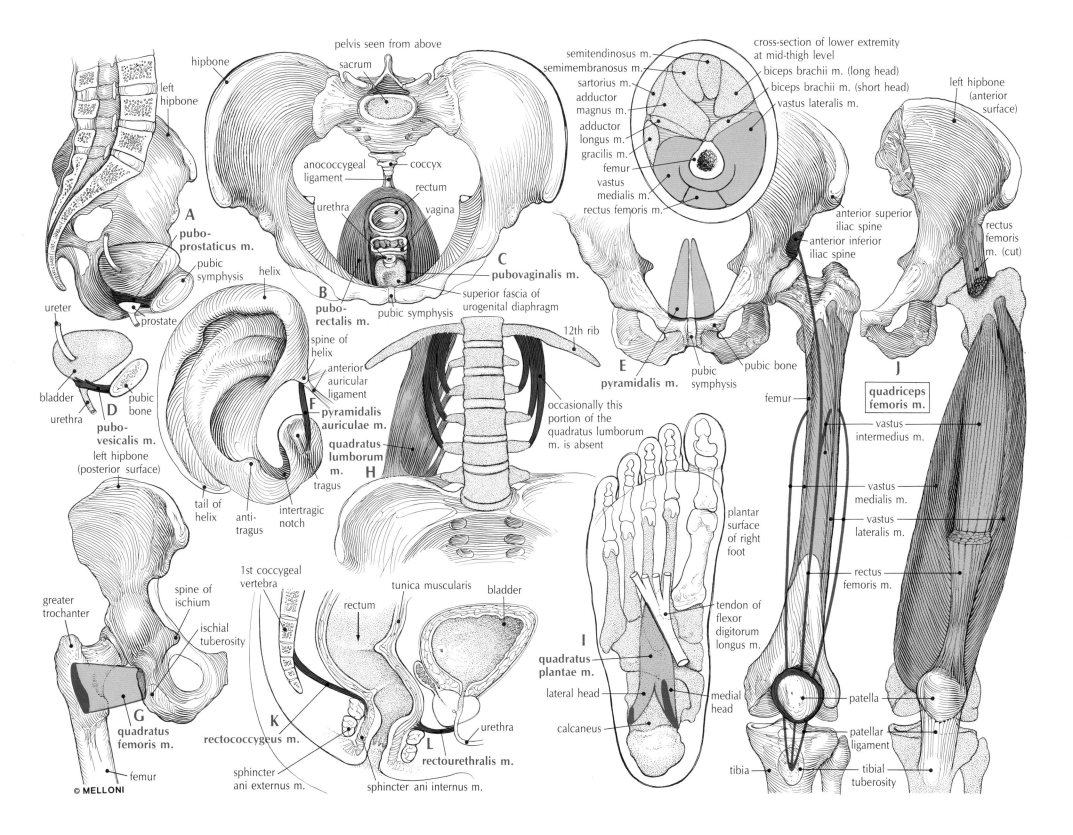

pelvis seen from above

hipbone

sacrum

A

**pubo-
prostaticus m.**

pubic
symphysis

left
hipbone

ureter

bladder

urethra

D

**pubo-
vesicalis m.**

left hipbone
(posterior surface)

greater
trochanter

spine of ischium

ischial
tuberosity

G

**quadratus
femoris m.**

femur

© MELLONI

anococcygeal
ligament

urethra

B

**pubo-
rectalis m.**

pubic symphysis

helix

spine of
helix

anterior
auricular
ligament

F

**pyramidalis
auriculae m.**

tragus

tail of
helix

anti-
tragus

intertragic
notch

coccyx

rectum

vagina

C

pubovaginalis m.

superior fascia of
urogenital diaphragm

12th rib

H

**quadratus
lumborum
m.**

occasionally this
portion of the
quadratus lumborum
m. is absent

1st coccygeal
vertebra

K

rectococcygeus m.

sphincter
ani externus m.

sphincter ani internus m.

rectum

tunica muscularis

bladder

L

rectourethralis m.

urethra

cross-section of lower extremity
at mid-thigh level

semitendinosus m.
semimembranosus m.
sartorius m.
adductor
magnus m.
adductor
longus m.
gracilis m.
femur
vastus
medialis m.
rectus femoris m.

E

pyramidalis m.

biceps brachii m. (long head)
biceps brachii m. (short head)
vastus lateralis m.

anterior superior
iliac spine
anterior inferior
iliac spine

pubic bone

pubic
symphysis

left hipbone
(anterior
surface)

rectus
femoris
m. (cut)

J

quadriceps
femoris m.

vastus
intermedius m.

vastus
medialis m.

vastus
lateralis m.

rectus
femoris m.

patella

patellar
ligament

tibia

tibial
tuberosity

plantar
surface
of right
foot

tendon of
flexor
digitorum
longus m.

I

**quadratus
plantae m.**

lateral head

medial
head

calcaneus

femur

	MUSCLE	ORIGIN	INSERTION	INNERVATION	ACTION
A	**m. rectouterinus** *rectouterine m.*	band of muscle fibers in rectouterine fold connecting the rectum with the cervix of the uterus		branches from inferior hypogastric plexus	secures uterus
B	**m. rectovesicalis** *rectovesical m.*	longitudinal musculature of anterior rectum	base of bladder	branches from vesical plexus	secures bladder
C	**m. rectus abdominis** *straight m. of abdomen*	crest and symphysis of pubis	xiphoid process; 5th to 7th costal cartilages	ventral rami of spinal nerves (T7 through T12)	tenses abdominal wall; flexes vertebral column; draws thorax downward
D	**m. rectus capitis anterior** *anterior rectus m. of head* *anterior straight m. of head*	lateral portion of 1st vertebra (atlas)	basilar portion of occipital bone just in front of foramen magnum	ventral branches of 1st and 2nd cervical spinal nerves	flexes and supports head
E	**m. rectus capitis lateralis** *lateral rectus m. of head* *lateral straight m. of head*	transverse process of 1st vertebra (atlas)	jugular process of occipital bone	ventral branches of 1st and 2nd cervical spinal nerves	aids in lateral movements of head; supports head
F	**m. rectus capitis posterior major** *greater posterior rectus m. of head* *greater posterior straight m. of head*	spinous process of 2nd vertebra (axis)	lateral part of inferior nuchal line of occipital	dorsal branches of 1st spinal nerve	extends head
G	**m. rectus capitis posterior minor** *smaller posterior rectus m. of head* *smaller posterior straight m. of head*	tubercle on posterior arch of 1st vertebra (atlas)	inferior nuchal line of occipital bone	dorsal branches of 1st spinal nerve	extends head
H	**m. rectus femoris** *rectus m. of thigh* *straight m. of thigh*	anterior, inferior iliac spine; upper margin of acetabulum	base of patella	femoral nerve (L2, L3, L4)	extends leg and flexes thigh
I	**m. rectus inferior bulbi** *inferior rectus m. of eyeball* *inferior straight m. of eyeball*	common tendinous ring around margins of optic canal	lower part of sclera 6.5 mm posterior to corneoscleral junction	oculomotor nerve (3rd cranial nerve)	rotates eyeball downward and somewhat medially
J	**m. rectus lateralis bulbi** *lateral rectus m. of eyeball* *lateral straight m. of eyeball*	common tendinous ring around margins of optic canal; orbital surface of greater wing of sphenoid	lateral part of sclera 7 mm posterior to corneoscleral junction	abducens nerve (6th cranial nerve)	rotates eyeball laterally (abduction)

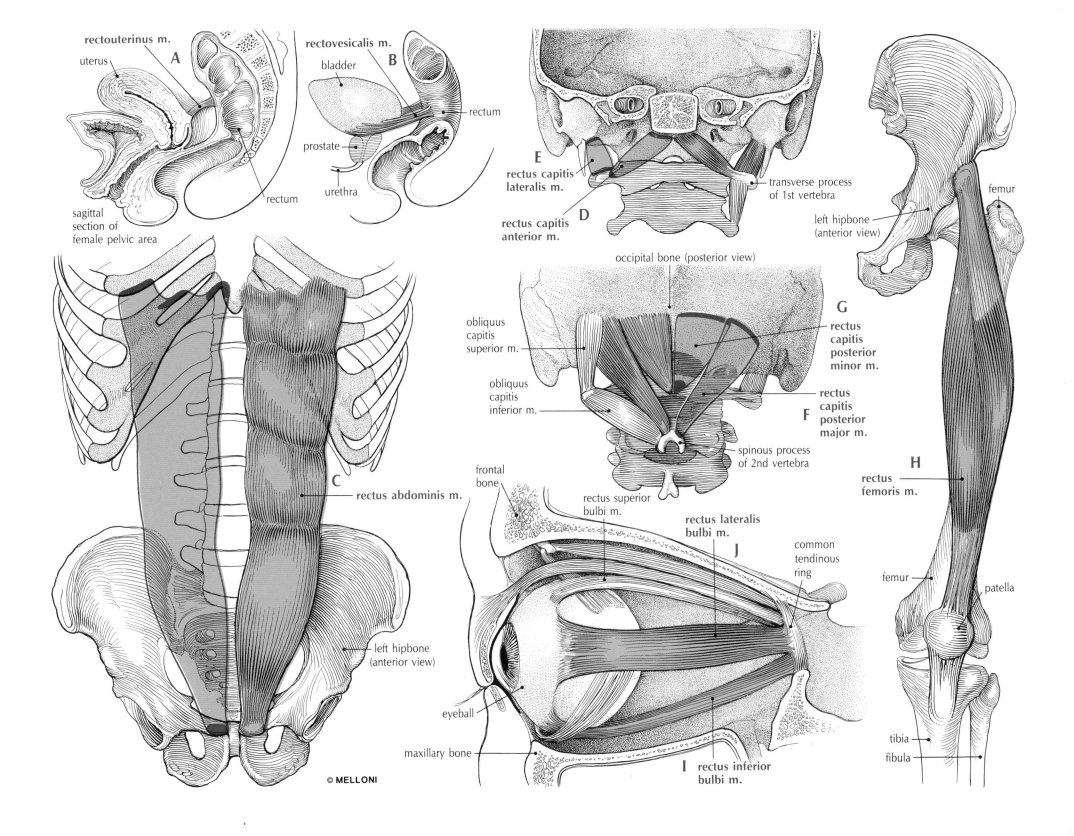

rectouterinus m. A

uterus

rectum

sagittal section of female pelvic area

rectovesicalis m. B

bladder

prostate

urethra

rectum

E

rectus capitis lateralis m.

rectus capitis anterior m. D

transverse process of 1st vertebra

left hipbone (anterior view)

femur

occipital bone (posterior view)

G

obliquus capitis superior m.

obliquus capitis inferior m.

rectus capitis posterior minor m.

rectus capitis posterior major m. F

spinous process of 2nd vertebra

rectus abdominis m. C

left hipbone (anterior view)

frontal bone

rectus superior bulbi m.

rectus lateralis bulbi m.

common tendinous ring

J

eyeball

maxillary bone

rectus inferior bulbi m. I

rectus femoris m. H

femur

patella

tibia

fibula

© MELLONI

	MUSCLE	ORIGIN	INSERTION	INNERVATION	ACTION
A	**m. rectus medialis bulbi** *medial rectus m. of eyeball* *medial straight m. of eyeball*	common tendinous ring around margins of optic canal	medial side of sclera 5.5 mm posterior to corneoscleral junction	oculomotor nerve (3rd cranial nerve)	rotates eyeball medially (adduction)
B	**m. rectus superior bulbi** *superior rectus m. of eyeball* *superior straight m. of eyeball*	common tendinous ring around margins of optic canal	upper aspect of sclera 7.5 mm posterior to corneoscleral junction	oculomotor nerve (3rd cranial nerve)	rotates eyeball upward and somewhat medially
C	**m. rhomboideus major** *greater rhomboid m.*	spinous processes of 2nd through 5th thoracic vertebrae; supraspinous ligament	lower two thirds of vertebral border of scapula	dorsal scapular nerve (4th and 5th cranial nerves)	rotates and draws scapula closer to midline
D	**m. rhomboideus minor** *smaller rhomboid m.*	lower part of nuchal ligament; spinous processes of 7th cervical and 1st thoracic vertebrae	vertebral margin of scapula at medial end of scapular spine	dorsal scapular nerve (4th and 5th cranial nerves)	rotates and draws scapula closer to midline
E	**m. risorius** *risorius m.*	fascia over parotid gland; platysma muscle	skin at angle of mouth	buccal branch of facial nerve (7th cranial nerve)	retracts angle of mouth
F	**mm. rotatores** *rotator muscles*	series of small muscles, each between the transverse process of the vertebra below and the lamina of the vertebra above, including mm. rotatores cervicis, mm. rotatores thoracis, and mm. rotatores lumborum			extend and rotate the vertebral column toward opposite side
G	**mm. rotatores cervicis** *rotator muscles of neck*	transverse process of cervical vertebrae	lamina of vertebra above	dorsal rami of spinal nerves	extend and rotate the cervical vertebral column toward the opposite side
H	**mm. rotatores lumborum** *rotator muscles of loins*	transverse processes of lumbar vertebrae	lamina of vertebra above	dorsal rami of spinal nerves	extend and rotate the lumbar vertebral column toward the opposite side
I	**mm. rotatores thoracis** *rotator muscles of thorax*	transverse process of thoracic vertebrae	lamina of vertebra above	dorsal rami of spinal nerves	extend and rotate the thoracic vertebral column toward the opposite side
J	**m. sacrococcygeus dorsalis** *posterior sacrococcygeal m.*	a muscular slip from the dorsal aspect of the sacrum to the coccyx		branch of spinal nerve (S5)	vestigial muscle; thought to feebly protect sacrococcygeal joint
K	**m. sacrococcygeus ventralis** *anterior sacrococcygeal m.*	a muscular slip from the ventral aspect of the sacrum to the coccyx		branch of spinal nerve (S5)	vestigial muscle; thought to feebly protect sacrococcygeal joint

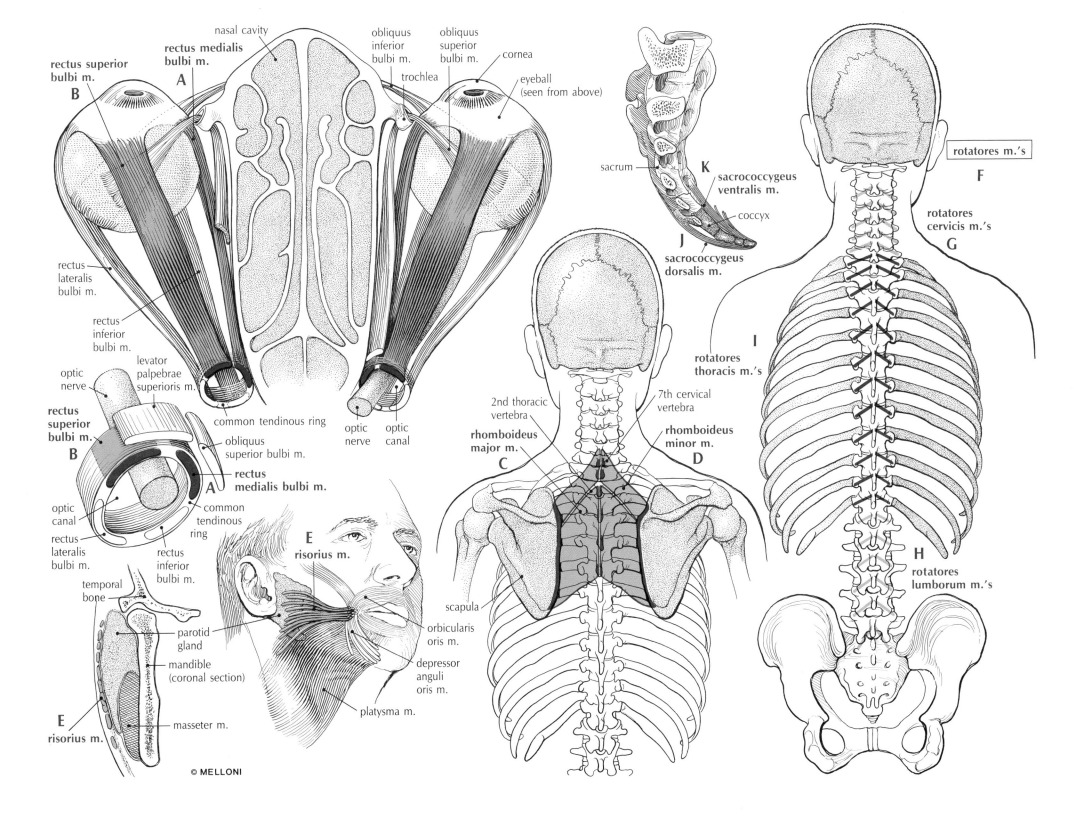

rectus superior bulbi m.

B

rectus medialis bulbi m.

A

nasal cavity

obliquus inferior bulbi m.

obliquus superior bulbi m.

trochlea

cornea

eyeball (seen from above)

rectus lateralis bulbi m.

rectus inferior bulbi m.

optic nerve

levator palpebrae superioris m.

optic nerve

obliquus superior bulbi m.

optic canal

common tendinous ring

rectus superior bulbi m.

B

optic canal

rectus lateralis bulbi m.

rectus inferior bulbi m.

A

obliquus superior bulbi m.

rectus medialis bulbi m.

common tendinous ring

temporal bone

parotid gland

mandible (coronal section)

E

risorius m.

masseter m.

E

risorius m.

orbicularis oris m.

depressor anguli oris m.

platysma m.

sacrum

K

sacrococcygeus ventralis m.

coccyx

J

sacrococcygeus dorsalis m.

2nd thoracic vertebra

7th cervical vertebra

rhomboideus major m.

C

rhomboideus minor m.

D

scapula

rotatores m.'s

F

rotatores cervicis m.'s

G

rotatores thoracis m.'s

I

rotatores lumborum m.'s

H

© MELLONI

	MUSCLE	ORIGIN	INSERTION	INNERVATION	ACTION
A	**m. salpingopharyngeus** *salpingopharyngeal m.*	bottom part of cartilage of auditory tube near its nasopharyngeal orifice	palatopharyngeal muscle in wall of pharynx	pharyngeal plexus of vagus nerve (10th cranial nerve)	elevates nasopharynx
B	**m. sartorius** *sartorius m.*	anterior superior iliac spine	medial side of upper tibia	femoral nerve (L2, L3)	flexes thigh and leg; rotates thigh laterally
C	**m. scalenus anterior** *anterior scalene m.* *anterior anticus m.*	transverse processes of 3rd to 6th cervical vertebrae	scalene tubercle of 1st rib	ventral branches of spinal nerves (4th, 5th, and 6th cranial nerves)	raises 1st rib; bends neck forward and rotates it toward opposite side
D	**m. scalenus medius** *middle scalene m.*	transverse processes of first six cervical vertebrae	upper surface of 1st rib	ventral branches of cervical spinal nerves (3rd through 8th cranial nerves)	raises 1st rib; bends neck to same side
E	**m. scalenus minimus** *smallest scalene m.*	transverse process of 7th cervical vertebra	1st rib; dome of pleura	ventral branches of cervical spinal nerves (5th and 6th cranial nerves)	tenses dome of pleura
F	**m. scalenus posterior** *posterior scalene m.*	transverse processes of 4th to 6th cervical vertebrae	outer aspect of 2nd rib	ventral branches of cervical spinal nerves (5th, 6th, and 7th cranial nerves)	raises 1st and 2nd ribs; bends neck to same side
G	**m. semimembranosus** *semimembranous m.*	lateral part of ischial tuberosity	medial condyle of tibia; oblique popliteal ligament	tibial part of sciatic nerve (L5, S1, S2)	extends thigh; flexes leg and rotates it medially
H	**mm. semispinales** *semispinal muscles*	a series of three muscles spanning four or more vertebrae including the m. semispinalis capitis, m. semispinalis cervicis, and the m. semispinalis thoracis		dorsal branches of cervical and thoracic spinal nerves	extend head and vertebral column and rotates them toward opposite side
I	**m. semispinalis capitis** *semispinal m. of head*	transverse processes of six upper thoracic and four lower cervical vertebrae	occipital bone between superior and inferior nuchal lines	dorsal branches of cervical and thoracic spinal nerves	extends head and turns it toward opposite side
J	**m. semispinalis cervicis** *semispinal m. of neck*	transverse processes of upper six thoracic vertebrae	spinous processes of 2nd through 6th cervical vertebrae	dorsal rami of cervical and thoracic spinal nerves	extends vertebral column and turns it toward the opposite side
K	**m. semispinalis thoracis** *semispinal m. of thorax*	transverse processes of lower six thoracic vertebrae	spinous processes of upper six thoracic and lower two cervical vertebrae	dorsal rami of thoracic spinal nerves	extends vertebral column and turns it toward opposite side
L	**m. semitendinosus** *semitendinous m.*	ischial tuberosity (in common with m. biceps femoris)	upper part of medial surface of tibia near tibial tuberosity	tibial part of sciatic nerve (L5, S1, S2)	flexes and rotates leg medially; extends thigh

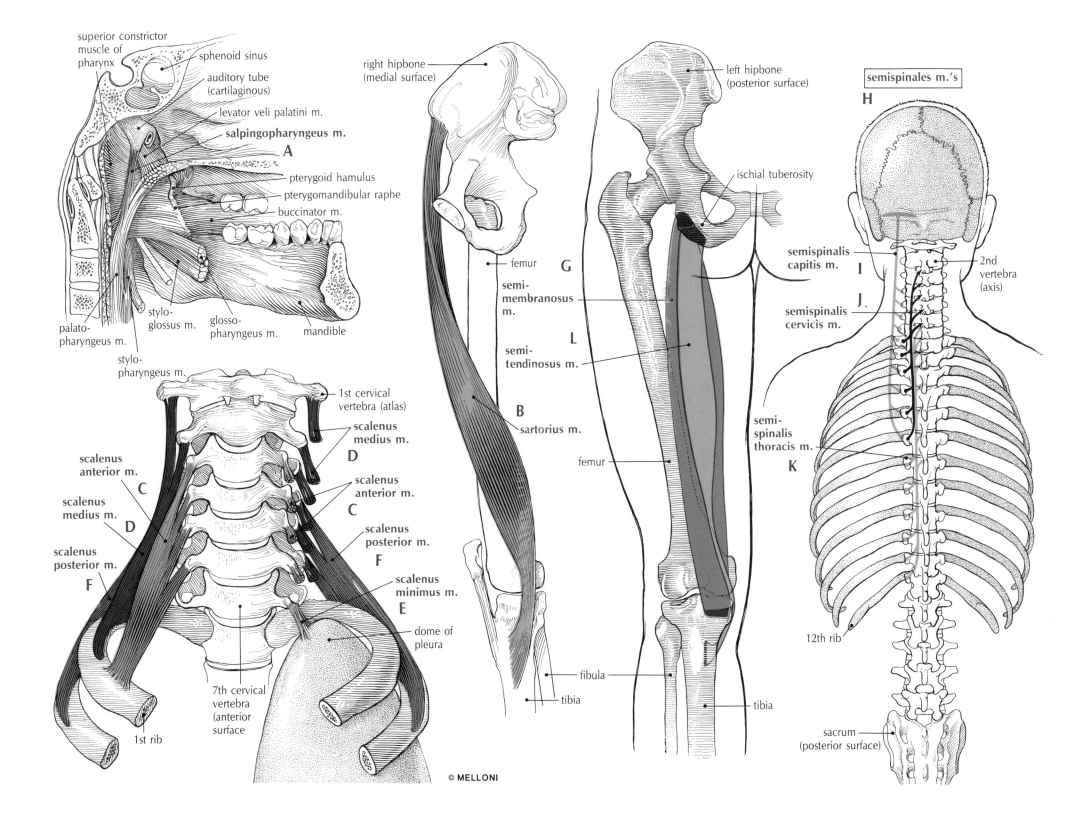

superior constrictor muscle of pharynx

sphenoid sinus

auditory tube (cartilaginous)

levator veli palatini m.

salpingopharyngeus m.

A

pterygoid hamulus

pterygomandibular raphe

buccinator m.

palatopharyngeus m.

styloglossus m.

glossopharyngeus m.

mandible

stylopharyngeus m.

1st cervical vertebra (atlas)

scalenus medius m.

D

scalenus anterior m.

C

scalenus anterior m.

C

scalenus medius m.

D

scalenus posterior m.

F

scalenus posterior m.

F

scalenus minimus m.

E

dome of pleura

7th cervical vertebra (anterior surface

1st rib

right hipbone (medial surface)

femur

G

semimembranosus m.

semitendinosus m.

B

sartorius m.

left hipbone (posterior surface)

ischial tuberosity

L

femur

semispinalis thoracis m.

K

fibula

tibia

tibia

semispinales m.'s

H

semispinalis capitis m.

I

semispinalis cervicis m.

J.

2nd vertebra (axis)

12th rib

sacrum (posterior surface)

© MELLONI

	MUSCLE	ORIGIN	INSERTION	INNERVATION	ACTION
A	**m. serratus anterior** *anterior serratus m.*	outer aspects of upper 8 to 10 ribs	anterior surface of vertebral (medial) border of scapula	long thoracic nerve (5th, 6th, and 7th cranial nerves)	draws scapula forward and laterally; rotates scapula in raising arm
B	**m. serratus posterior inferior** *inferior posterior serratus m.*	spinous processes of last two thoracic and first two lumbar vertebrae; supraspinous ligament	inferior borders of last four ribs, slightly beyond their angles	ventral rami of thoracic spinal nerves (T9 through T12)	draws ribs outward and downward (counteracting the inward pull of the diaphragm)
C	**m. serratus posterior superior** *superior posterior serratus m.*	lower part of nuchal ligament; spinous processes of 7th cervical and first two or three thoracic vertebrae; supraspinous ligament	upper borders of 2nd, 3rd, 4th, and 5th ribs, slightly beyond their angles	2nd, 3rd, 4th, and 5th intercostal nerves	raises the ribs
D	**m. soleus** *soleus m.*	proximal ends of tibia and fibula; popliteal fascia	calcaneus by calcaneal tendon (in common with m. gastrocnemius)	branches from tibial nerve (S1, S2)	plantarflexes foot
E	**m. sphincter ampullae hepatopancreaticae** *sphincter m. of hepatopancreatic ampulla* *sphincter of Oddi*	a sphincter of smooth circular muscle around terminal part of main pancreatic duct and common bile duct including duodenal ampulla (papilla of Vater)		branches from celiac plexus	constricts both lower part of common bile duct and main pancreatic duct
F	**m. sphincter ani externus** *(surrounds entire length of anal canal)* *external sphincter m. of anus*	subcutaneous part: anococcygeal ligament superficial part: posterior surface of last coccyx; anococcygeal raphe deep part: circular fibers surrounding the upper part of m. sphincter ani internus	subcutaneous part: perineal body (central tendon of perineum); skin superficial part: perineal body	perineal branch of 4th sacral spinal nerve; inferior rectal branch of pudendal nerve (S2, S3)	closes anal canal and anus
G	**m. sphincter ani internus** *internal sphincter m. of anus*	1 cm thick muscular ring surrounding the upper part (2.5 cm) of the anal canal, about 6 mm from the orifice of the anus		branches from inferior hypogastric plexus	closes anal canal and anus
H	**m. sphincter ductus choledochi** *sphincter m. of bile duct*	a sphincter of smooth muscle around lower part of the bile duct within the wall of the duodenum (part of the m. sphincter ampullae hepatopancreaticae)		branches from celiac plexus	constricts lower part of common bile duct
I	**m. sphincter pancreaticus** *sphincter m. of pancreas*	a sphincter of smooth circular muscle fibers around the terminal part of main pancreatic duct where it joins the common bile duct before entering into the duodenum		branches from ciliac plexus	constricts terminal part of main pancreatic duct

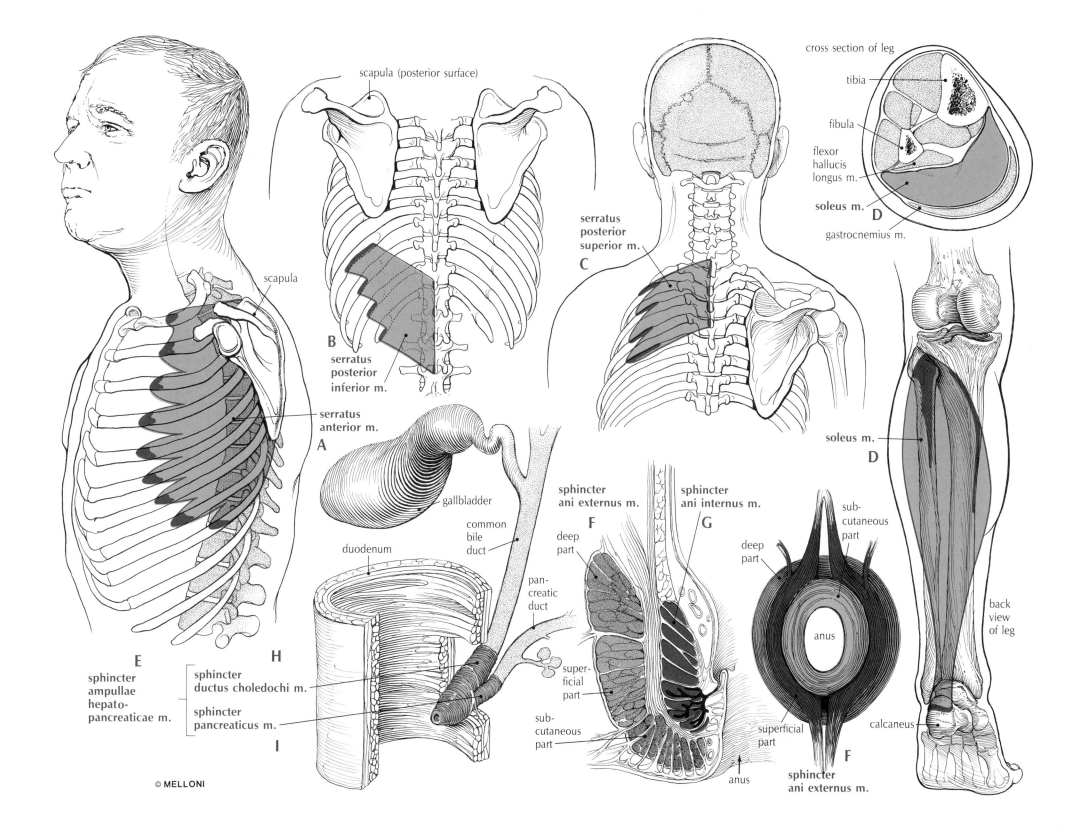

scapula (posterior surface)

scapula

serratus
anterior m.

A

B **serratus
posterior
inferior m.**

serratus
posterior
superior m.

C

cross section of leg

tibia

fibula

flexor
hallucis
longus m.

soleus m.

D

gastrocnemius m.

soleus m.

D

back
view
of leg

calcaneus

gallbladder

common
bile
duct

duodenum

pan-
creatic
duct

E

H

I

sphincter
ampullae
hepato-
pancreaticae m.

sphincter
ductus choledochi m.

sphincter
pancreaticus m.

**sphincter
ani externus m.**

F

deep
part

superficial
part

sub-
cutaneous
part

anus

**sphincter
ani internus m.**

G

sub-
cutaneous
part

deep
part

anus

superficial
part

F

**sphincter
ani externus m.**

© MELLONI

	MUSCLE	ORIGIN	INSERTION	INNERVATION	ACTION
A	**m. sphincter pupillae** *sphincter m. of pupil*	circular fibers of iris arranged in a narrow band about 1 mm wide and 0.20 mm thick		parasympathetic fibers of oculomotor nerve (3rd cranial nerve) by way of ciliary ganglion; long ciliary branch of nasociliary nerve	constricts pupil
B	**m. sphincter pylori** *sphincter m. of pylorus* *sphincter m. of stomach*	thick muscular ring at lower part of stomach near opening into duodenum		sympathetic branches from celiac plexus; para-sympathetic branches from vagus nerve (10th cranial nerve)	acts as valve to close lumen
C	**m. sphincter urethrae** *(part of urogenital diaphragm)* *sphincter m. of urethra*	ischiopubic rami; transverse perineal ligament; surrounding fascia	perineal body (central tendon of perineum)	perineal branch of pudendal nerve (S2, S3, S4)	compresses urethra; aids ejaculation
D	**m. sphincter vaginae** *sphincter m. of vagina*	pubic symphysis	interdigitates around and interlaces into vaginal barrel	inferior hypogastric plexus; uterovaginal plexus	constricts vaginal orifice
E	**m. sphincter vesicae urinariae** *sphincter m. of urinary bladder*	thick muscular ring toward the lower part of bladder surrounding the internal urethral orifice		vesical nerve (para-sympathetic; S2, S3, S4) (sympathetic; T11, T12, L1, L2)	acts as valve to close internal urethral orifice
F	**m. spinalis** *spinal m.*	the medial division of the m. erector spinae, including the m. spinalis capitis, m. spinalis cervicis, and m. spinalis thoracic		dorsal branches of lower cervical and thoracic spinal nerves	extend vertebral column
G	**m. spinalis capitis** *spinal m. of head* *diventer cervicis m.*	spinous processes of vertebrae C6 to C7, T1 to T2	occipital bone between superior and inferior nuchal lines	dorsal branches of cervical and upper thoracic spinal nerves	extends head
H	**m. spinalis cervicis** *spinal m. of neck*	spinous processes of vertebrae C6 to C7, T1 to T2	spinous processes of vertebrae C2 to C4	dorsal branches of lower cervical and thoracic spinal nerves	extends vertebral column
I	**m. spinalis thoracis** *spinal m. of thorax* *spinal m. of back*	spinous processes of vertebrae T11 to T12, L1 to L2	spinous processes of vertebrae T2 to T7	dorsal branches of thoracic spinal nerves	extends vertebral column
J	**m. splenius capitis** *splenius m. of head*	bottom portion of nuchal ligament; spinous processes of vertebrae C7, T1, T2, and T3	mastoid process of temporal bone; lateral portion of superior nuchal line	dorsal branch of middle cervical spinal nerves	inclines and rotates head

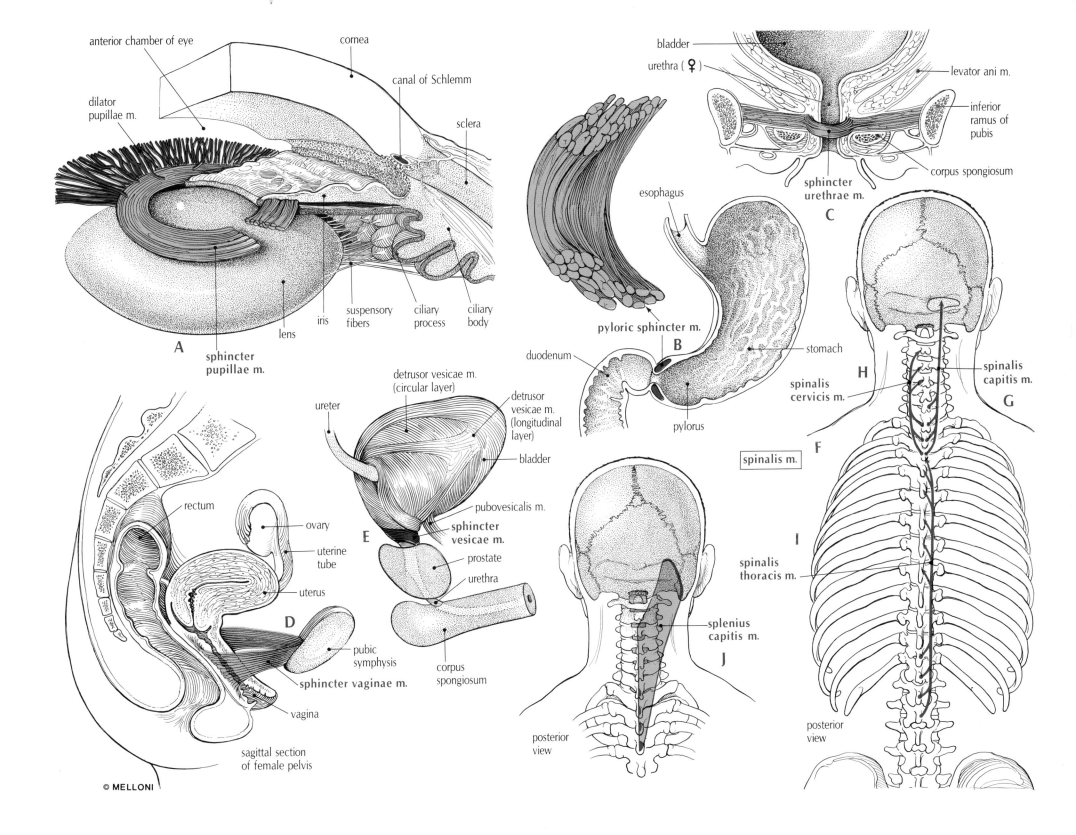

anterior chamber of eye

cornea

canal of Schlemm

dilator pupillae m.

sclera

sphincter pupillae m.

lens

iris

suspensory fibers

ciliary process

ciliary body

A

bladder

urethra (♀)

levator ani m.

inferior ramus of pubis

corpus spongiosum

sphincter urethrae m.

C

esophagus

pyloric sphincter m.

duodenum

stomach

pylorus

B

spinalis cervicis m.

spinalis capitis m.

H

G

F

spinalis m.

rectum

ovary

uterine tube

uterus

pubic symphysis

sphincter vaginae m.

vagina

sagittal section of female pelvis

D

detrusor vesicae m. (circular layer)

ureter

detrusor vesicae m. (longitudinal layer)

bladder

pubovesicalis m.

sphincter vesicae m.

prostate

urethra

corpus spongiosum

E

spinalis thoracis m.

I

splenius capitis m.

posterior view

J

posterior view

© MELLONI

	MUSCLE	ORIGIN	INSERTION	INNERVATION	ACTION
A	**m. splenius cervicis** *splenius m. of neck* *splenius colli m.*	nuchal ligament; spinous processes 3rd to 6th thoracic vertebrae	posterior tubercles of transverse processes of upper two or three cervical vertebrae	dorsal branches of the lower cervical spinal nerves	extends head and neck; turns head toward the same side
B	**m. stapedius** *stapedius m.*	bony canal in pyramidal eminence on posterior wall of middle ear chamber	posterior surface of neck of stapes	stapedial branch of facial nerve (7th cranial nerve)	dampens excessive vibrations of stapes by tilting the baseplate
C	**m. sternalis** *(in 5% of individuals)* *sternal m.*	a muscular band occasionally seen at the sternal end of m. pectoralis major, parallel to the margin of the sternum		branch of anterior thoracic nerve	protects sternum
D	**m. sternocleidomastoideus** *sternocleidomastoid m.*	sternal head: anterior surface of manubrium clavicular head: medial third of clavicle	mastoid process; superior nuchal line of occipital bone	accessory nerve (11th cranial nerve); ventral branch of 2nd cervical spinal nerve	rotates and extends head; flexes vertebral column
E	**m. sternohyoideus** *sternohyoid m.*	medial end of clavicle; upper and posterior part of manubrium	lower border of body of hyoid bone	branches from ansa cervicalis	draws hyoid bone and larynx down from elevated position during swallowing
F	**m. sternothyroideus** *sternothyroid m.*	posterior surface of manubrium; medial edge of 1st costal cartilage	oblique line on lamina of thyroid cartilage	branches from ansa cervicalis	draws the larynx down from elevated position during swallowing
G	**m. styloglossus** *styloglossus m.*	lower end of styloid process; upper end of stylomandibular ligament	longitudinal part: side of tongue near dorsal surface oblique part: over the m. hyoglossus	hypoglossal nerve (12th cranial nerve)	raises and retracts tongue
H	**m. stylohyoideus** *stylohyoid m.*	posterior surface of styloid process of temporal bone	hyoid bone at junction of greater horn with body	branch from posterior trunk of facial nerve (7th cranial nerve)	draws hyoid bone upward and backward
I	**m. stylopharyngeus** *stylopharyngeus m.*	base of styloid process of temporal bone	wall of pharynx; thyroid cartilage	branch of glossopharyngeal nerve (9th cranial nerve)	elevates and opens pharynx
J	**m. subclavius** *subclavius m.*	junction of 1st rib and costal cartilage	lower surface of clavicle	nerve to subclavius, a branch of brachial plexus (5th and 6th cranial nerves)	depresses lateral end of clavicle; protects sternoclavicular joint from physical abuse
K	**mm. subcostales** *subcostal muscles*	inner surface of ribs of lower thorax, near their angles	lower inner surface of 2nd or 3rd rib below rib of origin	intercostal nerves	depresses lower ribs and draws them closer together

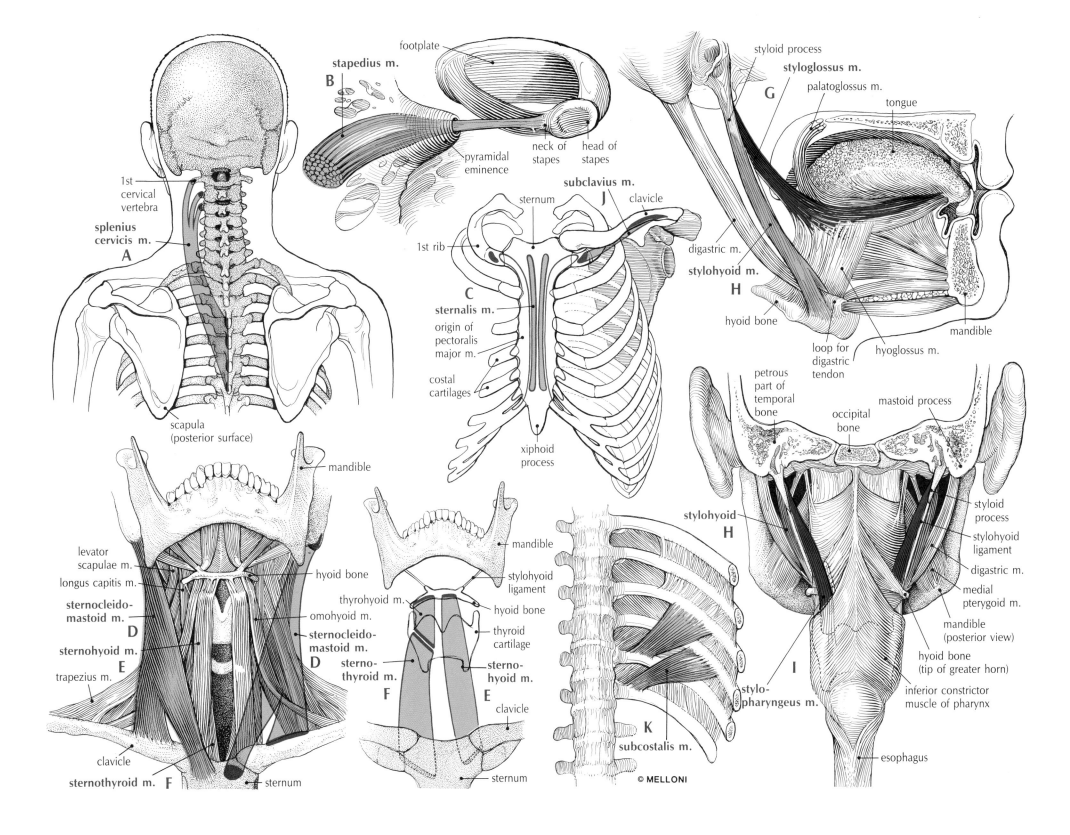

splenius cervicis m.
A

1st cervical vertebra

scapula (posterior surface)

stapedius m.
B

footplate

neck of stapes

head of stapes

pyramidal eminence

sternalis m.
C

sternum

1st rib

origin of pectoralis major m.

costal cartilages

xiphoid process

subclavius m.
J

clavicle

styloid process

styloglossus m.
G

palatoglossus m.

tongue

digastric m.

stylohyoid m.
H

hyoid bone

loop for digastric tendon

hyoglossus m.

mandible

levator scapulae m.

longus capitis m.

sternocleido-mastoid m.
D

sternohyoid m.
E

trapezius m.

clavicle

sternothyroid m. **F**

sternum

mandible

hyoid bone

omohyoid m.

sternocleido-mastoid m.
D

mandible

stylohyoid ligament

thyrohyoid m.

hyoid bone

thyroid cartilage

sterno-thyroid m.
F

sterno-hyoid m.
E

clavicle

sternum

stylohyoid
H

petrous part of temporal bone

occipital bone

mastoid process

styloid process

stylohyoid ligament

digastric m.

medial pterygoid m.

mandible (posterior view)

hyoid bone (tip of greater horn)

inferior constrictor muscle of pharynx

stylo-pharyngeus m.

subcostalis m.
K

esophagus

© MELLONI

	MUSCLE	ORIGIN	INSERTION	INNERVATION	ACTION
A	**m. subscapularis** *subscapular m.*	medial two thirds of subscapular fossa of scapula	lesser tubercle of humerus; front of capsule of shoulder joint	upper and lower subscapular nerves of the brachial plexus (5th, 6th, and 7th cranial nerves)	rotates arm medially
B	**m. supinator** *supinator m.*	lateral epicondyle of humerus; radial collateral ligament; supinator crest of ulna	upper third of radius	posterior intercostal nerve (deep branch of radial nerve; 5th and 6th cranial nerves)	supinates hand by rotating radius
C	**mm. suprahyoidei** *suprahyoid muscles*	a group of muscles attached to the upper part of the hyoid bone from the skull; it includes the m. digastricus, m. stylohoideus, m. mylohoideus, and m. geniohyoideus			elevate hyoid bone
D	**m. supraspinatus** *supraspinous m.*	medial two thirds of supraspinous fossa of scapula	superior surface of greater tubercle of humerus and capsule of shoulder joint	suprascapular nerve (4th, 5th, and 6th cranial nerves)	abducts arm
E	**m. suspensorius duodeni** *suspensory m. of duodenum* *ligament of Treitz*	connective tissue around celiac artery and right crus of diaphragm	superior border of duodenojejunal curve; part of ascending duodenum	branches from celiac plexus	acts as suspensory ligament of duodenum
F	**m. tarsalis inferior** *inferior tarsal m.*	fascial sheath of inferior rectus muscle of eyeball	lower border of inferior tarsus	sympathetic innervation	depresses lower eyelid widening palpebral fissure
G	**m. tarsalis superior** *superior tarsal m.* *lamina profundus*	fascial sheath of levator muscle of upper eyelid	upper border of superior tarsus	sympathetic innervation	raises upper eyelid, widening palpebral fissure
H	**m. temporalis** *temporal m.*	temporal fossa on side of cranium	coronoid process of mandible	mandibular division of trigeminal nerve (5th cranial nerve)	closes mouth; clenches teeth; moves mandible backward
I	**m. temporoparietalis** *temporoparietal m.*	temporal fascia above and anterior to ear	lateral border of frontal part of epicranial aponeurosis	temporal branches of facial nerve (7th cranial nerve)	tightens scalp
J	**m. tensor fasciae latae** *tensor m. of fascia lata*	upper lip of iliac crest; lateral part of anterior superior iliac spine; fascia lata	between two layers of iliotibial tract of fascia lata	superior gluteal nerve (L4, L5)	extends knee with lateral rotation of leg
K	**m. tensor tympani** *tensor tympani m.* *tensor m. of tympanic membrane*	cartilaginous portion of auditory tube and adjoining part of great wing of sphenoid bone	base of handle of malleus (most lateral ossicle of the ear)	branch of nerve to medial pterygoid, part of mandibular division of trigeminal nerve (5th cranial nerve)	draws tympanic membrane medially, thus increasing its tension

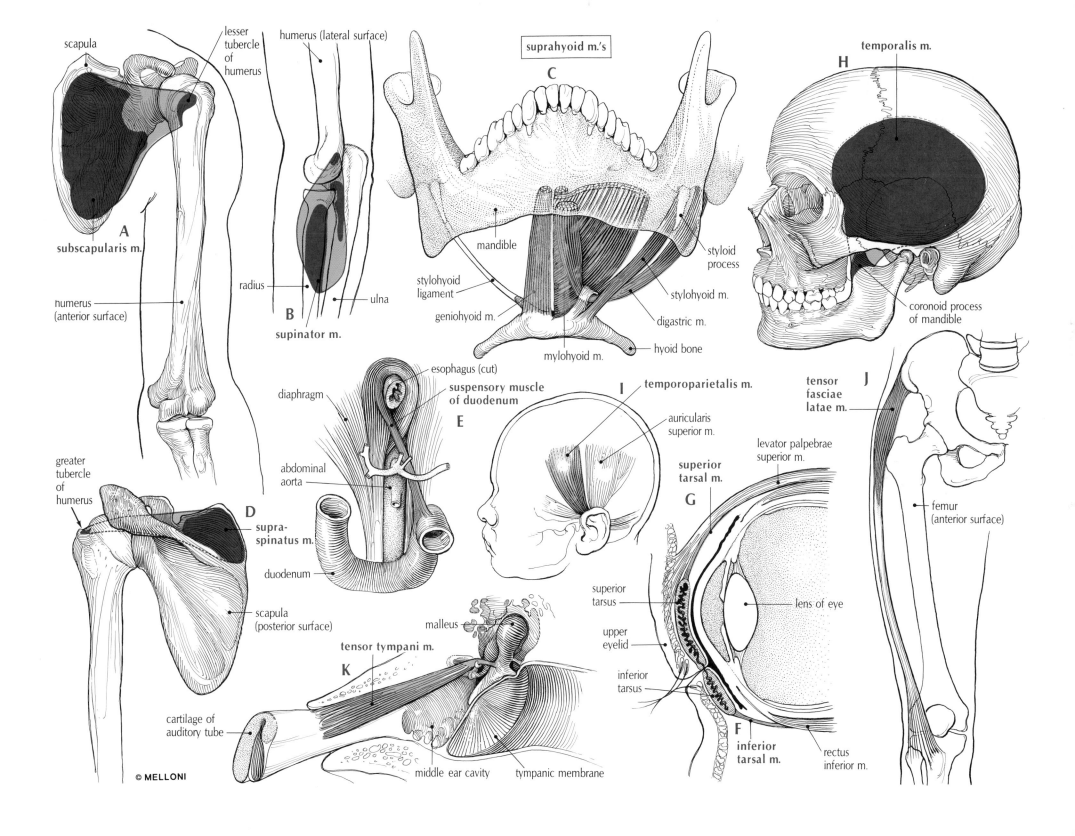

A

scapula

lesser tubercle of humerus

subscapularis m.

humerus (anterior surface)

B

humerus (lateral surface)

radius

ulna

supinator m.

C

suprahyoid m.'s

mandible

stylohyoid ligament

geniohyoid m.

mylohyoid m.

styloid process

stylohyoid m.

digastric m.

hyoid bone

H

temporalis m.

coronoid process of mandible

D

greater tubercle of humerus

supra-spinatus m.

scapula (posterior surface)

E

esophagus (cut)

diaphragm

suspensory muscle of duodenum

abdominal aorta

duodenum

I

temporoparietalis m.

auricularis superior m.

G

superior tarsal m.

levator palpebrae superior m.

superior tarsus

upper eyelid

inferior tarsus

inferior tarsal m.

lens of eye

rectus inferior m.

J

tensor fasciae latae m.

femur (anterior surface)

K

tensor tympani m.

cartilage of auditory tube

malleus

middle ear cavity

tympanic membrane

F

© MELLONI

	MUSCLE	ORIGIN	INSERTION	INNERVATION	ACTION
A	**m. tensor veli palatini** *tensor m. of palatine velum* *tensor m. of soft palate*	spine and scaphoid fossa of sphenoid bone; cartilage and membrane of auditory tube	midline of aponeurosis of soft palate; horizontal plate of palatine bone	mandibular division of trigeminal nerve (5th cranial nerve)	tenses soft palate; opens auditory tube
B	**m. teres major** *teres major m.*	lower one third of posterior surface of lateral border of scapula	medial lip of intertubercular (bicipital) groove of humerus	lower scapular nerve of brachial plexus (6th and 7th cranial nerves)	adducts and rotates arm medially
C	**m. teres minor** *teres minor m.*	upper two thirds of posterior surface of lateral border of scapula	lower facet of greater tubercle of humerus; posterior surface of capsule of shoulder joint	axillary nerve from brachial plexus (4th, 5th, and 6th cranial nerves)	rotates arm laterally and weakly adducts it
D	**m. thyroarytenoideus** *thyroarytenoid m.*	inside of thyroid cartilage	lateral surface of arytenoid cartilage	recurrent laryngeal nerve	relaxes vocal ligaments; aids in closure of glottis
E	**m. thyroepiglotticus** *thyroepiglottic m.*	inside of thyroid cartilage	margin of epiglottis	recurrent laryngeal nerve	widens inlet of larynx
F	**m. thyrohyoideus** *thyrohyoid m.*	oblique line of thyroid cartilage	greater horn of hyoid bone	branch of hypoglossal nerve (12th cranial nerve), containing fibers from 1st cervical spinal nerve	elevates larynx while depressing hyoid bone
G	**m. tibialis anterior** *anterior tibial m.*	lateral surface of upper two thirds of tibia; interosseous membrane	medial surface of medial cuneiform; base of 1st metatarsal bone	deep peroneal nerve (L4, L5)	dorsiflexes and inverts foot
H	**m. tibialis posterior** *posterior tibial m.*	tibia; fibula; interosseous membrane	navicular, with slips to three cuneiform bones; cuboid, 2nd, 3rd, and 4th metatarsals	tibial nerve (L4, L5)	principal invertor of foot; aids plantarflexion of foot
I	**m. trachealis** *tracheal m.*	anastomosing transverse muscular bands connecting the free ends of the tracheal rings		branches of vagus nerve (10th cranial nerve); recurrent laryngeal nerve; sympathetic chain	reduces size of tracheal lumen
J	**m. tragicus** *tragus m.*	a short, flat band of vertical muscular fibers on the lateral surface of the tragus of the ear		temporal branches of facial nerve (7th cranial nerve)	slightly alters the shape of ear
K	**m. transversospinalis** *transversospinal m.*	a general term for a group of seven muscles that run upwardly from the transverse processes to the spinous processes of the vertebrae; it includes the m. semispinalis capitis, m. semispinalis cervicis, m. semispinalis thoracic, m. multifidus, m. rotatores cervicis, m. rotatores lumborum, and m. rotatores thoracis			extend and rotate vertebral column toward opposite side

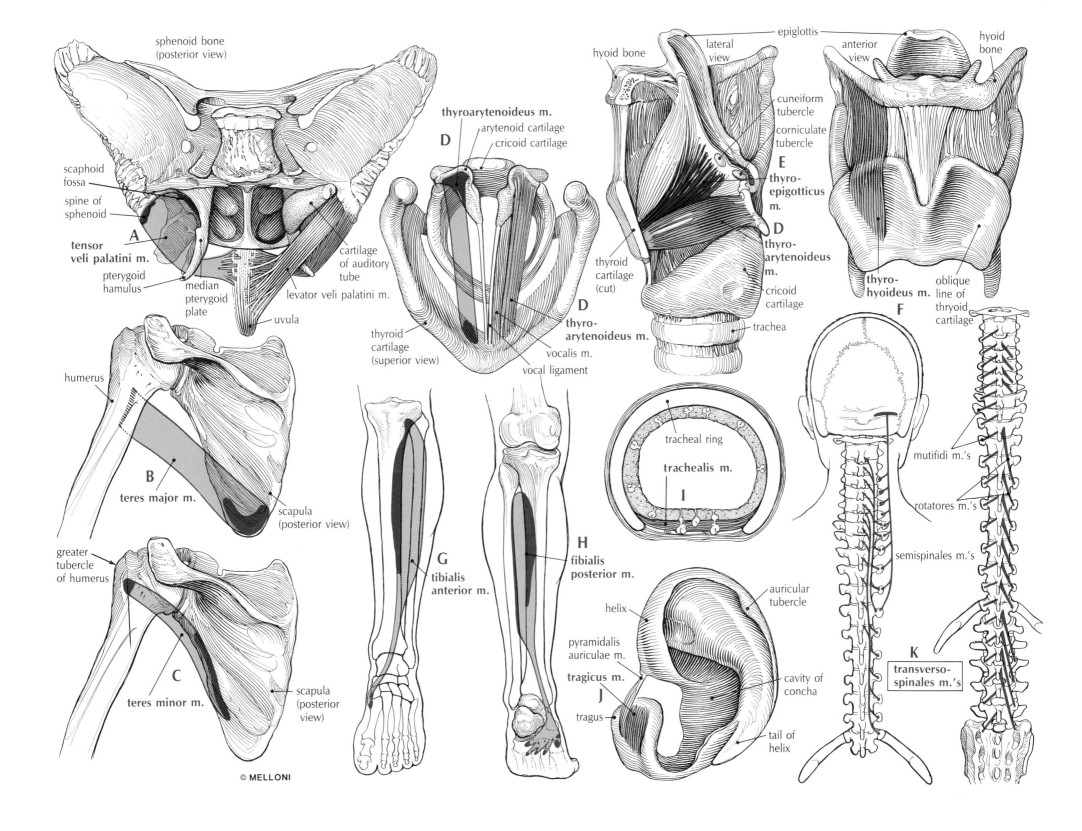

sphenoid bone
(posterior view)

scaphoid
fossa

spine of
sphenoid

**tensor
veli palatini m.**

A

pterygoid
hamulus

median
pterygoid
plate

uvula

levator veli palatini m.

cartilage
of auditory
tube

humerus

B

teres major m.

scapula
(posterior view)

greater
tubercle
of humerus

C

teres minor m.

scapula
(posterior
view)

thyroarytenoideus m.
arytenoid cartilage
cricoid cartilage

D

thyroid
cartilage
(superior view)

**thyro-
arytenoideus m.**

vocalis m.

vocal ligament

D

epiglottis

hyoid bone

lateral
view

cuneiform
tubercle

corniculate
tubercle

E

**thyro-
epigotticus
m.**

D

**thyro-
arytenoideus
m.**

thyroid
cartilage
(cut)

cricoid
cartilage

trachea

anterior
view

hyoid
bone

**thyro-
hyoideus m.**

F

oblique
line of
thryoid
cartilage

G

tibialis
anterior m.

H

**fibialis
posterior m.**

tracheal ring

trachealis m.

I

mutifidi m.'s

rotatores m.'s

semispinales m.'s

K

transverso-
spinales m.'s

auricular
tubercle

helix

pyramidalis
auriculae m.

tragicus m.

J

tragus

cavity of
concha

tail of
helix

© MELLONI

	MUSCLE	ORIGIN	INSERTION	INNERVATION	ACTION
A	**m. transversus abdominis** *transverse m. of abdomen*	inner surface of 7th to 12th costal cartilages; thoracolumbar fascia; iliac crest; lateral part of inguinal ligament	conjoined tendon to pubis; linea alba through sheath of m. rectus abdominis	lower six thoracic and 1st lumbar spinal nerves	tenses abdominal wall and supports abdominal contents
B	**m. transversus auriculae** *transverse m. of auricle*	conchal eminence on posterior surface of auricular cartilage	scaphal eminence on posterior surface of auricular cartilage	posterior auricular branch of facial nerve (7th cranial nerve)	retracts helix feebly
C	**m. transversus linguae** *transverse m. of tongue*	median fibrous septum of tongue	submucous fibrous tissue at sides of tongue	hypoglossal nerve (12th cranial nerve)	narrows and elongates tongue
D	*transverse m. of chin*	superficial muscular slips below the chin connecting the m. depressor anguli oris of either side		mandibular branch of facial nerve (7th cranial nerve)	aids in drawing angle of mouth downward
E	**m. transversus nuchae** *(in 20% of individuals)* *transverse m. of nape*	external occipital protuberance or superior nuchal line of occipital bone	posterior edge of upper end of m. sternocleidomastoideus or mastoid process of temporal bone	posterior auricular branch of facial nerve (7th cranial nerve)	
F	**m. transversus perinei profundus** *(part of urogenital diaphragm)* *deep transverse m. of perineum*	ramus of ischium	perineal body (central tendon of perineum)	perineal branch of pudendal nerve (S2, S3, S4)	supports pelvic viscera
G	**m. transversus perinei superficialis** *(inconstant part of urogenital diaphragm)* *superficial transverse m. of perineum*	ramus of ischium near tuberosity	perineal body (central tendon of perineum)	perineal branch of pudendal nerve	aids in support of pelvic viscera
H	**m. transversus thoracis** *transverse m. of thorax* *sternocostal m.*	posterior surface of xiphoid process; lower half of posterior surface of sternum and adjacent costal cartilages	inner surface of 2nd to 6th costal cartilages	intercostal nerves	draws costal cartilages downward; narrows chest
I	**m. trapezius** *trapezius m.*	superior nuchal line of occipital bone; external occipital protuberance; nuchal ligament; spinous processes of 7th cervical and all thoracic vertebrae	superior part: posterior border of lateral third of clavicle middle part: medial margin of acromion; superior lip of posterior border of scapular spine inferior part: tubercle at apex of medial end of scapular spine	accessory nerve (11th cranial nerve); ventral branches of 3rd and 4th cervical spinal nerves	elevates, rotates, and retracts scapula

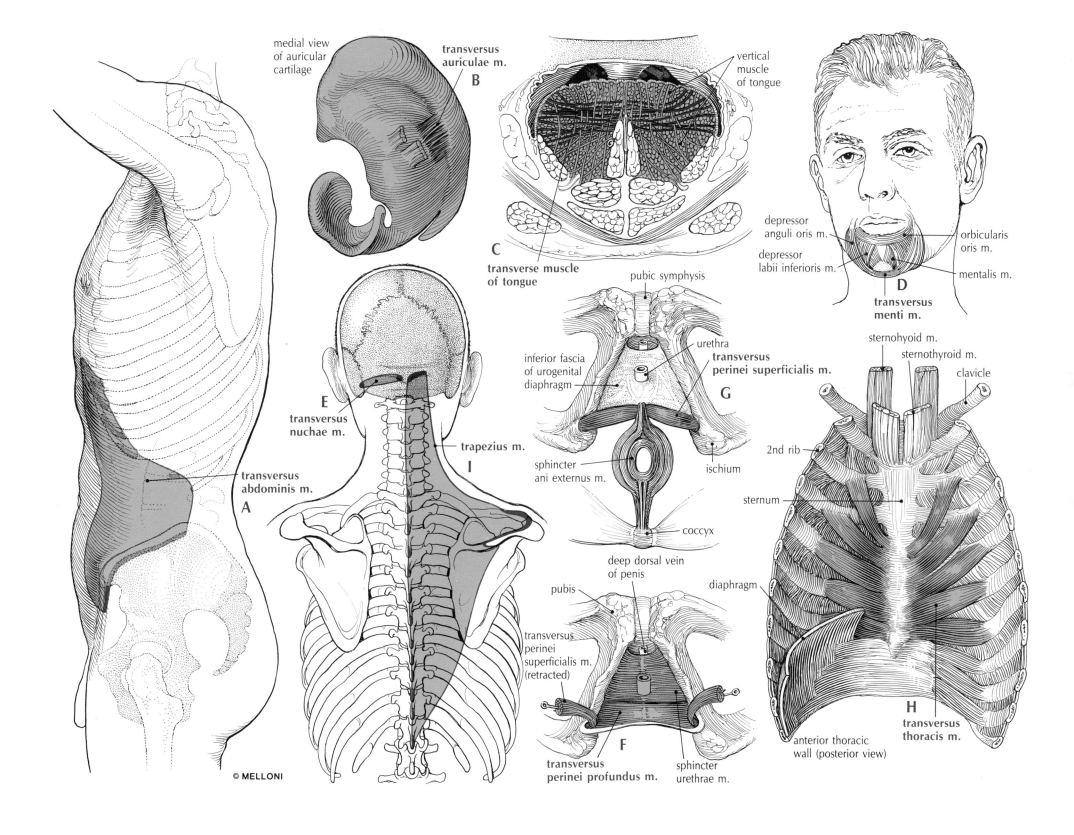

medial view of auricular cartilage

transversus auriculae m. B

vertical muscle of tongue

transverse muscle of tongue C

depressor anguli oris m.

depressor labii inferioris m.

orbicularis oris m.

mentalis m.

D

transversus menti m.

transversus abdominis m. A

transversus nuchae m. E

trapezius m. I

pubic symphysis

inferior fascia of urogenital diaphragm

urethra

transversus perinei superficialis m.

sphincter ani externus m.

ischium

coccyx G

sternohyoid m.

sternothyroid m.

clavicle

2nd rib

sternum

diaphragm

deep dorsal vein of penis

pubis

transversus perinei superficialis m. (retracted)

transversus perinei profundus m. F

sphincter urethrae m.

anterior thoracic wall (posterior view)

transversus thoracis m. H

© MELLONI

	MUSCLE	ORIGIN	INSERTION	INNERVATION	ACTION
A	**m. triceps brachii** *triceps m. of arm*	long head: infraglenoid tubercle of scapula lateral head: upper one third of posterior surface of humerus medial head: distal half of humerus (distal to groove for radial nerve)	posterior part of superior surface of olecranon process of ulna; adjacent deep fascia; articular capsule of elbow joint	radial nerve (6th, 7th, and 8th cranial nerves)	main extensor of forearm
B	**m. triceps surae** *triceps m. of calf*	combined gastrocnemius and soleus muscles possessing a common tendon that is attached to the calcaneus of the foot			plantarflexes foot
C	**m. uvulae** *uvula m.*	palatine aponeurosis and posterior nasal spine of palatine bone	mucous membrane and connective tissue of uvula	pharyngeal plexus of vagus nerve (10th cranial nerve)	elevates uvula
D	**m. vastus intermedius** *intermediate vastus m.* *intermediate great m.*	anterior and lateral surfaces of the upper two thirds of femur	common tendon of m. quadriceps femoris; patella	femoral nerve (L2, L3, L4)	extends leg
E	**m. vastus lateralis** *lateral vastus m.* *lateral great m.*	lateral aspect of upper part of femur	common tendon of m. quadriceps femoris; patella	femoral nerve (L2, L3, L4)	extends leg
F	**m. vastus medialis** *medial vastus m.* *medial great m.*	medial aspect of femur	common tendon of m. quadriceps femoris; patella	femoral nerve (L2, L3, L4)	extends leg
G	**m. verticalis linguae** *vertical m. of tongue*	dorsal surface of tongue	undersurface of tongue	hypoglossal nerve (12th cranial nerve)	aids in mastication, swallowing, and speech by altering shape of tongue
H	**m. vocalis** *vocal m.*	inner surface of thyroid cartilage near midline	vocal process of arytenoid cartilage	recurrent laryngeal nerve	adjusts tension of vocal cords
I	**m. zygomaticus major** *greater zygomatic m.*	lateral surface of zygomatic part of zygomatic arch	angle of mouth	buccal branch of facial nerve (7th cranial nerve)	draws angle of mouth upward and laterally
J	**m. zygomaticus minor** *smaller zygomatic m.*	lateral surface of zygomatic bone	muscular substance of upper lip	buccal branches of facial nerve (7th cranial nerve)	aids in forming nasolabial furrow; muscle of facial expression

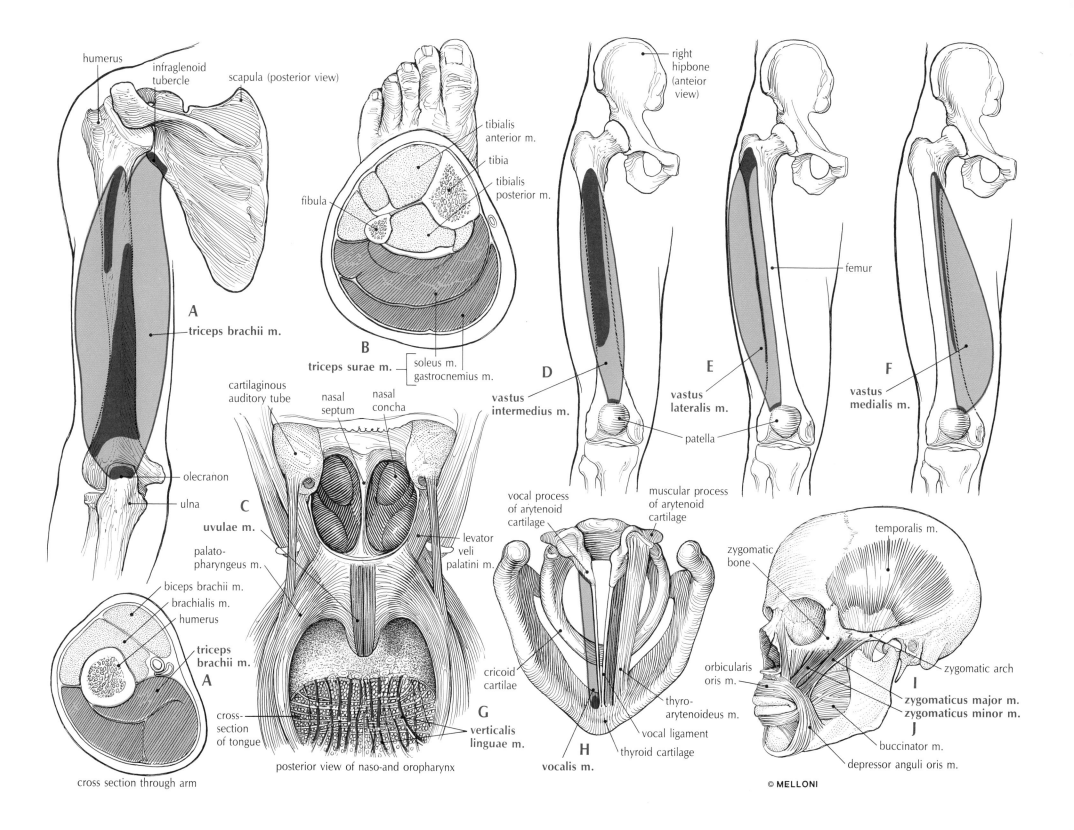

humerus
infraglenoid tubercle
scapula (posterior view)

A

triceps brachii m.

olecranon
ulna

biceps brachii m.
brachialis m.
humerus

triceps brachii m.

A

cross section through arm

tibialis anterior m.
tibia
tibialis posterior m.

fibula

B

triceps surae m.
soleus m.
gastrocnemius m.

cartilaginous auditory tube
nasal septum
nasal concha

uvulae m.
palato-pharyngeus m.

levator veli palatini m.

C

cross-section of tongue

verticalis linguae m.

posterior view of naso-and oropharynx

G

right hipbone (anteior view)

femur

D

vastus intermedius m.

patella

E

vastus lateralis m.

F

vastus medialis m.

vocal process of arytenoid cartilage
muscular process of arytenoid cartilage

cricoid cartilae

thyro-arytenoideus m.
vocal ligament
thyroid cartilage

H

vocalis m.

temporalis m.
zygomatic bone

zygomatic arch

I

orbicularis oris m.

zygomaticus major m.
zygomaticus minor m.

J

buccinator m.
depressor anguli oris m.

© MELLONI

NERVES

	NERVE	ORIGIN	BRANCHES	DISTRIBUTION
A	**n. abducens** *abducent n.* *sixth cranial n.*	nucleus in the pons located in the front part of the floor of the fourth ventricle	none	lateral rectus muscle of eyeball
B	**n. accessorius** *accessory n.* *spinal accessory n.* *eleventh cranial n.*	cranial roots: side of medulla oblongata spinal roots: anterolateral part of first five cervical segments of the spinal cord	internal external	muscles of pharynx, larynx, and soft palate sternocleidomastoid and trapezius muscles
C	**n. alveolaris inferior** *alveolar n., inferior* *inferior dental n.*	mandibular n.	mylohyoid, inferior dental, mental	mandibular teeth, periosteum, and gingiva of lower jaw; skin of lower lip and chin
D	**n. alveolaris superior medius** *alveolar n., middle superior* *middle superior dental n.*	infraorbital n.	superior dental, filaments	maxillary bicuspid teeth
E	**nn. alveolares superiores** *alveolar n.'s, superior* *superior dental n's*	They include the posterior, the middle, and the anterior superior alveolar (dental) nerves		
F	**nn. alveolares superiores anteriores** *alveolar n.'s, anterior superior* *anterior superior dental n.'s*	infraorbital n.	superior dental, nasal, filaments	anterior teeth (incisors and cuspids); mucous membrane of anterior walls and floor of nasal cavity; nasal septum
G	**nn. alveolares superiores posteriores** *alveolar n.'s, posterior superior* *posterior superior dental n.'s*	maxillary n.	superior dental, filaments	maxillary sinus, cheek, gums, molar teeth
H	**n. ampullaris lateralis** *ampullary n., lateral* *horizontal ampullary n.*	utriculoampullar n.	none	ampulla of lateral semicircular duct
I	**n. ampullaris posterior** *ampullary n., posterior* *inferior ampullary n.*	utriculoampullar n.	none	ampulla of posterior semicircular duct

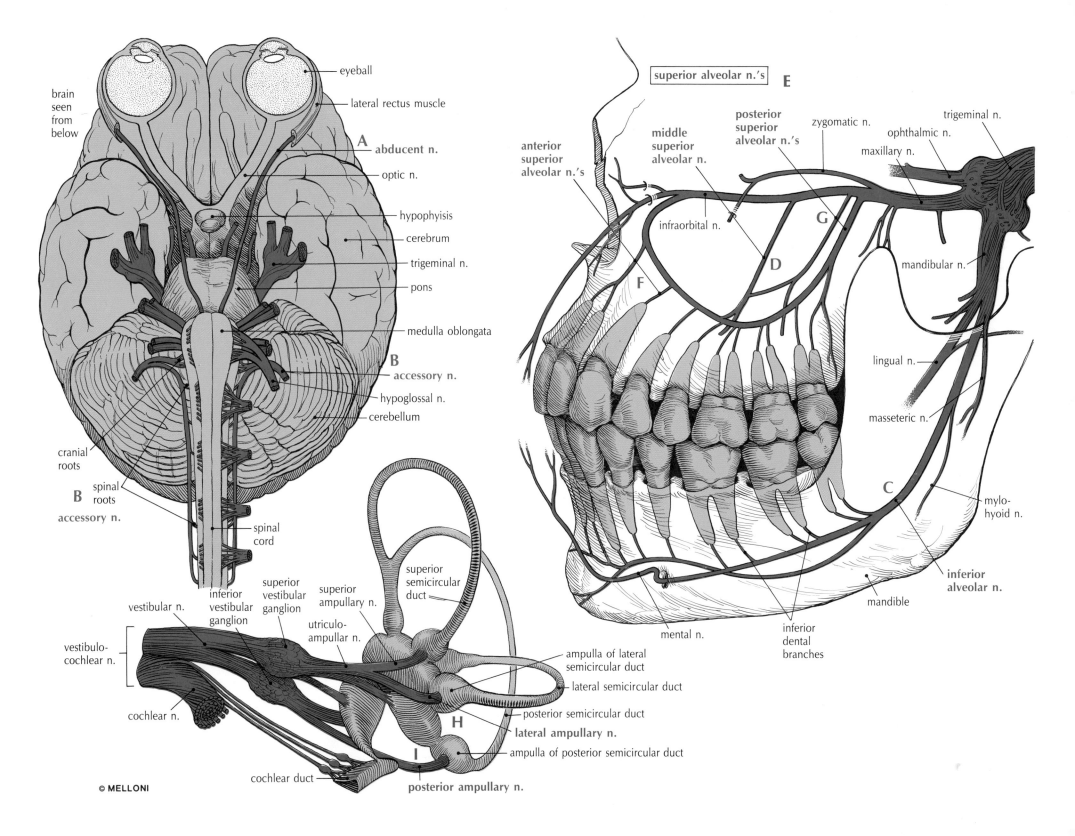

brain seen from below

eyeball

lateral rectus muscle

A **abducent n.**

optic n.

hypophyisis

cerebrum

trigeminal n.

pons

medulla oblongata

B

accessory n.

hypoglossal n.

cerebellum

cranial roots

spinal roots

B

accessory n.

spinal cord

vestibulo-cochlear n.

vestibular n.

inferior vestibular ganglion

superior vestibular ganglion

superior ampullary n.

utriculo-ampullar n.

inferior ampullary n.

superior semicircular duct

cochlear n.

cochlear duct

H

I

ampulla of lateral semicircular duct

lateral semicircular duct

posterior semicircular duct

lateral ampullary n.

ampulla of posterior semicircular duct

posterior ampullary n.

superior alveolar n.'s   **E**

anterior superior alveolar n.'s

middle superior alveolar n.

posterior superior alveolar n.'s

zygomatic n.

trigeminal n.

ophthalmic n.

maxillary n.

infraorbital n.

G

D

F

mandibular n.

lingual n.

masseteric n.

C

mylo-hyoid n.

mental n.

inferior dental branches

mandible

inferior alveolar n.

© MELLONI

	NERVE	ORIGIN	BRANCHES	DISTRIBUTION
A	**n. ampullaris superior** *ampullary n., superior* *anterior ampullary n.*	utriculoampullar n.	none	ampulla of superior semicircular duct
B	**nn. anococcygei** *anococcygeal n.'s*	coccygeal plexus	filaments	skin over coccyx
C	**ansa cervicalis** *ansa cervicalis* *ansa hypoglossi*	branches from the first three cervical segments of the spinal cord (forming a loop)	filaments	omohyoid, sternothyroid, and sternohyoid muscles
D	**nn. auriculares anterior** (usually two in number) *auricular n.'s, anterior*	auriculotemporal n.	filaments	skin over the upper part of the external ear
E	**n. auricularis magnus** *auricular n., great*	second and third cervical n.'s	anterior, posterior	skin over mastoid process and parotid gland, and around part of the external ear
F	**n. auricularis posterior** *auricular n., posterior*	facial n.	auricular, occipital	auricularis posterior and occipito-frontalis muscles, and the intrinsic muscles on the upper surface of the external ear
G	**n. auriculotemporalis** *auriculotemporal n.*	mandibular n. (by two roots)	anterior auricular, external acoustic meatus, parotid, superficial temporal, branch to tympanic membrane, branches communicating with facial nerve	skin of external acoustic meatus, upper part of external ear and surrounding temporal region, parotid gland and facial nerve
H	**n. axillaris** *axillary n.* *circumflex n.*	posterior cord of brachial plexus	anterior, posterior, cutaneous, articular	deltoid and teres minor muscles, skin
I	**n. buccalis** *buccal n.* *buccinator n.* *long buccal n.*	mandibular n.	branches communicating with buccal branches of the facial n., occasionally the anterior deep temporal n.	skin and mucous membrane of anterior part of cheek, gums

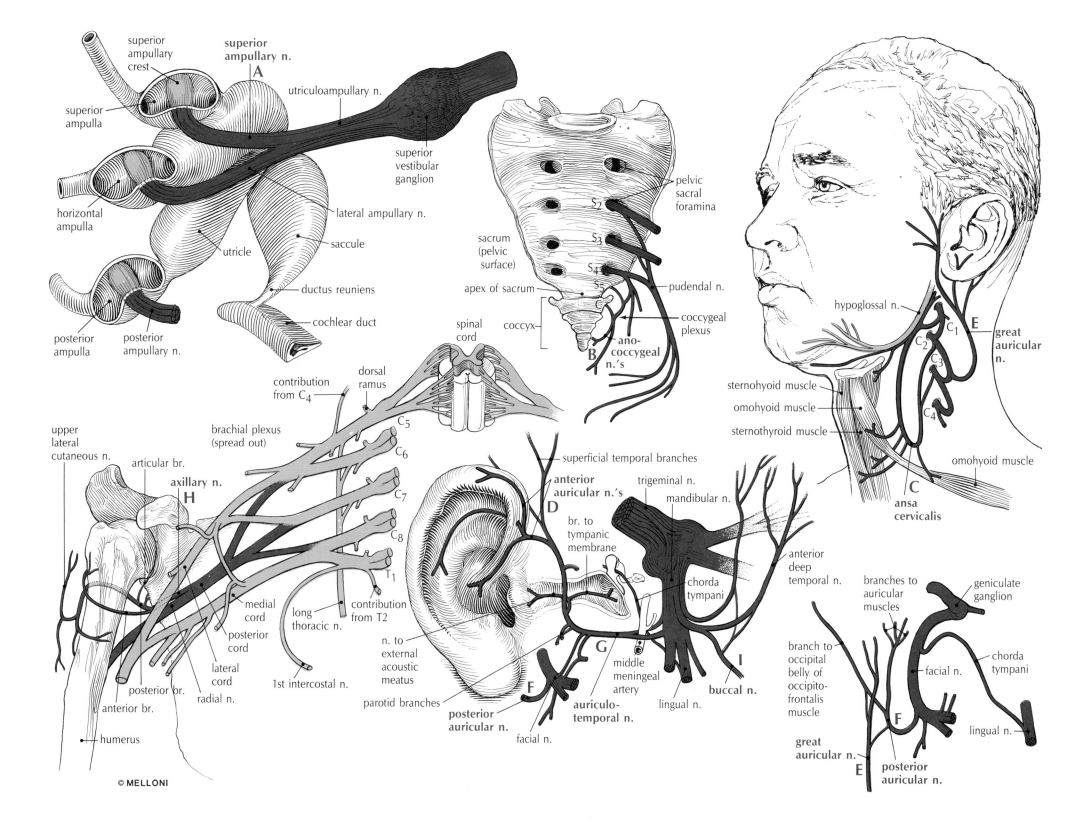

A

superior ampullary crest

superior ampulla

superior **superior ampullary n.**

utriculoampullary n.

superior vestibular ganglion

lateral ampullary n.

horizontal ampulla

utricle

saccule

ductus reuniens

cochlear duct

posterior ampulla

posterior ampullary n.

B

pelvic sacral foramina

sacrum (pelvic surface)

S₂

S₃

S₄

S₅

apex of sacrum

C

pudendal n.

coccygeal plexus

coccyx

ano-coccygeal n.'s

spinal cord

hypoglossal n.

C₁

C₂

C₃

C₄

E

great auricular n.

sternohyoid muscle

omohyoid muscle

sternothyroid muscle

C

ansa cervicalis

omohyoid muscle

H

contribution from C₄

dorsal ramus

brachial plexus (spread out)

C₅

C₆

C₇

C₈

T₁

upper lateral cutaneous n.

articular br.

axillary n.

medial cord

long thoracic n.

contribution from T2

posterior cord

lateral cord

radial n.

1st intercostal n.

posterior br.

anterior br.

humerus

© MELLONI

D

superficial temporal branches

anterior auricular n.'s

br. to tympanic membrane

n. to external acoustic meatus

parotid branches

F

posterior auricular n.

facial n.

G

auriculo-temporal n.

middle meningeal artery

trigeminal n.

mandibular n.

anterior deep temporal n.

chorda tympani

I

buccal n.

lingual n.

branches to auricular muscles

geniculate ganglion

branch to occipital belly of occipito-frontalis muscle

facial n.

chorda tympani

F

lingual n.

great auricular n.

E

posterior auricular n.

	NERVE	ORIGIN	BRANCHES	DISTRIBUTION
A	**n. canalis pterygoidei** *pterygoid canal, n. of Vidian n.*	union of greater petrosal and deep petrosal n.'s	filaments	glands of nose and pharynx, pterygopalatine ganglion
B	**nn. cardiaci thoracici** *cardiac n.'s, thoracic*	second to fourth or fifth thoracic ganglia of the sympathetic trunk	filaments	deep part of cardiac plexus
C	**n. cardiacus cervicalis inferior** *cardiac n., inferior cervical*	cervicothoracic (stellate) ganglion (fusion of inferior cervical ganglion with 1st thoracic ganglion)	filaments	deep part of cardiac plexus
D	**n. cardiacus cervicalis medius** *cardiac n., middle cervical* *great cardiac n.*	middle cervical ganglion	filaments	deep part of cardiac plexus
E	**n. cardiacus cervicalis superior** *cardiac n., superior cervical*	superior cervical ganglion, and occasionally a branch from the trunk joining the superior and middle cervical ganglia	filaments	right side: deep part of cardiac plexus left side: superficial part of cardiac plexus
F	**nn. carotici externi** *carotid n.'s, external*	superior cervical ganglion	filaments	external carotid plexus
G	**nn. caroticotympanici** *caroticotympanic n.'s*	internal carotid plexus of the sympathetic	superior, inferior	tympanic plexus
H	**n. caroticus** *carotid sinus n.* *carotid n.*	glossopharyngeal n. just below the skull	filaments	carotid sinus, carotid body
I	**n. caroticus internus** *carotid n., internal*	superior cervical ganglion	lateral, medial	internal carotid plexus

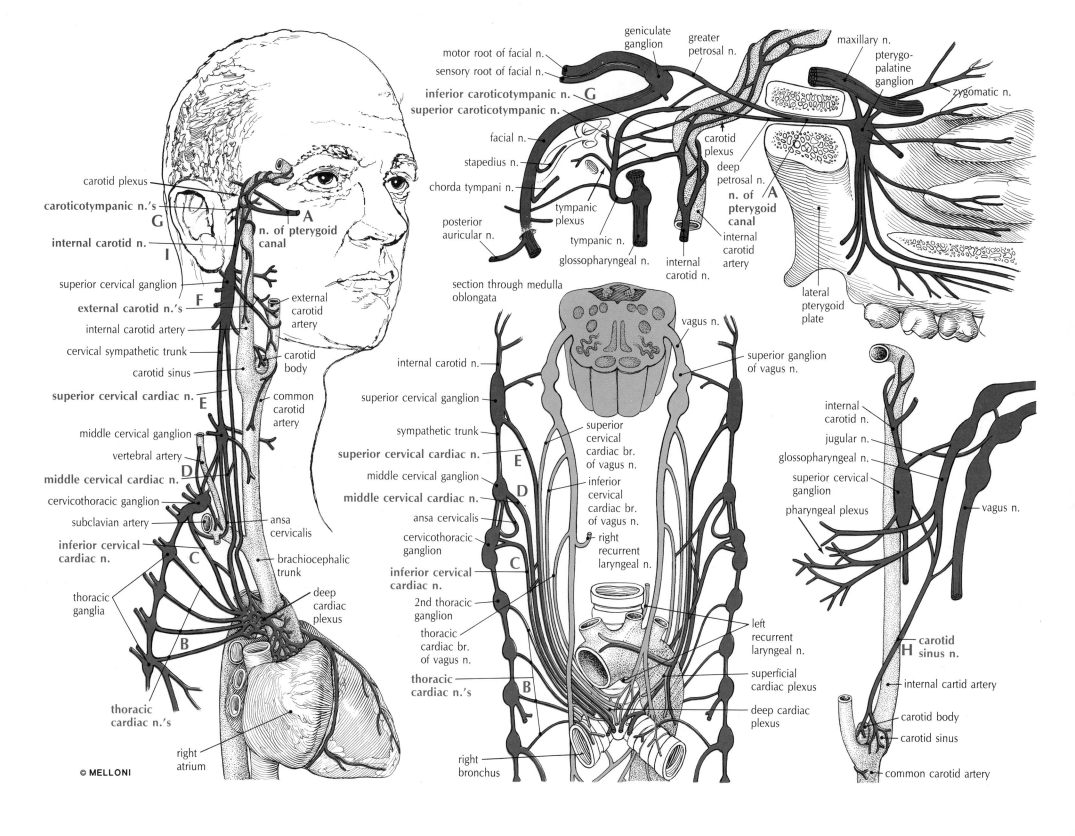

carotid plexus

caroticotympanic n.'s

G

internal carotid n.

I

superior cervical ganglion

F

external carotid n.'s

internal carotid artery

cervical sympathetic trunk

carotid sinus

superior cervical cardiac n.

E

middle cervical ganglion

vertebral artery

D

middle cervical cardiac n.

cervicothoracic ganglion

subclavian artery

inferior cervical cardiac n.

C

thoracic ganglia

G

B

thoracic cardiac n.'s

© MELLONI

A

n. of pterygoid canal

external carotid artery

carotid body

common carotid artery

ansa cervicalis

brachiocephalic trunk

deep cardiac plexus

right atrium

motor root of facial n.

sensory root of facial n.

inferior caroticotympanic n.

G

superior caroticotympanic n.

facial n.

stapedius n.

chorda tympani n.

posterior auricular n.

tympanic plexus

tympanic n.

glossopharyngeal n.

geniculate ganglion

greater petrosal n.

carotid plexus

deep petrosal n.

n. of pterygoid canal

A

internal carotid n.

internal carotid artery

maxillary n.

pterygo-palatine ganglion

zygomatic n.

lateral pterygoid plate

section through medulla oblongata

internal carotid n.

superior cervical ganglion

sympathetic trunk

superior cervical cardiac n.

E

middle cervical ganglion

middle cervical cardiac n.

D

ansa cervicalis

cervicothoracic ganglion

C

inferior cervical cardiac n.

2nd thoracic ganglion

thoracic cardiac br. of vagus n.

thoracic cardiac n.'s

B

right bronchus

vagus n.

superior ganglion of vagus n.

superior cervical cardiac br. of vagus n.

inferior cervical cardiac br. of vagus n.

right recurrent laryngeal n.

left recurrent laryngeal n.

superficial cardiac plexus

deep cardiac plexus

internal carotid n.

jugular n.

glossopharyngeal n.

superior cervical ganglion

pharyngeal plexus

vagus n.

H **carotid sinus n.**

internal cartid artery

carotid body

carotid sinus

common carotid artery

NERVE	ORIGIN	BRANCHES	DISTRIBUTION
A **nn. cavernosi clitorides minor** *cavernous n.'s of clitoris, lesser*	uterovaginal plexus	filaments	corpus cavernosum of clitoris
B **nn. cavernosi penis minor** *cavernous n.'s of penis, lesser*	prostatic plexus	filaments	corpus spongiosum of penis, penile urethra
C **n. cavernosus clitoridis major** *cavernous n. of clitoris, greater*	uterovaginal plexus	filaments	corpus cavernosum of clitoris
D **n. cavernosus penis major** *cavernous n. of penis, greater*	prostatic plexus	filaments	corpus cavernosum of penis
E **nn. cervicales** (eight pairs) *cervical n.'s*	cervical segments of spinal cord	filaments	cervical plexus, brachial plexus
F **n. chorda tympani** *chorda tympani n.*	facial n. just above the stylomastoid foramen	filaments	submandibular and sublingual glands, mucous membrane covering the anterior part of the tongue
G **nn. ciliares breves** (6–10 in number) *ciliary n.'s, short*	ciliary ganglion	filaments	ciliary body, sphincter pupillae, iris, cornea, and choroid layer of eyeball
H **nn. ciliares longi** (two or three in number) *ciliary n.'s, long*	nasociliary n.	filaments	ciliary body, iris, cornea
I **nn. clunium inferior** *clunial n.'s, inferior*	posterior femoral cutaneous n.	filaments	skin of lower gluteal region
J **nn. clunium medii** *clunial n.'s, middle*	lateral branches of dorsal rami of upper sacral n.'s	filaments	skin over middle gluteal region

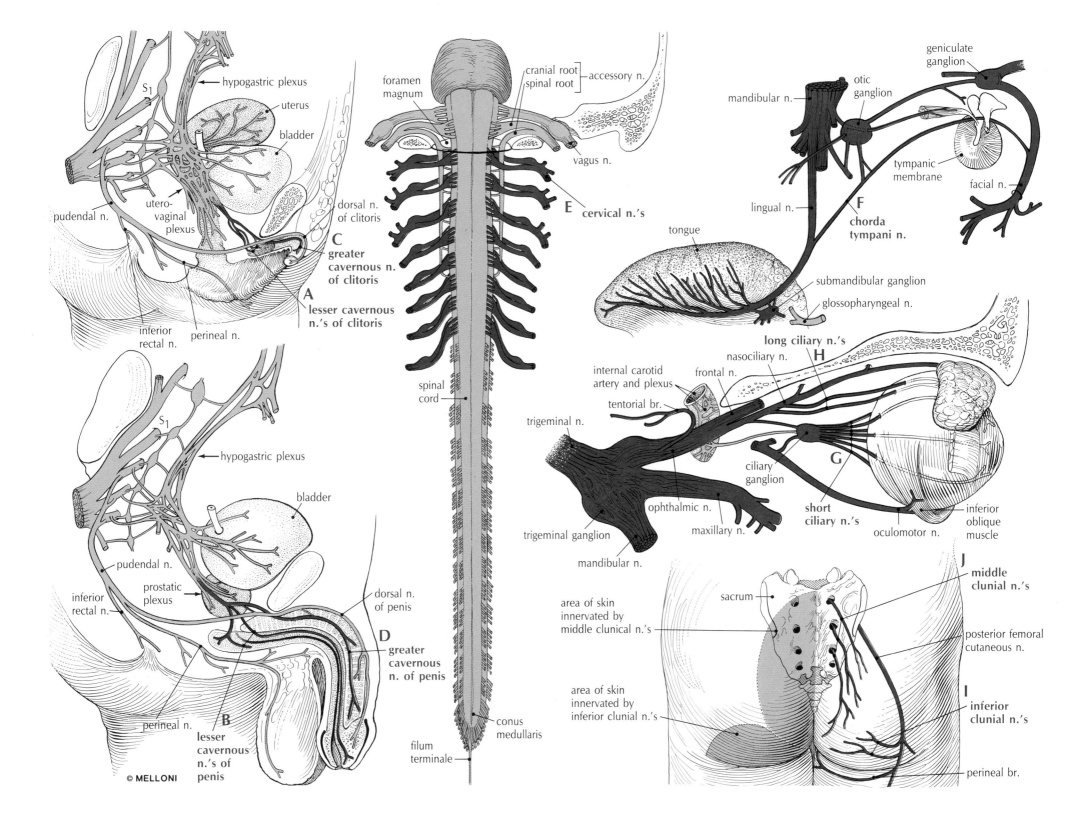

A

hypogastric plexus

S₁

uterus

bladder

pudendal n.

utero-vaginal plexus

dorsal n. of clitoris

C greater cavernous n. of clitoris

A lesser cavernous n.'s of clitoris

inferior rectal n.

perineal n.

B

S₁

hypogastric plexus

bladder

pudendal n.

prostatic plexus

inferior rectal n.

perineal n.

dorsal n. of penis

D greater cavernous n. of penis

B lesser cavernous n.'s of penis

© MELLONI

E

foramen magnum

cranial root
spinal root] accessory n.

vagus n.

E cervical n.'s

spinal cord

conus medullaris

filum terminale

F

geniculate ganglion

mandibular n.

otic ganglion

tympanic membrane

lingual n.

facial n.

F chorda tympani n.

tongue

submandibular ganglion

glossopharyngeal n.

H

long ciliary n.'s

nasociliary n.

internal carotid artery and plexus

frontal n.

tentorial br.

trigeminal n.

ciliary ganglion

G

ophthalmic n.

G short ciliary n.'s

trigeminal ganglion

maxillary n.

inferior oblique muscle

oculomotor n.

mandibular n.

J middle clunial n.'s

sacrum

area of skin innervated by middle clunial n.'s

posterior femoral cutaneous n.

area of skin innervated by inferior clunial n.'s

I inferior clunial n.'s

perineal br.

	NERVE	ORIGIN	BRANCHES	DISTRIBUTION
A	**nn. clunium superior** *clunial n.'s, superior*	lateral branches of dorsal rami of upper three lumbar n.'s	filaments	skin over upper gluteal region
B	**n. coccygeus** *coccygeal n.*	lowest segment of spinal cord	filaments	coccygeal plexus
C	**n. cochlearis** *cochlear n.* *n. of hearing*	vestibulocochlear n.	vestibular, filaments	spiral organ of Corti, cochlea
D	**nn. craniales** *cranial n.'s* *cerebral n.'s*	12 pairs of nerves that are continuous with the brain. The paired nerves include (I) olfactory; (II) optic; (III) oculomotor; (IV) trochlear; (V) trigeminal; (VI) abducent; (VII) facial; (VIII) vestibulocochlear; (IX) glossopharyngeal; (X) vagus; (XI) accessory; (XII) hypoglossal		
E	**n. cutaneus antebrachii lateralis** *cutaneous n. of forearm, lateral* *lateral antebrachial cutaneous n.*	terminal branch of musculocutaneous n.	anterior, posterior, filaments	skin on radial side of forearm
F	**n. cutaneus antebrachii medialis** *cutaneous n. of forearm, medial* *medial antebrachial cutaneous n.*	medial cord of brachial plexus	anterior, ulnar, filaments	skin over biceps muscle and anterior and ulnar surfaces of forearm
G	**n. cutaneus antebrachii posterior** *cutaneous n. of forearm, posterior* *posterior antebrachial cutaneous n.*	radial n.	filaments	skin on dorsal region of forearm
H	**n. cutaneus brachii lateralis inferior** *cutaneous n. of arm, lower lateral* *lower lateral brachial cutaneous n.*	radial n.	filaments	skin on lateral surface of lower half of arm
I	**n. cutaneus brachii lateralis superior** *cutaneous n. of arm, upper lateral* *upper lateral brachial cutaneous n.*	axillary n.	filaments	skin over lower part of deltoid and upper part of triceps muscles
J	**n. cutaneus brachii medialis** *cutaneous n. of arm, medial* *medial brachial cutaneous n.*	medial cord of brachial plexus	filaments	skin on medial side of arm

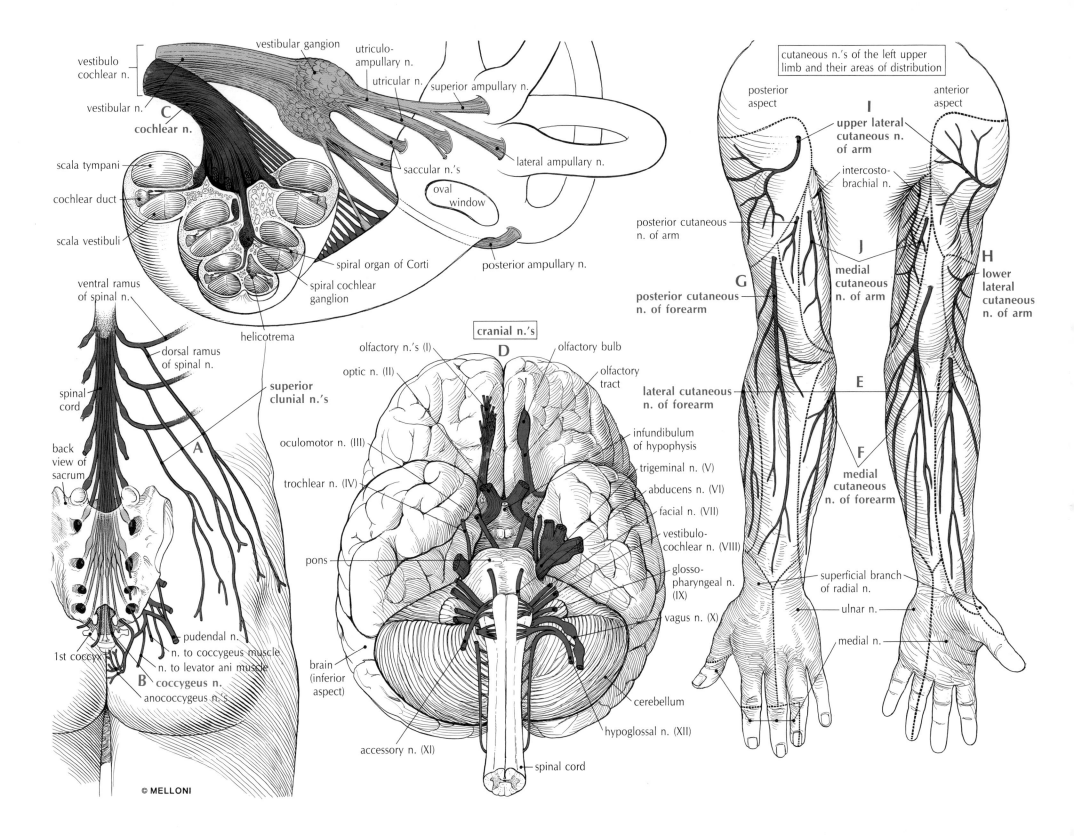

vestibulo cochlear n.

vestibular ganglion

utriculo-ampullary n.

utricular n.

superior ampullary n.

vestibular n.

C

cochlear n.

saccular n.'s

lateral ampullary n.

scala tympani

cochlear duct

scala vestibuli

oval window

spiral organ of Corti

spiral cochlear ganglion

posterior ampullary n.

helicotrema

ventral ramus of spinal n.

dorsal ramus of spinal n.

spinal cord

superior clunial n.'s

back view of sacrum

A

1st coccyx

pudendal n.

n. to coccygeus muscle

n. to levator ani muscle

B coccygeus n.

anococcygeus n.'s

cranial n.'s

D

olfactory n.'s (I)

olfactory bulb

optic n. (II)

olfactory tract

oculomotor n. (III)

infundibulum of hypophysis

trochlear n. (IV)

trigeminal n. (V)

abducens n. (VI)

facial n. (VII)

vestibulo-cochlear n. (VIII)

pons

glosso-pharyngeal n. (IX)

brain (inferior aspect)

vagus n. (X)

cerebellum

accessory n. (XI)

hypoglossal n. (XII)

spinal cord

cutaneous n.'s of the left upper limb and their areas of distribution

posterior aspect

anterior aspect

I

upper lateral cutaneous n. of arm

intercosto-brachial n.

posterior cutaneous n. of arm

J

G

medial cutaneous n. of arm

H

lower lateral cutaneous n. of arm

posterior cutaneous n. of forearm

lateral cutaneous n. of forearm

E

F

medial cutaneous n. of forearm

superficial branch of radial n.

ulnar n.

medial n.

© MELLONI

	NERVE	ORIGIN	BRANCHES	DISTRIBUTION
A	**n. cutaneus brachii posterior** *cutaneous n. of arm, posterior* *posterior brachial cutaneous n.*	radial n.	filaments	skin on posterior surface of upper arm
B	**n. cutaneus colli** *cutaneous n., transverse cervical* *cervical cutaneous n.* *anterior cutaneous n.* *transverse cutaneous n. of neck*	second and third cervical n.'s	ascending, descending	skin of front and side of neck
C	**n. cutaneus dorsalis intermedius pedis** *cutaneous n. of foot, intermediate* *dorsal*	superficial peroneal n.	dorsal digital	skin on lateral side of ankle and dorsum of foot; adjacent sides of third, fourth, and fifth toes
D	**n. cutaneus dorsalis lateralis pedis** *cutaneous n. of foot, lateral dorsal*	continuation of sural n.	filaments	skin on lateral sides and dorsum of foot
E	**n. cutaneus dorsalis medialis pedis** *cutaneous n. of foot, medial dorsal*	superficial peroneal n.	filaments	skin on medial sides and dorsum of foot, adjacent sides of second and third toes
F	**n. cutaneus femoris lateralis** *cutaneous n., lateral femoral* *cutaneous n. of thigh, lateral* *external cutaneous n.*	second and third lumbar n.'s	anterior, posterior, filaments	skin on anterior and lateral surfaces of thigh, occasionally skin of the gluteal region
G	**n. cutaneus femoris posterior** *cutaneous n., posterior femoral* *cutaneous n. of thigh, posterior* *small sciatic n.*	first, second, and third sacral n.'s	perineal, filaments	skin of gluteal region, external genitalia, perineum, posterior surface of thigh and calf
H	**n. cutaneus surae lateralis** *cutaneous n., lateral sural* *cutaneous n. of calf, lateral*	common peroneal n.	filaments	skin on lateral and posterior parts of calf
I	**n. cutaneus surae medialis** *cutaneous n., medial sural* *cutaneous n. of calf, medial*	tibial n.	forms sural n. after joining the communicating branch of the common peroneal n.	skin on medial and posterior part of calf

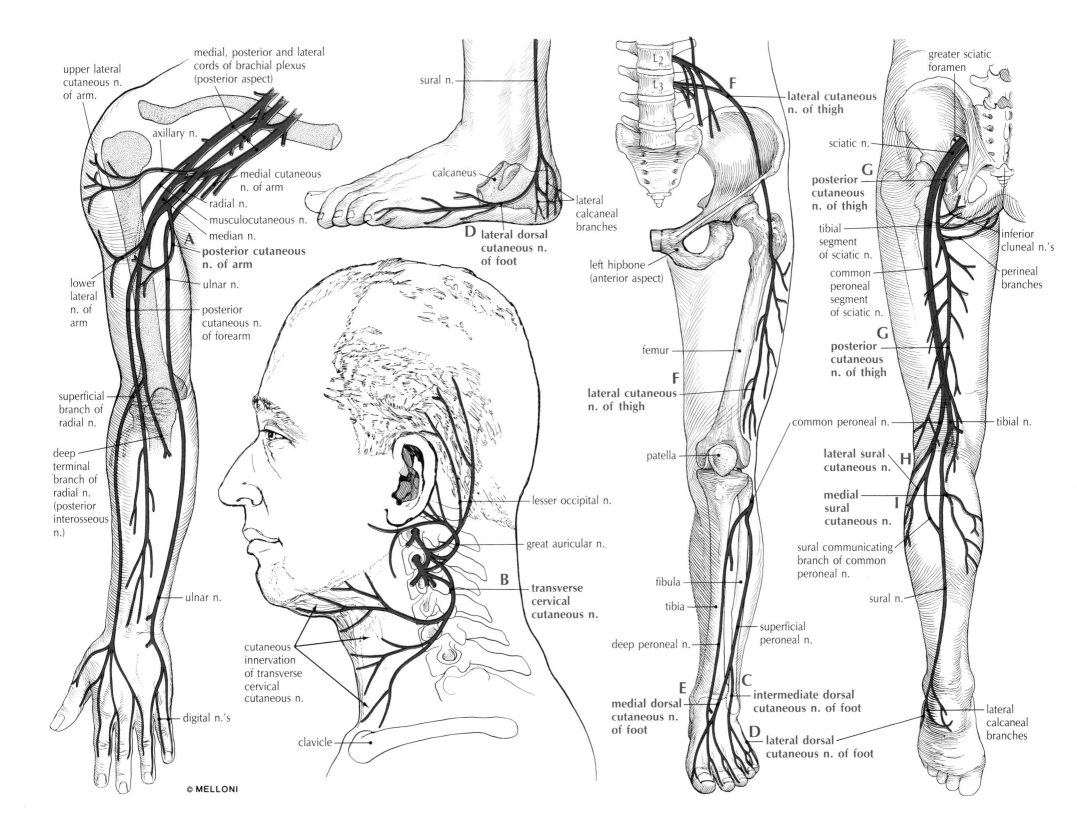

upper lateral cutaneous n. of arm.

medial, posterior and lateral cords of brachial plexus (posterior aspect)

axillary n.

medial cutaneous n. of arm

radial n.

musculocutaneous n.

median n.

A **posterior cutaneous n. of arm**

lower lateral n. of arm

ulnar n.

posterior cutaneous n. of forearm

superficial branch of radial n.

deep terminal branch of radial n. (posterior interosseous n.)

ulnar n.

digital n.'s

© MELLONI

sural n.

calcaneus

lateral calcaneal branches

D **lateral dorsal cutaneous n. of foot**

lesser occipital n.

great auricular n.

B **transverse cervical cutaneous n.**

cutaneous innervation of transverse cervical cutaneous n.

clavicle

L2
L3

F

lateral cutaneous n. of thigh

left hipbone (anterior aspect)

femur

F

lateral cutaneous n. of thigh

patella

fibula

tibia

deep peroneal n.

superficial peroneal n.

E **medial dorsal cutaneous n. of foot**

C **intermediate dorsal cutaneous n. of foot**

D **lateral dorsal cutaneous n. of foot**

greater sciatic foramen

sciatic n.

G **posterior cutaneous n. of thigh**

tibial segment of sciatic n.

common peroneal segment of sciatic n.

G **posterior cutaneous n. of thigh**

inferior cluneal n.'s

perineal branches

common peroneal n.

tibial n.

lateral sural cutaneous n. **H**

medial sural cutaneous n. **I**

sural communicating branch of common peroneal n.

sural n.

lateral calcaneal branches

	NERVE	ORIGIN	BRANCHES	DISTRIBUTION
A	**nn. digitales dorsales hallucis lateralis et digiti secundi medialis** *digital n.'s of lateral side of great toe and medial side of second toe, dorsal*	deep peroneal n.	none	adjacent surfaces of great and second toes
B	**nn. digitales dorsales pedis** *digital n.'s of foot, dorsal*	intermediate dorsal cutaneous n.	none	skin over adjacent sides of third, fourth, and fifth toes
C	**nn. digitales dorsales nervi radialis** *(4 or 5 in number)* *digital n.'s of radial n., dorsal* *radial dorsal digital n.'s*	superficial branch of radial n.	none	skin on lateral side of thumb, adjoining sides of thumb, second, third, and fourth (inconstant) fingers
D	**nn. digitales dorsales nervi ulnaris** *(2 or 3 in number)* *digital n.'s of ulnar n., dorsal* *ulnar dorsal digital n.'s*	dorsal branch of ulnar n.	none	skin on adjoining sides of third (inconstant), fourth, and fifth fingers
E	**nn. digitales palmares communes** *digital n.'s, common palmar*	median n., ulnar n.	proper palmar digital	skin on adjacent sides of digits, first two lumbrical muscles
F	**nn. digitales palmares communes nervi ulnaris** *digital n.'s of ulnar n., common palmar*	superficial branch of ulnar n.	proper palmar digital (two)	adjacent sides of third and fourth fingers
G	**nn. digitales palmares proprii** *digital n.'s, proper palmar* *digital collaterals*	common palmar digital n.'s	none	skin over distal phalanx of the digits, first two lumbrical muscles
H	**nn. digitales palmares proprii nervi ulnaris** *digital n.'s of ulnar n., proper palmar*	common palmar digital n.'s of ulnar n.	none	adjacent sides of fourth and fifth fingers and lateral side of third finger
I	**nn. digitales plantares communes nervi plantaris lateralis** *digital n.'s of lateral plantar n., common plantar*	superficial branch of lateral plantar n.	proper plantar digital (medial and lateral)	lateral branch: flexor digiti minimi brevis and two interosseous muscles medial branch: adjacent sides of fourth and fifth toes

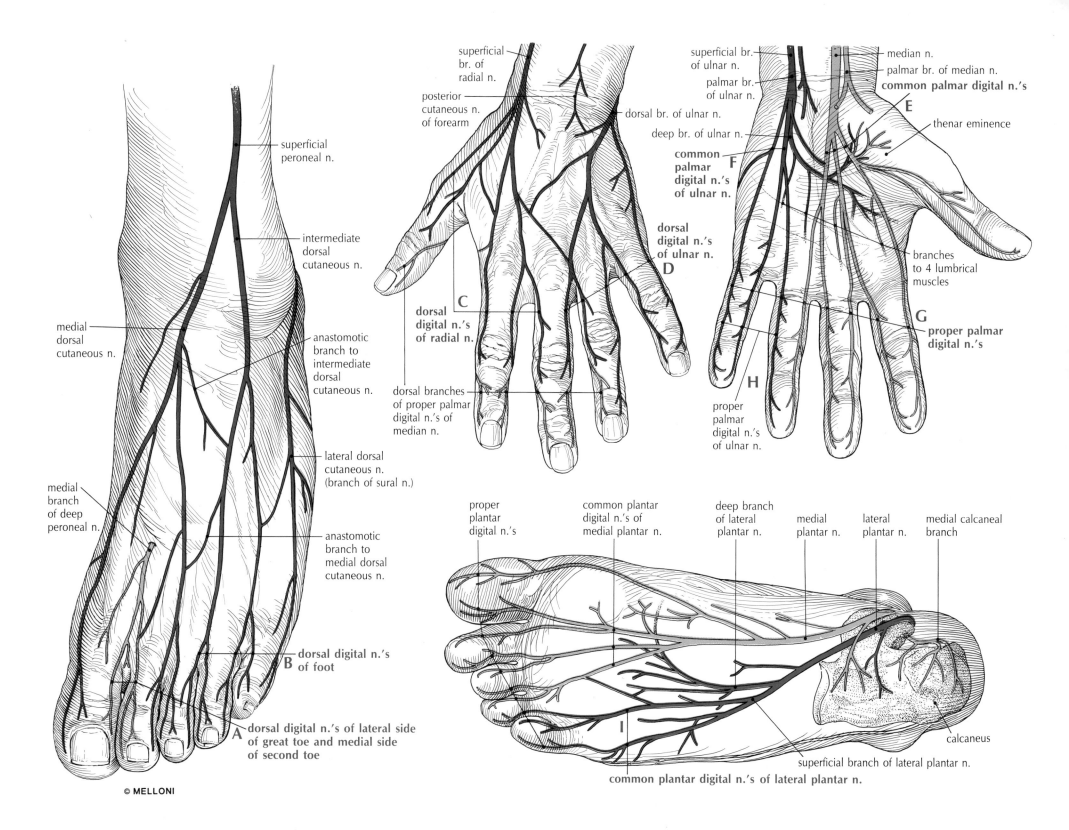

superficial peroneal n.

intermediate dorsal cutaneous n.

medial dorsal cutaneous n.

anastomotic branch to intermediate dorsal cutaneous n.

lateral dorsal cutaneous n. (branch of sural n.)

medial branch of deep peroneal n.

anastomotic branch to medial dorsal cutaneous n.

A

B dorsal digital n.'s of foot

A dorsal digital n.'s of lateral side of great toe and medial side of second toe

© MELLONI

superficial br. of radial n.

posterior cutaneous n. of forearm

dorsal br. of ulnar n.

C

D dorsal digital n.'s of ulnar n.

dorsal digital n.'s of radial n.

dorsal branches of proper palmar digital n.'s of median n.

superficial br. of ulnar n.

palmar br. of ulnar n.

deep br. of ulnar n.

F common palmar digital n.'s of ulnar n.

median n.

palmar br. of median n.

common palmar digital n.'s

E

thenar eminence

branches to 4 lumbrical muscles

G proper palmar digital n.'s

H proper palmar digital n.'s of ulnar n.

proper plantar digital n.'s

common plantar digital n.'s of medial plantar n.

deep branch of lateral plantar n.

medial plantar n.

lateral plantar n.

medial calcaneal branch

calcaneus

I

superficial branch of lateral plantar n.

common plantar digital n.'s of lateral plantar n.

	NERVE	ORIGIN	BRANCHES	DISTRIBUTION
A	**nn. digitales plantares communes nervi plantaris medialis** *digital n.'s of medial plantar n., common plantar*	medial plantar n.	proper plantar digital n.'s, muscular	adjacent sides of great, second, third, and fourth toes; flexor hallucis brevis and first lumbrical muscles
B	**nn. digitales plantares proprii nervi plantaris lateralis** *digital n.'s of lateral plantar n., proper plantar*	common plantar digital n.'s	none	skin on lateral surface of sole, adjacent sides of fourth and fifth toes, flexor digiti minimi brevis muscle
C	**nn. digitales plantares proprii nervi plantaris medialis** *digital n.'s of medial plantar n., proper plantar*	common plantar digital n.'s	none	adjacent sides of first, second, third, and fourth toes
D	**n. dorsalis clitoridis** *clitoris, dorsal n. of*	pudendal n.	filaments	clitoris and urethra
E	**n. dorsalis penis** *penis, dorsal n. of*	pudendal n.	filaments	corpus cavernosum penis; skin, prepuce, and glans of penis
F	**n. dorsalis scapulae** *scapular n., dorsal*	fifth cervical n.	filaments	major and minor rhomboid and occasionally levator scapulae muscles
G	**n. ethmoidalis anterior** *ethmoidal n., anterior*	continuation of nasociliary n.	lateral internal nasal, medial internal nasal, exteral nasal	mucous membrane of anterior surface of nasal septum, anterior part of nasal cavity, skin on anterior surface of nose
H	**n. ethmoidalis posterior** *(inconstant)* *ethmoidal n., posterior*	nasociliary n.	filaments	posterior ethmoidal and sphenoidal sinuses
I	**n. facialis** *facial n* *seventh cranial n.*	lower border of pons	stapedius, posterior auricular, parotid plexus, temporal, buccal, zygomatic, marginal mandibular, cervical, communicating branch to tympanic plexus, chorda tympani, digastric (posterior belly), stylohyoid	motor root: muscles of face and neck including the buccinator, platysma, stylohyoid, stapedius, and posterior belly of the digastric; scalp; external ear sensory root: anterior part of tongue, soft palate parasympathetic innervation: sub-mandibular, sublingual, lacrimal, nasal, and palatine glands

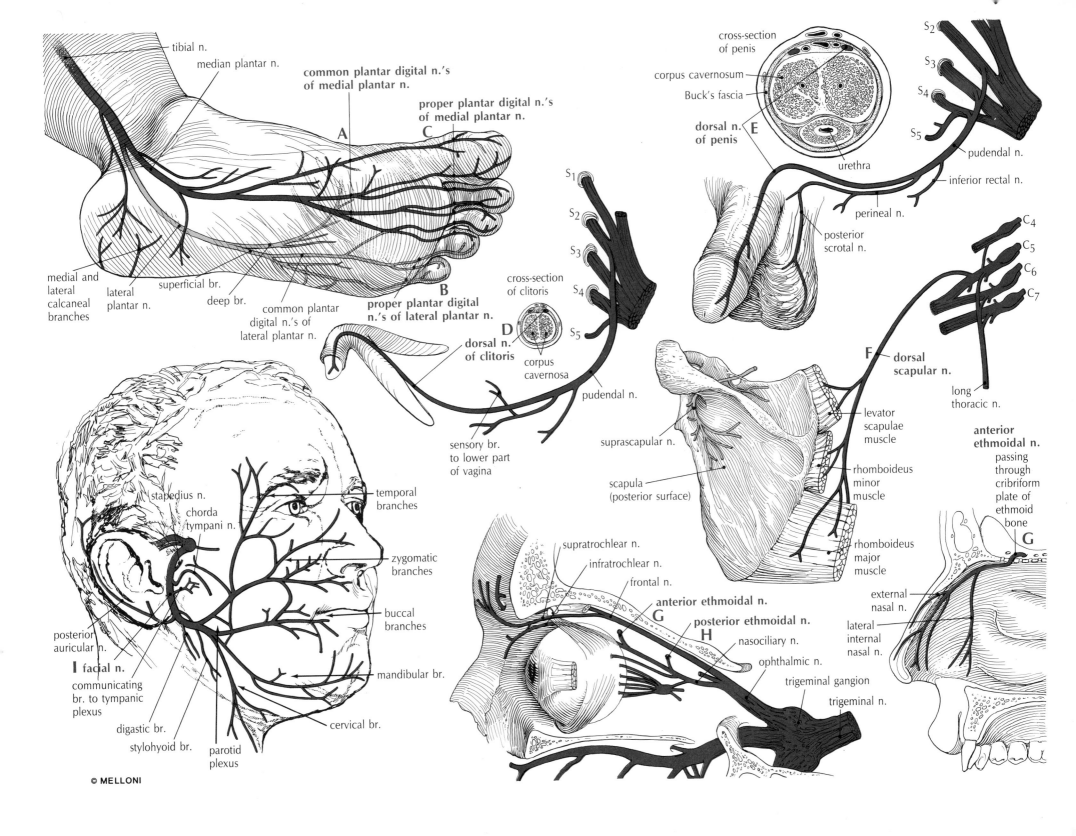

tibial n.

median plantar n.

common plantar digital n.'s of medial plantar n.

proper plantar digital n.'s of medial plantar n.

A

C

medial and lateral calcaneal branches

lateral plantar n.

superficial br.

deep br.

common plantar digital n.'s of lateral plantar n.

B

proper plantar digital n.'s of lateral plantar n.

D

dorsal n. of clitoris

cross-section of clitoris

corpus cavernosa

sensory br. to lower part of vagina

pudendal n.

S1
S2
S3
S4
S5

cross-section of penis

corpus cavernosum

Buck's fascia

dorsal n. of penis

E

urethra

S2
S3
S4
S5

pudendal n.

inferior rectal n.

perineal n.

posterior scrotal n.

C4
C5
C6
C7

dorsal scapular n.

F

long thoracic n.

levator scapulae muscle

suprascapular n.

scapula (posterior surface)

rhomboideus minor muscle

rhomboideus major muscle

anterior ethmoidal n. passing through cribriform plate of ethmoid bone

G

external nasal n.

lateral internal nasal n.

stapedius n.

chorda tympani n.

temporal branches

zygomatic branches

buccal branches

posterior auricular n.

I facial n.

communicating br. to tympanic plexus

digastic br.

stylohyoid br.

parotid plexus

cervical br.

mandibular br.

supratrochlear n.

infratrochlear n.

frontal n.

anterior ethmoidal n.

G

posterior ethmoidal n.

H

nasociliary n.

ophthalmic n.

trigeminal ganglion

trigeminal n.

© MELLONI

	NERVE	ORIGIN	BRANCHES	DISTRIBUTION
A	**n. femoralis** *femoral n.* *anterior crural n.*	second, third, and fourth lumbar n.'s	muscular, anterior cutaneous, saphenous, articular	muscles and skin of anterior thigh, knee, and hip joints
B	**n. frontalis** *frontal n.*	ophthalmic n.	supraorbital, supratrochlear	upper eyelid and conjunctiva, skin of the scalp, corrugator and occipito-frontalis muscles, and frontal sinus
C	**radix genitalis nervi genitofemoralis** *genital branch of genitofemoral n.*	genitofemoral n.	filaments	cremaster muscle, skin of scrotum (male) and labium majus (female), skin on surrounding part of thigh
D	**n. genitofemoralis** *genitofemoral n.* *genitocrural n.*	first and second lumbar n.'s	genital, femoral	genital branch: skin of scrotum (male), skin of mons pubis and labium majus (female), cremaster muscle femoral branch: skin over upper part of anterior surface of thigh
E	**n. glossopharyngeus** *glossopharyngeal n.* *ninth cranial n.*	upper part of medulla oblongata	tympanic, pharyngeal, stylo-pharyngeal, carotid sinus, tonsillar, lingual	proximal part of tongue, stylo-pharyngeus muscle, parotid gland, pharynx, and tonsil
F	**n. gluteus inferior** *gluteal n., inferior*	fifth lumbar and first and second sacral n.'s	none	gluteus maximus muscle
G	**n. gluteus superior** *gluteal n., superior*	fourth and fifth lumbar and first sacral n.'s	superior, inferior	tensor fascia lata, gluteus medius and minimus muscles
H	**n. hypogastricus** *hypogastric n.*	One of two nerve trunks (right and left) that descends from the superior hypogastric plexus into the pelvis to join the inferior hypogastric plexus		
I	**n. hypoglossus** *hypoglossal n.* *twelfth cranial n.*	emerges as several rootlets from the medulla oblongata between the olive and the pyramid	lingual, n. of thyrohyoid, filaments	intrinsic muscles of the tongue; styloglossus, genioglossus, and hyoglossus muscles

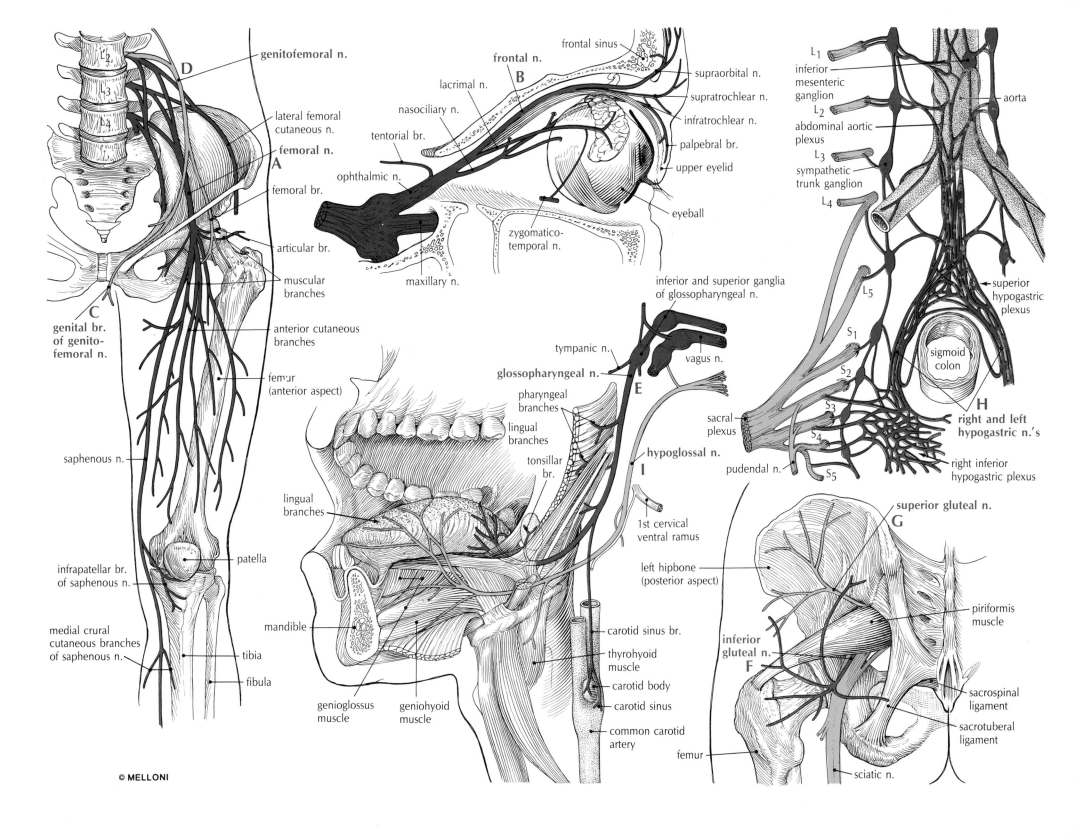

genitofemoral n.

lateral femoral
cutaneous n.

femoral n.

A

D

L₂

L₃

L₄

femoral br.

articular br.

muscular
branches

anterior cutaneous
branches

C

**genital br.
of genito-
femoral n.**

femur
(anterior aspect)

saphenous n.

infrapatellar br.
of saphenous n.

patella

medial crural
cutaneous branches
of saphenous n.

tibia

fibula

frontal n.

B

frontal sinus

supraorbital n.

supratrochlear n.

lacrimal n.

nasociliary n.

infratrochlear n.

tentorial br.

palpebral br.

upper eyelid

ophthalmic n.

eyeball

zygomatico-
temporal n.

maxillary n.

inferior and superior ganglia
of glossopharyngeal n.

tympanic n.

vagus n.

glossopharyngeal n.

E

pharyngeal
branches

lingual
branches

tonsillar
br.

hypoglossal n.

I

sacral
plexus

1st cervical
ventral ramus

lingual
branches

pudendal n.

mandible

genioglossus
muscle

geniohyoid
muscle

carotid sinus br.

thyrohyoid
muscle

carotid body

carotid sinus

common carotid
artery

L₁

inferior
mesenteric
ganglion

L₂

abdominal aortic
plexus

L₃

sympathetic
trunk ganglion

L₄

aorta

L₅

S₁

S₂

S₃

S₄

S₅

superior
hypogastric
plexus

sigmoid
colon

H

**right and left
hypogastric n.'s**

right inferior
hypogastric plexus

superior gluteal n.

G

left hipbone
(posterior aspect)

piriformis
muscle

**inferior
gluteal n.**

F

sacrospinal
ligament

sacrotuberal
ligament

femur

sciatic n.

© MELLONI

	NERVE	ORIGIN	BRANCHES	DISTRIBUTION
A	**n. iliohypogastricus** *iliohypogastric n.*	first lumbar n.	lateral cutaneous, anterior cutaneous, muscular	skin on the lateral side of the buttock, and on the abdomen above the pubis; internal oblique and transversus muscle
B	**n. ilioinguinalis** *ilioinguinal n.*	first lumbar n.	anterior scrotal (male), anterior labial (female), muscular	internal oblique muscle, skin of the upper medial part of the thigh, skin on the root of the penis and adjoining part of scrotum (male), skin on the mons pubis and adjoining part of the labium majus (female)
C	**n. infraorbitalis** *infraorbital n.*	continuation of the maxillary n. after entering the orbit through the inferior orbital tissue	anterior superior alveolar, middle superior alveolar, inferior palpebral, superior labial, nasal	upper teeth, part of nose, lower eyelid, upper lip, skin and mucous membrane of face
D	**n. infratrochlearis** *infratrochlear n.*	nasociliary n.	palpebral	skin of eyelids and sides of nose, conjunctiva, caruncle, lacrimal sac and duct
E	**nn. intercostales** (ventral rami of upper 11 thoracic nerves) *intercostal n.'s*	thoracic segments of spinal cord	anterior cutaneous, lateral cutaneous, collateral	first two supply skin of axilla and medial side of arm; next four supply thoracic wall; last five supply lower thoracic and upper abdominal walls
F	**nn. intercostobrachiales** *intercostobrachial n.'s*	second and third intercostal n.'s	filaments	skin on medial and posterior parts of upper arm; axilla
G	**n. interosseus antebrachii anterior** *interosseous n. of forearm, anterior*	median n.	filaments	deep anterior muscles of forearm, including flexor pollicus longus, flexor digitorum profundus, and pronator quadratus muscles; wrist and carpal joints
H	**n. interosseus antebrachii posterior** *interosseous n. of forearm, posterior*	deep branch of radial n.	muscular, articular	supinator, abductor pollicis longus, and extensor muscles of forearm; intercarpal joints
I	**n. interosseus cruris** *interosseous n. of leg*	tibial n.	filaments	tibia and fibula articulations, interosseous membrane

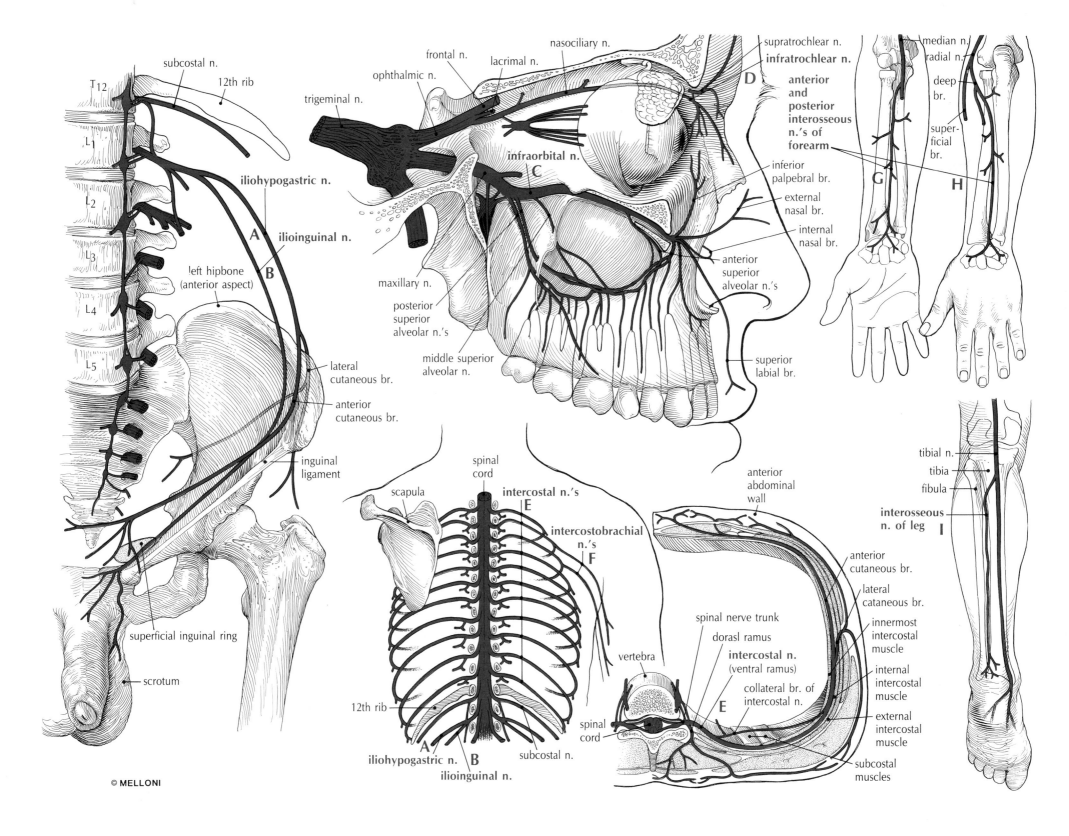

subcostal n.

12th rib

T₁₂

L₁

L₂

L₃

L₄

L₅

iliohypogastric n.

A

ilioinguinal n.

B

left hipbone (anterior aspect)

lateral cutaneous br.

anterior cutaneous br.

inguinal ligament

superficial inguinal ring

scrotum

© MELLONI

trigeminal n.

ophthalmic n.

frontal n.

lacrimal n.

nasociliary n.

supratrochlear n.

infratrochlear n.

D

anterior and posterior interosseous n.'s of forearm

inferior palpebral br.

external nasal br.

internal nasal br.

anterior superior alveolar n.'s

infraorbital n.

C

maxillary n.

posterior superior alveolar n.'s

middle superior alveolar n.

superior labial br.

median n.

radial n.

deep br.

superficial br.

G

H

scapula

spinal cord

intercostal n.'s

E

intercostobrachial n.'s

F

12th rib

A

iliohypogastric n.

B

ilioinguinal n.

subcostal n.

anterior abdominal wall

vertebra

spinal cord

spinal nerve trunk

dorasl ramus

intercostal n. (ventral ramus)

E

collateral br. of intercostal n.

anterior cutaneous br.

lateral cataneous br.

innermost intercostal muscle

internal intercostal muscle

external intercostal muscle

subcostal muscles

tibial n.

tibia

fibula

interosseous n. of leg

I

	NERVE	ORIGIN	BRANCHES	DISTRIBUTION
A	**n. ischiadicus** (largest nerve in body) *sciatic n.* *great sciatic n.*	fourth and fifth lumbar and first, second, and third sacral n.'s	common peroneal, tibial, articular	semimembranosus and semitendinosus muscles, knee and tibiofibular joints, muscles and skin of calf, skin of plantar surface of foot and toes, tibialis anterior and short and long heads of biceps femoris muscles
B	**n. jugularis** *jugular n.*	superior cervical ganglion	filaments	superior ganglion of the vagus n., and inferior ganglion of the glossopharyngeal n.
C	**nn. labiales anterior** *labial n.'s, anterior*	ilioinguinal n.	filaments	skin of anterior part of labium majus
D	**nn. labiales posterior** *labial n.'s, posterior*	perineal n.	filaments	skin of posterior part of labium majus and vestibule of vagina
E	**n. lacrimalis** *lacrimal n.*	ophthalmic n.	superior palpebral, filaments	skin of upper eyelid, lacrimal gland, and conjunctiva
F	**n. laryngeus inferior** *laryngeal n., inferior*	recurrent laryngeal n.	filaments	intrinsic muscles of larynx except the cricothyroid muscle
G	**n. laryngeus recurrens** *recurrent laryngeal n.*	vagus n.	inferior laryngeal, tracheal, esophageal, cardiac	mucous membrane and muscles of larynx (excluding the cricothyroid), mucous membrane of esophagus and trachea, cardiac plexus, inferior constrictor muscle
H	**n. laryngeus superior** *laryngeal n., superior*	vagus n. at the inferior ganglion	external branch, internal branch	inferior constrictor and cricothyroid muscles, pharyngeal plexus, mucous membrane of the larynx, epiglottis, and aryepiglottic fold
I	**n. lingualis** *lingual n.* *small hypoglossal n.*	mandibular n.	sublingual, lingual, branches to the isthmus of the fauces, branches communicating with hypoglossal and chorda tympani n.'s	mucous membrane of the floor of the mouth and anterior part of the tongue; gums

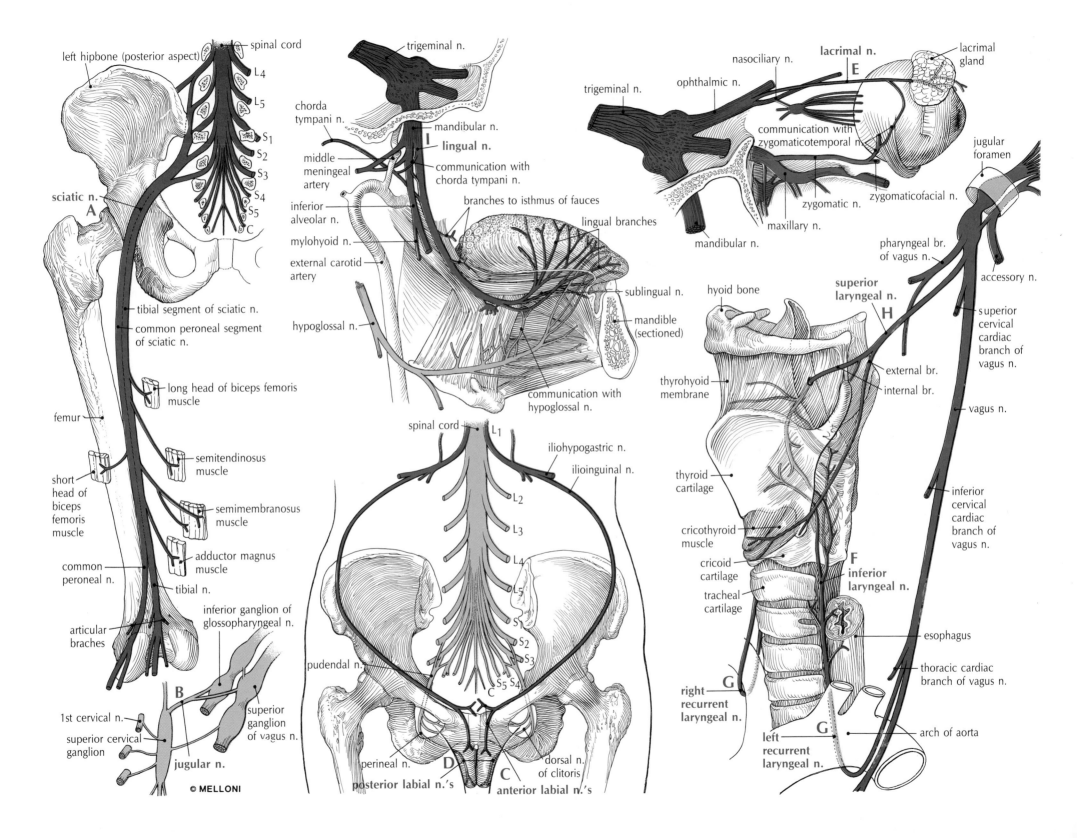

left hipbone (posterior aspect)

spinal cord

L4

L5

S1

S2

S3

S4

S5

C

sciatic n.

A

tibial segment of sciatic n.

common peroneal segment of sciatic n.

long head of biceps femoris muscle

femur

semitendinosus muscle

short head of biceps femoris muscle

semimembranosus muscle

adductor magnus muscle

common peroneal n.

tibial n.

articular braches

inferior ganglion of glossopharyngeal n.

1st cervical n.

superior cervical ganglion

B

superior ganglion of vagus n.

jugular n.

trigeminal n.

chorda tympani n.

mandibular n.

I

lingual n.

middle meningeal artery

communication with chorda tympani n.

inferior alveolar n.

branches to isthmus of fauces

mylohyoid n.

lingual branches

external carotid artery

hypoglossal n.

sublingual n.

mandible (sectioned)

communication with hypoglossal n.

spinal cord

L1

iliohypogastric n.

L2

ilioinguinal n.

L3

L4

L5

S1

S2

S3

pudendal n.

S5 S4

C

perineal n.

D

C

posterior labial n.'s

dorsal n. of clitoris

anterior labial n.'s

trigeminal n.

nasociliary n.

lacrimal n.

lacrimal gland

ophthalmic n.

E

communication with zygomaticotemporal n.

zygomaticofacial n.

zygomatic n.

mandibular n.

maxillary n.

jugular foramen

pharyngeal br. of vagus n.

accessory n.

superior cervical cardiac branch of vagus n.

hyoid bone

superior laryngeal n.

H

external br.

internal br.

thyrohyoid membrane

thyroid cartilage

vagus n.

cricothyroid muscle

inferior cervical cardiac branch of vagus n.

cricoid cartilage

F

inferior laryngeal n.

tracheal cartilage

esophagus

G

right recurrent laryngeal n.

G

left recurrent laryngeal n.

thoracic cardiac branch of vagus n.

arch of aorta

© MELLONI

	NERVE	ORIGIN	BRANCHES	DISTRIBUTION
A	**nn. lumbales** (five pairs) *lumbar n.'s*	five lumbar segments of the spinal cord	ventral, dorsal	lumbar and sacral plexuses, deep muscles of lower back, and skin of gluteal region
B	**n. mandibularis** *mandibular n.* *inferior maxillary n.*	trigeminal n.	masseteric, meningeal, deep temporal, medial pterygoid, lateral pterygoid, buccal, auriculotemporal, lingual, inferior alveolar	muscles of mastication, teeth, gums, mucous membrane of floor of mouth and anterior part of tongue, skin of temporal region, lower half of face, and external ear, temporomandibular joint
C	**n. massetericus** *masseteric n.*	mandibular n.	filaments	temporomandibular joint, masseter muscle
D	**n. maxillaris** *maxillary n.* *superior maxillary n.*	trigeminal n.	middle meningeal, zygomatic, posterior superior alveolar, branches of pterygopalatine ganglion, infraorbital	skin of face and temple, maxillary sinus, teeth, gums, lower eyelid, mucous membrane of nose and pharynx
E	**n. meatus acustici externi** *acoustic meatus n., external*	auriculotemporal n.	none	external acoustic meatus
F	**n. medianus** *median n.*	lateral and medial cords of brachial plexus	muscular, anterior interosseous, common palmar digital, communicating branch with the ulnar n., palmar cutaneous	skin of hand, flexor muscles of forearm (excluding flexor carpi ulnaris), elbow and hand joints, short muscles of thumb
G	**n. meningeus medius** *meningeal n., middle*	maxillary n.	filaments	dura mater of middle cranial fossa
H	**n. mentalis** *mental n.*	inferior alveolar n.	filaments	skin over chin, mucous membrane of lower lip
I	**n. musculocutaneus** *musculocutaneous n.*	lateral cord of brachial plexus	muscular, lateral cutaneous n. of forearm	coracobrachialis, brachialis, and biceps muscles; skin over lateral side of forearm

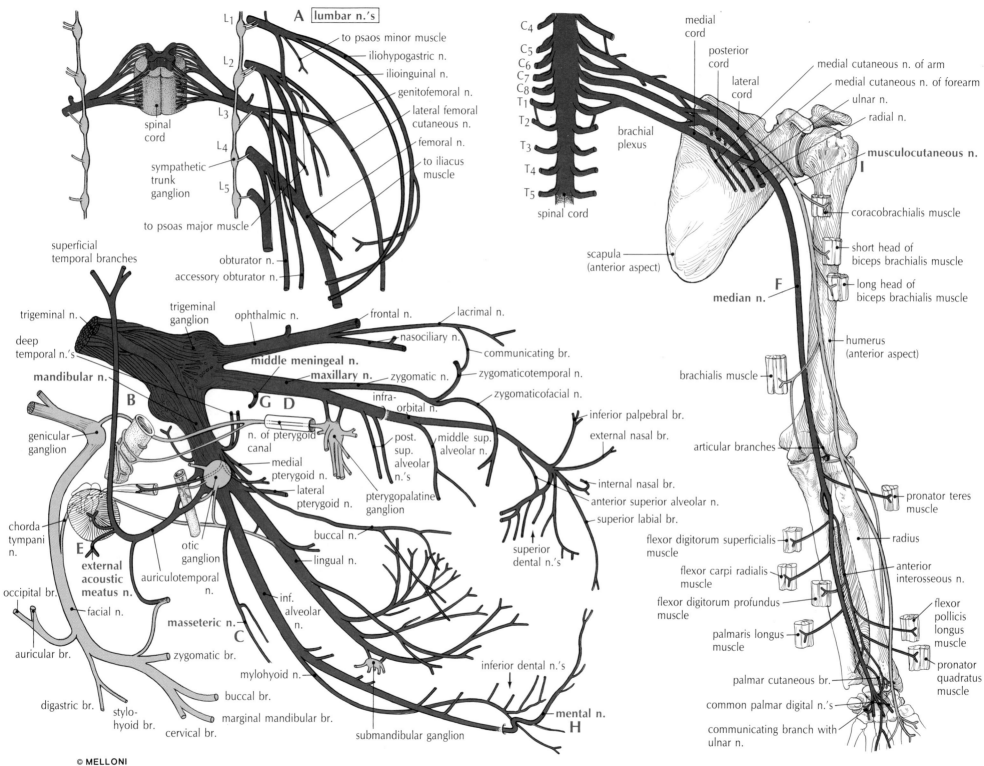

A lumbar n.'s

spinal cord

L₁
L₂
L₃
L₄
L₅

sympathetic trunk ganglion

to psaos minor muscle
iliohypogastric n.
ilioinguinal n.
genitofemoral n.
lateral femoral cutaneous n.
femoral n.
to iliacus muscle

to psoas major muscle

obturator n.
accessory obturator n.

C₄
C₅
C₆
C₇
C₈
T₁
T₂
T₃
T₄
T₅

brachial plexus

spinal cord

medial cord
posterior cord
lateral cord

medial cutaneous n. of arm
medial cutaneous n. of forearm
ulnar n.
radial n.

musculocutaneous n.

I

scapula (anterior aspect)

coracobrachialis muscle

short head of biceps brachialis muscle

long head of biceps brachialis muscle

median n.   **F**

brachialis muscle

humerus (anterior aspect)

articular branches

pronator teres muscle

radius

anterior interosseous n.

flexor digitorum superficialis muscle

flexor carpi radialis muscle

flexor digitorum profundus muscle

palmaris longus muscle

flexor pollicis longus muscle

pronator quadratus muscle

palmar cutaneous br.

common palmar digital n.'s

communicating branch with ulnar n.

superficial temporal branches

trigeminal n.

deep temporal n.'s

mandibular n.

B

genicular ganglion

chorda tympani n.

E

external acoustic meatus n.

occipital br.

facial n.

auricular br.

digastric br.

stylo-hyoid br.

cervical br.

buccal br.

marginal mandibular br.

zygomatic br.

mylohyoid n.

otic ganglion

auriculotemporal n.

trigeminal ganglion

ophthalmic n.

middle meningeal n.

maxillary n.

G   **D**

n. of pterygoid canal

medial pterygoid n.

lateral pterygoid n.

pterygopalatine ganglion

buccal n.

lingual n.

inf. alveolar n.

masseteric n.   **C**

frontal n.   lacrimal n.

nasociliary n.

communicating br.

zygomatic n.   zygomaticotemporal n.

zygomaticofacial n.

infra-orbital n.

post. sup. alveolar n.'s

middle sup. alveolar n.

inferior palpebral br.

external nasal br.

internal nasal br.

anterior superior alveolar n.

superior labial br.

superior dental n.'s

submandibular ganglion

inferior dental n.'s

mental n.

H

© MELLONI

	NERVE	ORIGIN	BRANCHES	DISTRIBUTION
A	**n. mylohyoideus** *mylohyoid n.*	inferior alveolar n.	filaments	mylohyoid muscle and anterior belly of digastric muscle
B	**nn. nasales externi** *nasal n.'s, external*	anterior ethmoidal n.	filaments	skin of nose
C	**n. nasociliaris** *nasociliary n.* *nasal n.*	opthalmic n.	anterior ethmoidal, posterior ethmoidal, long ciliary, infratrochlear, communicating branch with ciliary ganglion	mucous membrane and skin of nose, ciliary body, iris, cornea, conjunctiva, lacrimal sac, caruncle, and eyelids
D	**n. nasopalatinus** *nasopalatine n.* *long sphenopalatine n.* *Scarpa's n.*	pterygopalatine ganglion	filaments	mucous membrane of anterior surface of hard palate, nasal septum
E	**n. obturatorius** *obturator n.*	second, third, and fourth lumbar n.'s	anterior, posterior	skin on medial surface of thigh; adductor magnus, longus, and brevis muscles; pectineus and obturator externus muscles; hip and knee joints
F	**n. obturatorius accessorius** (sometimes absent) *obturator n., accessory*	third and fourth lumbar n.'s	articular, muscular	hip joint, pectineus muscle
G	**n. obturatorius internus** *n. of obturator, internal*	fifth lumbar and first and second sacral n.'s	muscular	obturator internus and gemellus superior muscles
H	**n. occipitalis major** *occipital n., greater*	medial branch of dorsal division of second cervical n.	muscular, auricular, medial, lateral	skin of scalp and semispinalis capitis muscle
I	**n. occipitalis minor** *occipital n., lesser*	second and occasionally third cervical n.	auricular filaments	skin on side of head and upper third of medial surface of external ear
J	**n. occipitalis tertius** *occipital n., third* *least occipital n.*	medial branch of dorsal division of third cervical n.	medial, lateral	skin on lower part of back of head

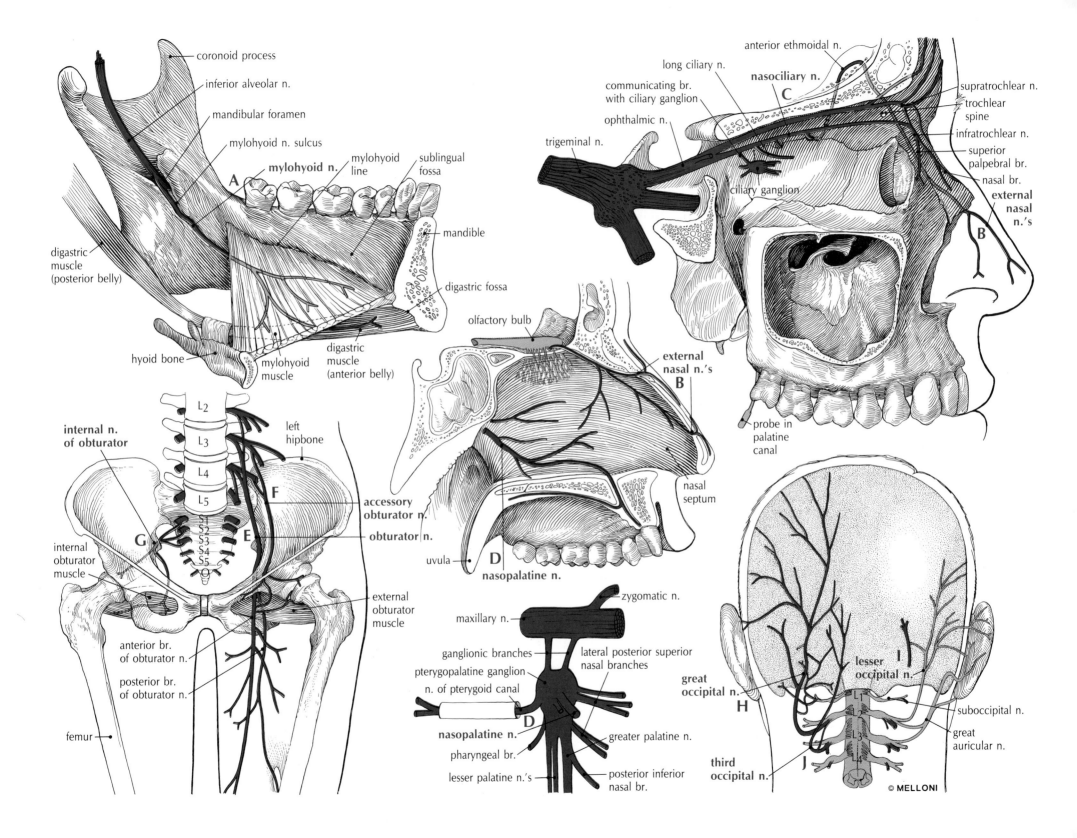

coronoid process

inferior alveolar n.

mandibular foramen

mylohyoid n. sulcus

mylohyoid n.

mylohyoid line

sublingual fossa

A

mandible

digastric muscle (posterior belly)

digastric fossa

hyoid bone

mylohyoid muscle

digastric muscle (anterior belly)

anterior ethmoidal n.

long ciliary n.

nasociliary n.

communicating br. with ciliary ganglion

ophthalmic n.

trigeminal n.

ciliary ganglion

C

supratrochlear n.

trochlear spine

infratrochlear n.

superior palpebral br.

nasal br.

external nasal n.'s

B

probe in palatine canal

olfactory bulb

external nasal n.'s

B

nasal septum

D

nasopalatine n.

uvula

internal n. of obturator

left hipbone

L2

L3

L4

L5

F

accessory obturator n.

S1
S2
S3
S4
S5

G

E

obturator n.

internal obturator muscle

external obturator muscle

anterior br. of obturator n.

posterior br. of obturator n.

femur

zygomatic n.

maxillary n.

ganglionic branches

lateral posterior superior nasal branches

pterygopalatine ganglion

n. of pterygoid canal

nasopalatine n.

D

pharyngeal br.

greater palatine n.

lesser palatine n.'s

posterior inferior nasal br.

great occipital n.

lesser occipital n.

I

H

L1

suboccipital n.

L3

great auricular n.

third occipital n.

L4

J

© MELLONI

	NERVE	ORIGIN	BRANCHES	DISTRIBUTION
A	**n. oculomotorius** *oculomotor n.* *third cranial n.*	brain stem	superior, inferior	extrinsic muscles of eye (excluding lateral rectus and superior oblique), levator palpebrae superioris and ciliary muscles, sphincter pupillae muscle
B	**nn. olfactorii** *olfactory n.'s* *first cranial n.'s*	olfactory mucosa in the nasal cavity	filaments	olfactory bulb
C	**n. ophthalmicus** *ophthalmic n.*	trigeminal n.	frontal, lacrimal, nasociliary, tentorial	eyeball, lacrimal gland, conjunctiva, skin and mucous membrane of nose, skin of eyelids and forehead, tentorium cerebelli
D	**n. opticus** *optic n.* *second cranial n.*	ganglionic layer of retina	filaments	optic chiasma
E	**nn. palatini minores** *palatine n.'s, lesser* *posterior palatine n.*	pterygopalatine ganglion	filaments	soft palate, tonsil, uvula
F	**n. palatinus major** *palatine n., greater* *anterior palatine n.*	pterygopalatine ganglion	posterior inferior nasal	gums, mucous membrane of hard palate and soft palate
G	**n. palpebralis inferior** *palpebral n., inferior*	infraorbital n.	filaments	skin of the lower eyelid
H	**n. palpebralis superior** *palpebral n., superior*	lacrimal n.	filaments	skin of the upper eyelid
I	**n. pectoralis lateralis** *pectoral n., lateral*	lateral cord of brachial plexus	filaments	pectoralis major and minor muscles
J	**n. pectoralis medialis** *pectoral n., medial*	medial cord of brachial plexus	filaments	pectoralis major and minor muscles

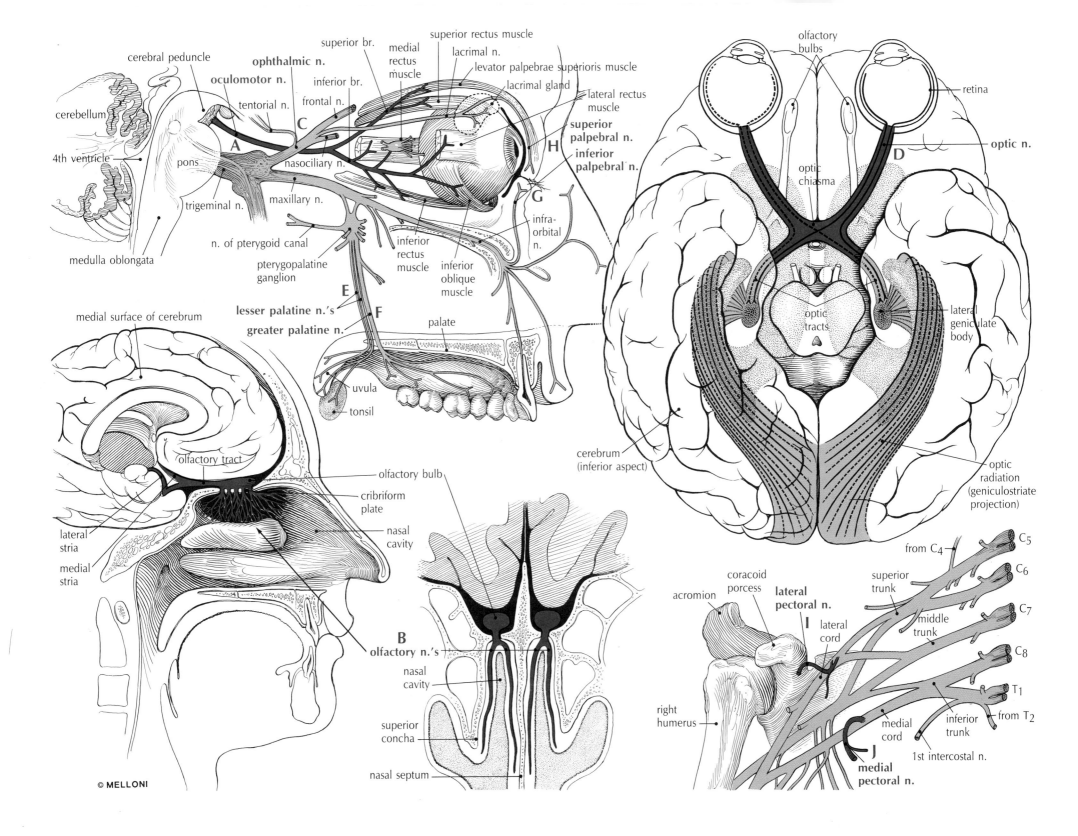

cerebral peduncle
cerebellum
4th ventricle
medulla oblongata
pons
ophthalmic n.
oculomotor n.
tentorial n.
A
C
superior br.
inferior br.
frontal n.
nasociliary n.
trigeminal n.
maxillary n.
n. of pterygoid canal
pterygopalatine ganglion
medial rectus muscle
superior rectus muscle
lacrimal n.
levator palpebrae superioris muscle
lacrimal gland
lateral rectus muscle
superior palpebral n.
inferior palpebral n.
H
G
infra-orbital n.
inferior rectus muscle
inferior oblique muscle
E
F
lesser palatine n.'s
greater palatine n.
palate

olfactory bulbs
retina
optic n.
D
optic chiasma
optic tracts
lateral geniculate body
cerebrum (inferior aspect)
optic radiation (geniculostriate projection)

medial surface of cerebrum
olfactory tract
lateral stria
medial stria
olfactory bulb
cribriform plate
nasal cavity
uvula
tonsil

B
olfactory n.'s
nasal cavity
superior concha
nasal septum

acromion
coracoid porcess
lateral pectoral n.
I
lateral cord
right humerus
medial cord
J
medial pectoral n.
1st intercostal n.
from C₄
C₅
C₆
C₇
C₈
T₁
from T₂
superior trunk
middle trunk
inferior trunk

© MELLONI

	NERVE	ORIGIN	BRANCHES	DISTRIBUTION
A	**n. perinei** *perineal n.*	pudendal n.	muscular, posterior scrotal (male) or labial (female), n. to urethral bulb	muscles of perineum, skin of scrotum (male) labium majus (female)
B	**n. peroneus communis** *peroneal n., common* *external popliteal n.* *peroneal n.*	sciatic n.	superficial peroneal, deep peroneal, lateral cutaneous n. of calf, sural communicating, articular	knee and superior tibiofibular joints; skin on anterior, posterior, and lateral parts of leg; short head of biceps femoris and tibialis anterior muscles
C	**n. peroneus profundus** *peroneal n., deep* *anterior tibial n.*	common peroneal n.	articular, muscular, lateral terminal, medial terminal, dorsal digital	tibialis anterior, extensor digitorum longus, extensor hallucis longus, extensor digitorum brevis, and peroneus tertius muscles; tarsal, metatarsophalangeal, and ankle joints; skin of adjacent sides of the big toe and the second toe
D	**n. peroneus superficialis** *peroneal n., superficial* *musculocutaneous n.*	common peroneal n.	muscular, medial dorsal cutaneous, intermediate dorsal cutaneous	peroneus longus and brevis muscles; skin of lower leg; skin of medial side of big toe and adjacent sides of toes; skin of lateral side of ankle
E	**n. petrosus major** *petrosal n., greater* *greater superficial petrosal n.*	geniculate ganglion of facial n.	joins deep petrosal nerve to form nerve of pterygoid canal	lacrimal, palatine, and nasal glands; mucous membrane of palate
F	**n. petrosus minor** *petrosal n., lesser* *lesser superficial petrosal n.*	tympanic plexus	filaments	otic ganglion, parotid gland
G	**n. petrosus profundus** *petrosal n., deep*	internal carotid plexus	joins greater petrosal nerve to form nerve of pterygoid canal	lacrimal, palatine, and nasal glands
H	**nn. phrenici accessorii** *phrenic n.'s, accessory*	fifth cervical n. or n. to subclavius	joins phrenic n.	diaphragm
I	**n. phrenicus** *phrenic n.*	third, fourth, and fifth cervical n.'s	pericardiac, phrenicoabdominal	diaphragm, pericardium, mediastinal pleura, sympathetic plexus

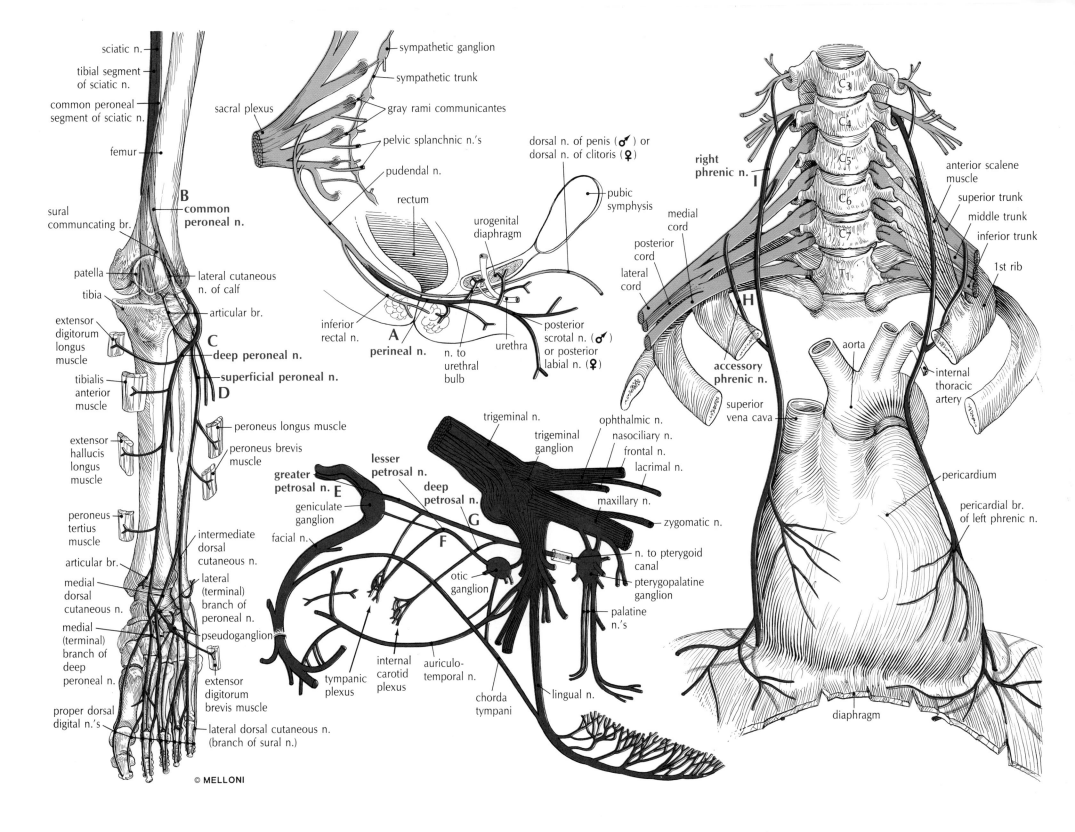

sciatic n.

tibial segment of sciatic n.

common peroneal segment of sciatic n.

femur

sural communcating br.

patella

tibia

extensor digitorum longus muscle

tibialis anterior muscle

extensor hallucis longus muscle

peroneus tertius muscle

articular br.

medial dorsal cutaneous n.

medial (terminal) branch of deep peroneal n.

proper dorsal digital n.'s

B common peroneal n.

lateral cutaneous n. of calf

articular br.

C deep peroneal n.

superficial peroneal n.

D

peroneus longus muscle

peroneus brevis muscle

intermediate dorsal cutaneous n.

lateral (terminal) branch of peroneal n.

pseudoganglion

extensor digitorum brevis muscle

lateral dorsal cutaneous n. (branch of sural n.)

© MELLONI

sacral plexus

sympathetic ganglion

sympathetic trunk

gray rami communicantes

pelvic splanchnic n.'s

pudendal n.

rectum

dorsal n. of penis (♂) or dorsal n. of clitoris (♀)

pubic symphysis

urogenital diaphragm

inferior rectal n.

A

perineal n.

n. to urethral bulb

urethra

posterior scrotal n. (♂) or posterior labial n. (♀)

trigeminal n.

trigeminal ganglion

ophthalmic n.

nasociliary n.

frontal n.

lacrimal n.

maxillary n.

zygomatic n.

lesser petrosal n.

greater petrosal n. E

deep petrosal n. G

geniculate ganglion

facial n.

F

otic ganglion

n. to pterygoid canal

pterygopalatine ganglion

palatine n.'s

tympanic plexus

internal carotid plexus

auriculo-temporal n.

chorda tympani

lingual n.

right phrenic n. **I**

anterior scalene muscle

superior trunk

middle trunk

inferior trunk

1st rib

medial cord

posterior cord

lateral cord

H

accessory phrenic n.

superior vena cava

aorta

internal thoracic artery

pericardium

pericardial br. of left phrenic n.

diaphragm

C_3

C_4

C_5

C_6

C_7

T_1

	NERVE	ORIGIN	BRANCHES	DISTRIBUTION
A	**n. piriformis** *n. of piriform*	first and second sacral n.'s	filaments	piriformis muscle
B	**n. plantaris lateralis** *plantar n., lateral* *external plantar n.*	tibial n.	superficial, deep, muscular	deep muscles of foot, skin of fifth and lateral aspect of fourth toe
C	**n. plantaris medialis** *plantar n., medial* *internal plantar n.*	tibial n.	common plantar digital, cutaneous, muscular	flexor digitorum brevis, flexor hallucis brevis, abductor hallucis, and first lumbrical muscles; skin of sole of foot, adjacent sides of toes, joints of tarsus and metatarsus
D	**plexus brachialis** *brachial plexus*	ventral rami of the fifth to eighth cervical and first thoracic n.'s	supraclavicular branches: dorsal scapular, subclavius, long thoracic, suprascapular infraclavicular branches: lateral pectoral, medial pectoral, musculo-cutaneous, medial cutaneous nerve of forearm, medial cutaneous nerve of arm, subscapular, thoracodorsal, axillary, median, ulnar, radial	upper limb
E	**plexus caroticus internus** *internal carotid plexus*	internal carotid n.	lateral part: caroticotympanic n.'s, deep petrosal n., abducent n., tympanic br. of glossopharyngeal n., communication to trigeminal ganglion medial part: trochlear n., ophthalmic n., abducent n., ciliary ganglion, communication to oculomotor n.	internal carotid artery, tympanic plexus, pterygopalatine ganglion, ciliary ganglion, oculomotor, abducens, and n.'s of the cavernous sinus
F	**plexus cervicalis** *cervical plexus*	ventral rami of first to fourth cervical n.'s	ansa cervicalis, greater auricular, lesser occipital, transverse nerve of neck, medial supraclavicular, intermediate supraclavicular, lateral supraclavicular, phrenic, communi-cating, muscular, cutaneous	muscles of neck; skin of parts of head, neck, and chest; diaphragm
G	**plexus coccygeus** *coccygeal plexus*	lower sacral n.'s and the coccygeal n.'s	anococcygeal	skin over coccyx

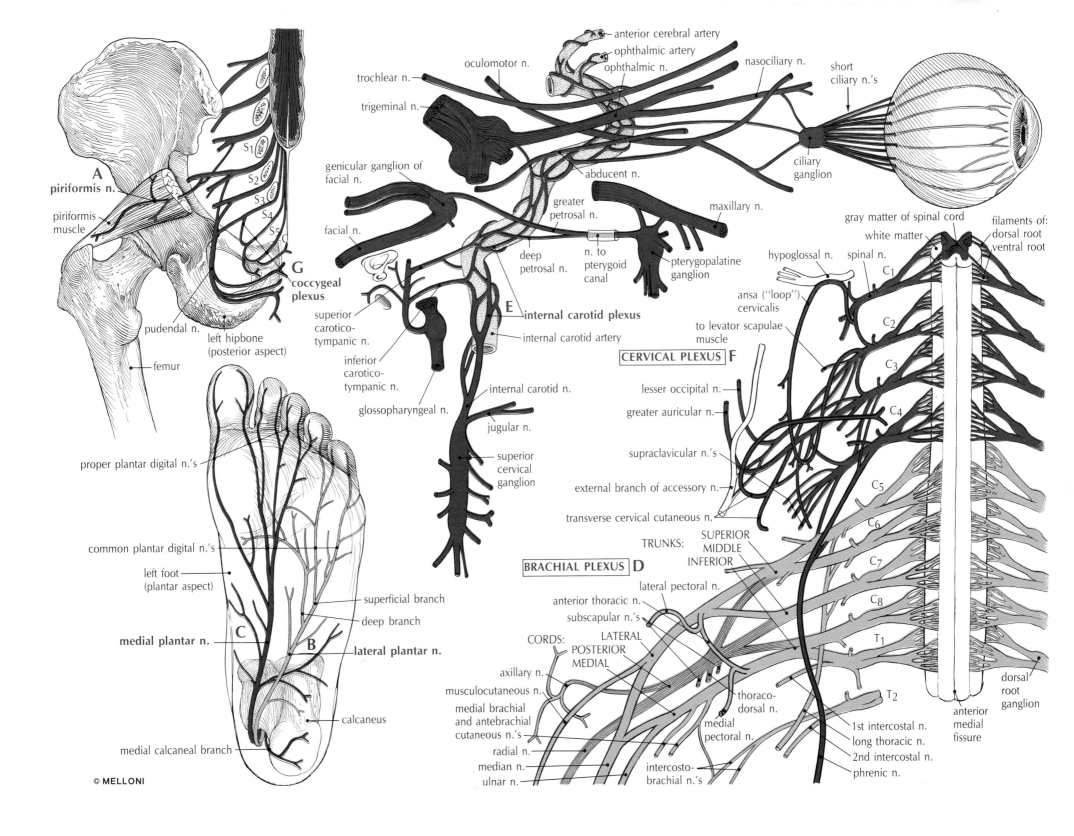

A
piriformis n.
piriformis muscle
pudendal n.
left hipbone (posterior aspect)
femur

S₁
S₂
S₃
S₄
S₅
C
G coccygeal plexus

proper plantar digital n.'s
common plantar digital n.'s
left foot (plantar aspect)
medial plantar n. **C**
B **lateral plantar n.**
superficial branch
deep branch
medial calcaneal branch
calcaneus

© MELLONI

anterior cerebral artery
ophthalmic artery
oculomotor n.
ophthalmic n.
nasociliary n.
short ciliary n.'s
trochlear n.
trigeminal n.
abducent n.
ciliary ganglion
genicular ganglion of facial n.
greater petrosal n.
maxillary n.
facial n.
n. to pterygoid canal
deep petrosal n.
pterygopalatine ganglion
superior carotico-tympanic n.
E **internal carotid plexus**
inferior carotico-tympanic n.
internal carotid artery
glossopharyngeal n.
internal carotid n.
jugular n.
superior cervical ganglion

gray matter of spinal cord
white matter
filaments of: dorsal root ventral root
hypoglossal n.
spinal n.
C₁
ansa ("loop") cervicalis
C₂
to levator scapulae muscle
C₃
CERVICAL PLEXUS **F**
lesser occipital n.
C₄
greater auricular n.
supraclavicular n.'s
C₅
external branch of accessory n.
transverse cervical cutaneous n.
C₆
TRUNKS: SUPERIOR MIDDLE INFERIOR
C₇
BRACHIAL PLEXUS **D**
lateral pectoral n.
C₈
anterior thoracic n.
subscapular n.'s
CORDS: LATERAL POSTERIOR MEDIAL
T₁
axillary n.
musculocutaneous n.
medial brachial and antebrachial cutaneous n.'s
thoraco-dorsal n.
medial pectoral n.
T₂
radial n.
median n.
ulnar n.
intercosto-brachial n.'s
1st intercostal n.
long thoracic n.
2nd intercostal n.
phrenic n.
anterior medial fissure
dorsal root ganglion

	NERVE	ORIGIN	BRANCHES	DISTRIBUTION
A	**plexus lumbalis** *lumbar plexus*	ventral rami of first four lumbar n.'s	iliohypogastric, ilioinguinal, genito-femoral, lateral femoral cutaneous, obturator, accessory obturator (occasionally), femoral	quadratus lumborum, psoas major and minor, and iliacus muscles; structures of perineum, muscles of abdomen, skin of lower abdomen, buttock, and thigh; adductor magnus, adductor longus, and adductor brevis muscles, pectineus and obturator externus muscles; hip and knee joints
B	**plexus prostaticus** *prostatic plexus*	inferior hypogastric plexus	greater cavernous n. of penis, lesser cavernous n.'s of penis, filaments	prostate, corpus cavernosum of penis, corpus spongiosum of penis, penile urethra, seminal vesicles, bulbo-urethral glands
C	**plexus sacralis** *sacral plexus*	fourth and fifth lumbar and first through fourth sacral n.'s	nerve to quadratus femoris, nerve to obturator internus, superior gluteal, inferior gluteal, nerve to piriformis, posterior femoral cutaneous, sciatic, pudendal, perforating cutaneous, nerve to levator ani, coccygeus, and sphincter ani externus muscles	skin and muscles of perineum, buttock, and lower limb
D	**plexus uterovaginalis** *uterovaginal plexus*	inferior hypogastric plexus	greater cavernous n. of clitoris, lesser cavernous n.'s of clitoris, vaginal n.'s	uterus, vagina, ovary, cervix, urethra, corpus cavernosum of clitoris
E	**n. pterygoideus lateralis** *pterygoid n., lateral*	mandibular n.	none	lateral pterygoid muscle
F	**n. pterygoideus medialis** *pterygoid n., medial*	mandibular n.	filaments, n. to tensor tympani, n. to tensor veli palatini	medial pterygoid, tensor tympani, and tensor veli palatini muscles
G	**nn. pterygopalatini** *pterygopalatine n.'s* *sphenopalatine n.'s*	Two nerves arising from the maxillary nerve and passing to the pterygopalatine ganglion		
H	**n. pudendus** *pudendal n.* *internal pudic n.*	second, third, and fourth sacral n.'s	perineal, inferior rectal, dorsal n. of penis (male) or dorsal n. of clitoris (female)	muscles of perineum; skin around anus, scrotum (male), and labium major (female); erectile tissue

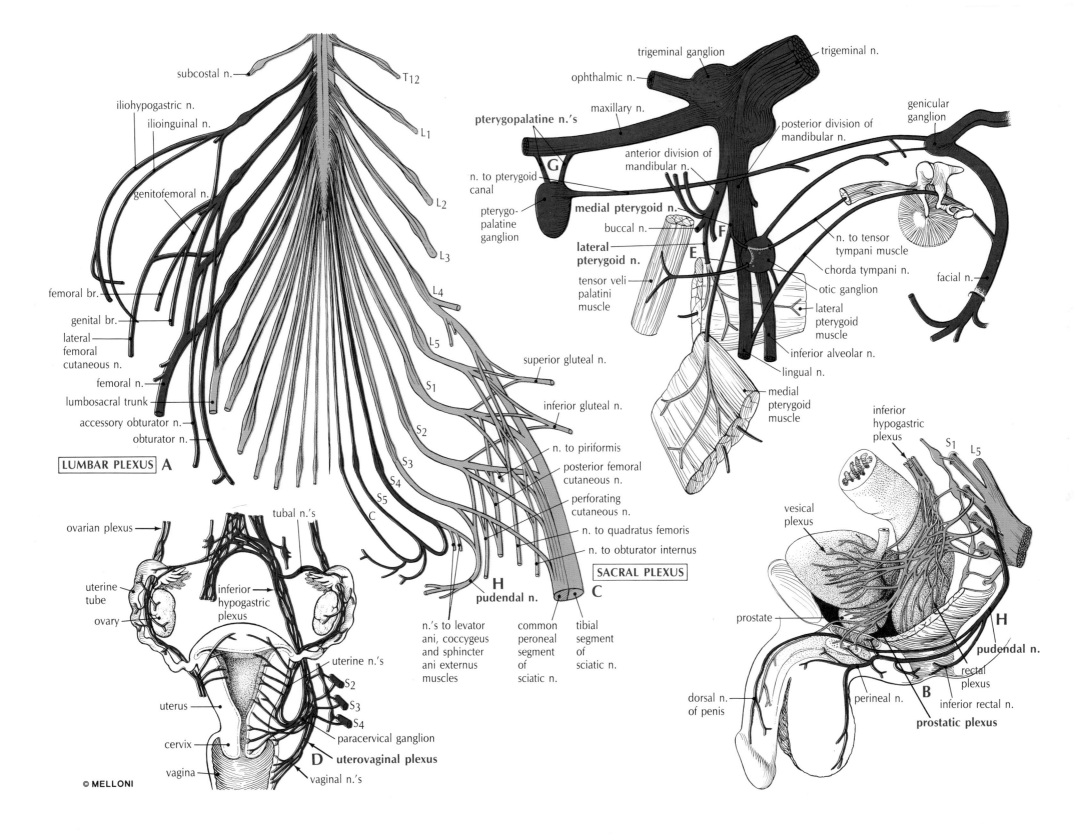

LUMBAR PLEXUS A

subcostal n.
iliohypogastric n.
ilioinguinal n.
genitofemoral n.
femoral br.
genital br.
lateral femoral cutaneous n.
femoral n.
lumbosacral trunk
accessory obturator n.
obturator n.

T12
L1
L2
L3
L4
L5
S1
S2
S3
S4
S5
C

superior gluteal n.
inferior gluteal n.
n. to piriformis
posterior femoral cutaneous n.
perforating cutaneous n.
n. to quadratus femoris
n. to obturator internus

SACRAL PLEXUS C

n.'s to levator ani, coccygeus and sphincter ani externus muscles

pudendal n. H

common peroneal segment of sciatic n.

tibial segment of sciatic n.

ovarian plexus
uterine tube
ovary
uterus
cervix
vagina

tubal n.'s
inferior hypogastric plexus
uterine n.'s
S2
S3
S4
paracervical ganglion
uterovaginal plexus D
vaginal n.'s

© MELLONI

trigeminal ganglion
ophthalmic n.
maxillary n.
pterygopalatine n.'s
n. to pterygoid canal
pterygopalatine ganglion
medial pterygoid n.
buccal n.
lateral pterygoid n.
tensor veli palatini muscle
medial pterygoid muscle

trigeminal n.
posterior division of mandibular n.
anterior division of mandibular n.
G
F
E
genicular ganglion
n. to tensor tympani muscle
chorda tympani n.
otic ganglion
lateral pterygoid muscle
inferior alveolar n.
lingual n.
facial n.

inferior hypogastric plexus
vesical plexus
prostate
dorsal n. of penis

S1
L5
pudendal n.
rectal plexus
inferior rectal n.
perineal n.
B
prostatic plexus
H

	NERVE	ORIGIN	BRANCHES	DISTRIBUTION
A	**n. quadratus femoris** *n. of quadrate muscle of thigh*	fourth and fifth lumbar and first sacral n.'s	filaments	quadratus femoris, gemellus inferior muscles and hip joint
B	**n. radialis** *(largest branch of brachial plexus)* *musculospiral n.*	posterior cord of brachial plexus C5, 6, 7, 8; (T1)	muscular, deep, superficial, posterior cutaneous, inferior lateral cutaneous, articular	skin on dorsal part of arm and forearm, skin on adjacent sides of fingers; extensor muscles of arm and forearm; elbow joint and joints of hand
C	**nn. rectales inferiores** *rectal n.'s, inferior* *inferior hemorrhoidal n.'s*	pudendal n.	filaments	sphincter ani externus muscle, skin around anus, lining of anal canal
D	**n. saccularis** *saccular n.*	vestibular ganglion	superior, major	macula of the saccule of internal ear
E	**nn. sacrales** *(five pairs)* *sacral n.'s*	sacral segments of spinal cord	dorsal, ventral, pelvic splanchnic	sacral and coccygeal plexuses
F	**n. sphenus** *saphenous n.*	femoral n.	infrapatellar, medial crural cutaneous	skin on medial surface of leg and foot, skin over patella, knee joint, subsartorial and patellar plexuses
G	**nn. scrotales anterior** *scrotal n.'s, anterior*	ilioinguinal n.	filaments	skin over anterior part of scrotum, root of penis
H	**nn. scrotales posterior** *scrotal n.'s, posterior*	perineal n.	filaments	skin over posterior part of scrotum
I	**nn. spinales** *spinal n.'s*	Thirty-one pairs of nerves that arise from the spinal cord and are formed by the union of ventral and dorsal spinal nerve roots. The 31 pairs of nerves include 8 cervical, 12 thoracic, 5 lumbar, 5 sacral, and 1 coccygeal.		
J	**nn. splanchnici lumbales** *(two to four in number)* *splanchnic n.'s, lumbar*	lumbar ganglia of sympathetic trunk	filaments	celiac, renal intermesenteric, and superior hypogastric plexuses

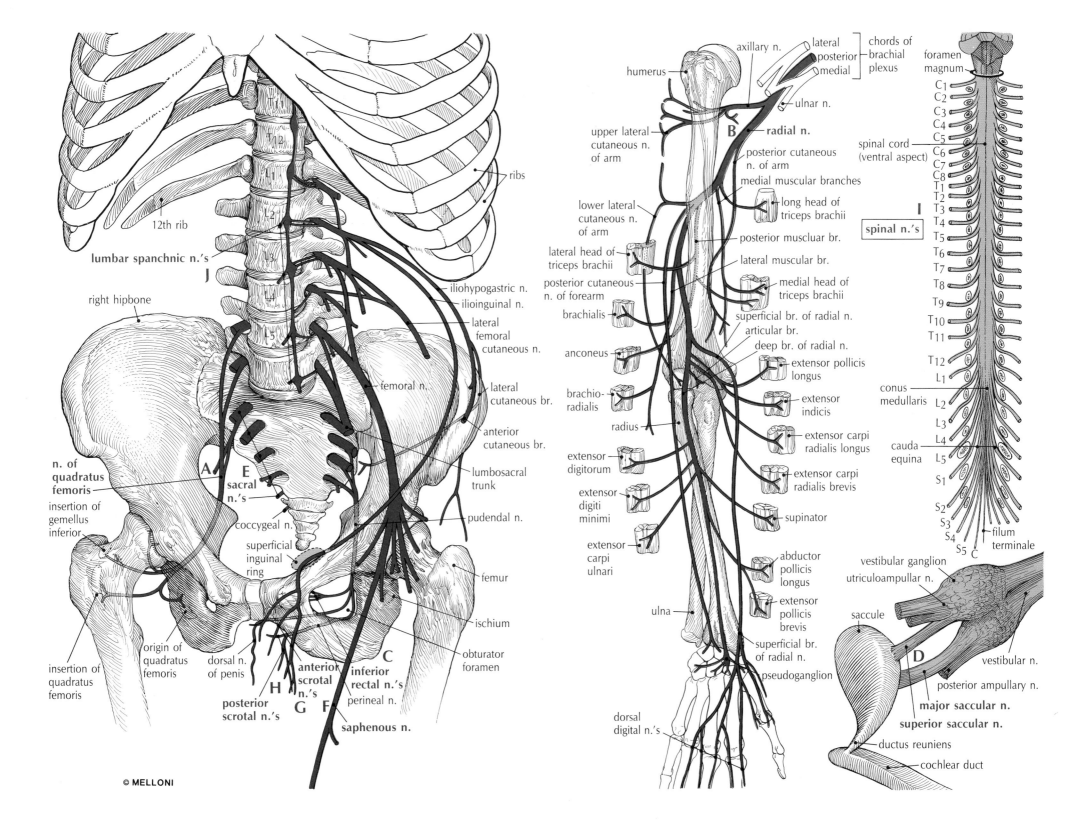

ribs

12th rib

lumbar spanchnic n.'s

J

right hipbone

A **E**
sacral
n.'s

coccygeal n.

n. of
quadratus
femoris

insertion of
gemellus
inferior

superficial
inguinal
ring

insertion of
quadratus
femoris

origin of
quadratus
femoris

dorsal n.
of penis

**posterior
scrotal n.'s**

H   **anterior
G **F** scrotal
n.'s**

perineal n.

saphenous n.

iliohypogastric n.
ilioinguinal n.
lateral
femoral
cutaneous n.

femoral n.

lateral
cutaneous br.

anterior
cutaneous br.

lumbosacral
trunk

pudendal n.

C
**inferior
rectal n.'s**

femur

ischium

obturator
foramen

© MELLONI

---

humerus

axillary n.

lateral
posterior   chords of
medial   brachial
plexus

ulnar n.

B   **radial n.**

upper lateral
cutaneous n.
of arm

posterior cutaneous
n. of arm

medial muscular branches

long head of
triceps brachii

lower lateral
cutaneous n.
of arm

posterior muscluar br.

lateral head of
triceps brachii

lateral muscular br.

posterior cutaneous
n. of forearm

medial head of
triceps brachii

brachialis

superficial br. of radial n.

articular br.

anconeus

deep br. of radial n.

extensor pollicis
longus

brachio-
radialis

extensor
indicis

radius

extensor carpi
radialis longus

extensor
digitorum

extensor carpi
radialis brevis

extensor
digiti
minimi

supinator

extensor
carpi
ulnari

abductor
pollicis
longus

ulna

extensor
pollicis
brevis

superficial br.
of radial n.

pseudoganglion

dorsal
digital n.'s

---

foramen
magnum

C1
C2
C3
C4
C5
C6
C7
C8
T1
T2
T3
T4
T5
T6
T7
T8
T9
T10
T11
T12
L1
L2
L3
L4
L5
S1
S2
S3
S4
S5 C

spinal cord
(ventral aspect)

I

spinal n.'s

conus
medullaris

cauda
equina

filum
terminale

---

vestibular ganglion

utriculoampullar n.

saccule

D

vestibular n.

posterior ampullary n.

major saccular n.

superior saccular n.

ductus reuniens

cochlear duct

	NERVE	ORIGIN	BRANCHES	DISTRIBUTION
A	**nn. splanchnici pelvini** *splanchnic n.'s, pelvic* *erigentes n.'s*	second, third, and fourth sacral n.'s of spinal cord	filaments	inferior hypogastric plexus
B	**nn. splanchnici sacrales** *splanchnic n.'s, sacral*	sacral portion of sympathetic trunk	filaments	inferior hypogastric plexus
C	**n. splanchnicus imus** *splanchnic n., lowest* *least splanchnic n.*	last thoracic ganglion of sympathetic trunk or lesser splanchnic n.	filaments	renal plexus
D	**n. splanchnicus major** *splanchnic n., greater*	fifth or sixth to ninth or tenth thoracic sympathetic ganglia	filaments	celiac ganglion, thoracic aorta, suprarenal gland, aorticorenal ganglion
E	**n. splanchnicus minor** *splanchnic n., lesser*	ninth and tenth, or occasionally tenth and eleventh thoracic ganglia of sympathetic trunk	renal	aorticorenal ganglion
F	**n. stapedius** *stapedius n.*	facial n.	filaments	stapedius muscle
G	**n. subclavius** *subclavian n.*	superior trunk of brachial plexus	filaments, accessory phrenic n. (occasionally)	subclavius muscle
H	**n. subcostalis** *subcostal n.*	twelfth thoracic n.	anterior cutaneous, lateral cutaneous	abdominal muscles, skin of lower abdominal wall and gluteal region
I	**n. sublingualis** *sublingual n.*	lingual n.	filaments	sublingual gland, mucous membrane of floor of mouth
J	**n. suboccipitalis** *suboccipital n.* *infraoccipital n.*	first cervical n.	filaments	three muscles that form the suboccipital triangle (rectus capitis posterior major, superior oblique, inferior oblique), rectus capitis posterior minor, and semispinalis capitis muscles

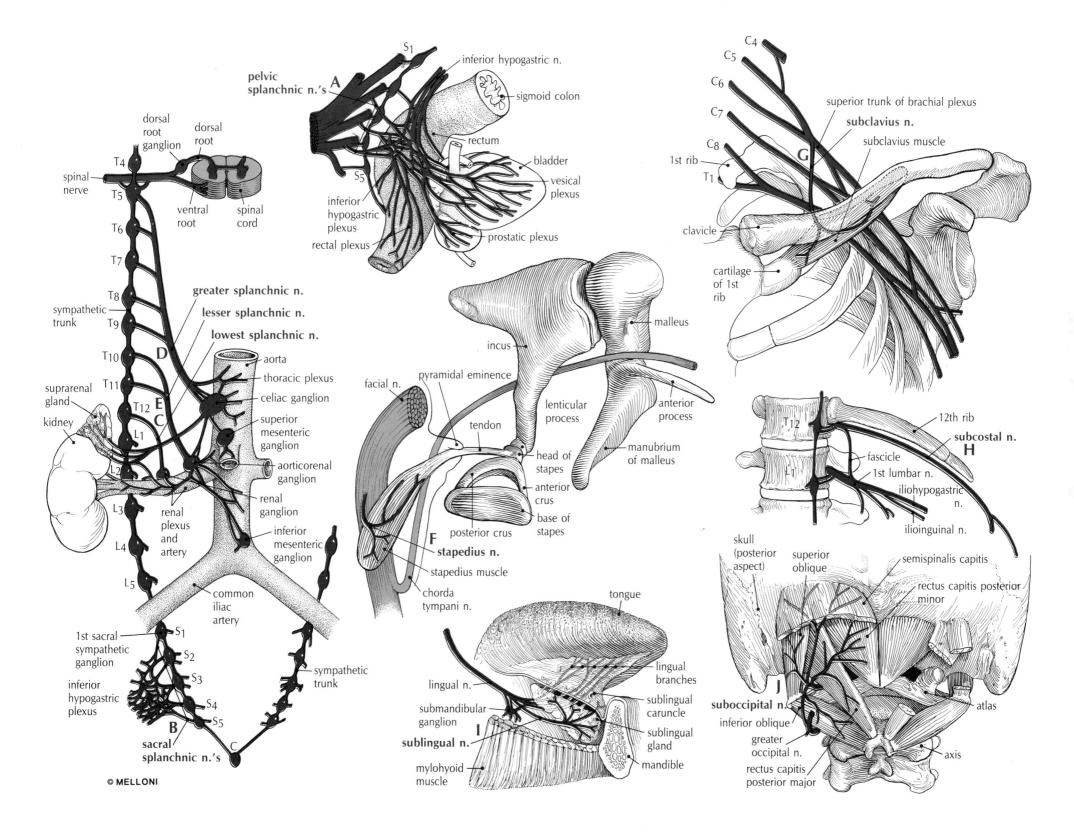

pelvic splanchnic n.'s A

S₁

inferior hypogastric n.

sigmoid colon

rectum

bladder

vesical plexus

inferior hypogastric plexus

S₅

prostatic plexus

rectal plexus

dorsal root ganglion

dorsal root

spinal nerve

T₄

ventral root

spinal cord

T₅

T₆

T₇

T₈

sympathetic trunk

greater splanchnic n.

lesser splanchnic n.

lowest splanchnic n.

T₉

T₁₀

D

aorta

thoracic plexus

celiac ganglion

superior mesenteric ganglion

T₁₁

suprarenal gland

E

C

T₁₂

kidney

L₁

aorticorenal ganglion

renal ganglion

L₂

renal plexus and artery

renal ganglion

inferior mesenteric ganglion

L₃

L₄

common iliac artery

L₅

1st sacral sympathetic ganglion

S₁

S₂

sympathetic trunk

inferior hypogastric plexus

S₃

S₄

S₅

B

sacral splanchnic n.'s

C

© MELLONI

C₄

C₅

C₆

C₇

C₈

superior trunk of brachial plexus

subclavius n.

subclavius muscle

1st rib

G

T₁

clavicle

cartilage of 1st rib

incus

malleus

facial n.

pyramidal eminence

lenticular process

anterior process

tendon

manubrium of malleus

head of stapes

anterior crus

base of stapes

posterior crus

F

stapedius n.

stapedius muscle

chorda tympani n.

12th rib

subcostal n.

T₁₂

H

fascicle

L₁

1st lumbar n.

iliohypogastric n.

ilioinguinal n.

skull (posterior aspect)

superior oblique

semispinalis capitis

rectus capitis posterior minor

tongue

lingual branches

lingual n.

sublingual caruncle

submandibular ganglion

sublingual gland

J

suboccipital n.

inferior oblique

atlas

greater occipital n.

sublingual n. I

mylohyoid muscle

mandible

rectus capitis posterior major

axis

	NERVE	ORIGIN	BRANCHES	DISTRIBUTION
A	**nn. subscapulares** (usually two in number) *subscapular n.'s*	posterior cord of brachial plexus	filaments	subscapularis and teres major muscles
B	**nn. supraclaviculares intermedii** *supraclavicular n.'s, intermediate* *middle supraclavicular n.'s*	common trunk formed by third and fourth cervical n.'s	filaments	skin over pectoralis major and deltoid muscles
C	**nn. supraclaviculares laterales** *supraclavicular n.'s, lateral* *posterior supraclavicular n.'s* *supra-acromial n.'s*	common trunk formed by third and fourth cervical n.'s	filaments	skin of upper and posterior surfaces of shoulder
D	**nn. supraclaviculares mediales** *supraclavicular n.'s, medial* *anterior supraclavicular n.'s*	common trunk formed by third and fourth cervical n.'s	filaments	skin of upper medial part of thorax as low as the second rib
E	**n. supraorbitalis** *supraorbital n.*	frontal n.	lateral, medial, filaments	skin of forehead and upper eyelid, frontal sinus, pericranium
F	**n. suprascapularis** *suprascapular n.*	superior trunk of brachial plexus	filaments, articular	supraspinatus and infraspinatus muscles, shoulder joint, scapula
G	**n. supratrochlearis** *supratrochlear n.*	frontal n.	ascending, descending	skin of forehead, upper eyelid, conjunctiva
H	**n. suralis** *sural n.* *short saphenous n.*	medial sural cutaneous branch of the tibial n., and sural communicating branch of the common peroneal n.	lateral dorsal cutaneous, lateral calcaneal	skin on posterior surface of leg and lateral side of plantar surface of foot
I	**nn. temporales profundi** *temporal n.'s, deep*	mandibular n. masseteric n. (occasionally) buccal n. (occasionally)	filaments	temporalis muscle

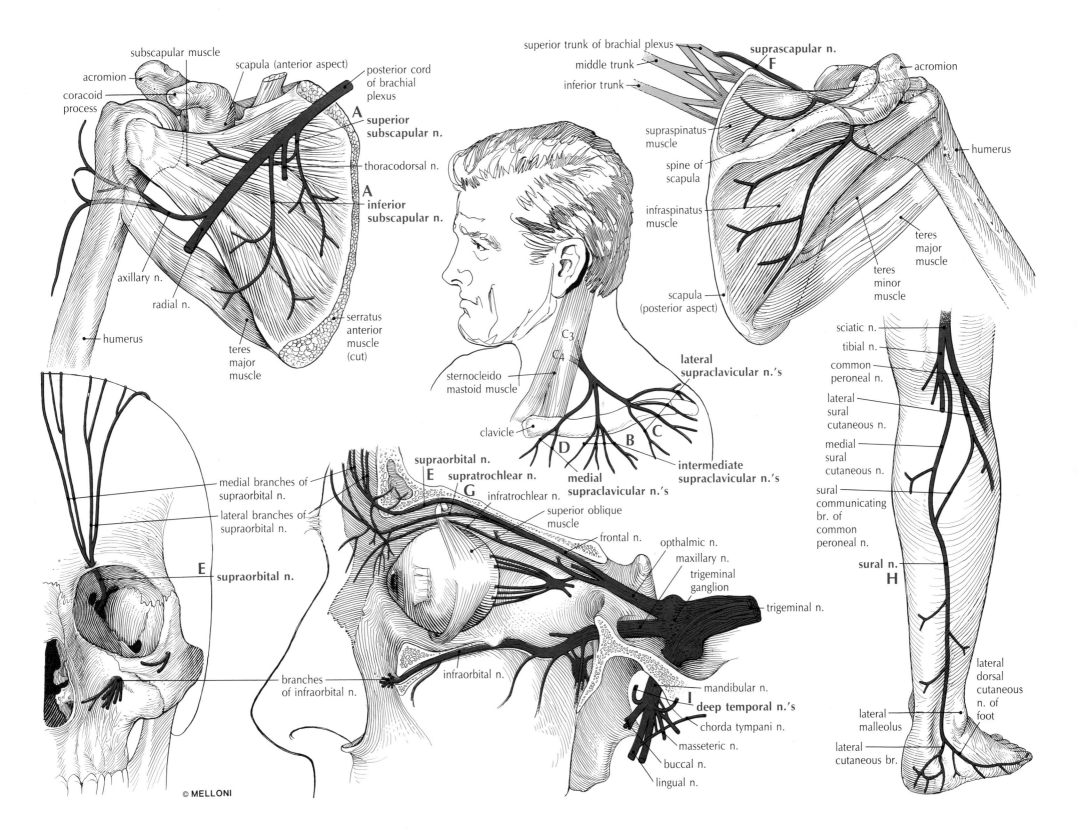

subscapular muscle

acromion

coracoid process

scapula (anterior aspect)

posterior cord of brachial plexus

A **superior subscapular n.**

thoracodorsal n.

A **inferior subscapular n.**

axillary n.

radial n.

humerus

teres major muscle

serratus anterior muscle (cut)

superior trunk of brachial plexus

middle trunk

inferior trunk

suprascapular n.

F

acromion

supraspinatus muscle

spine of scapula

infraspinatus muscle

humerus

teres major muscle

teres minor muscle

scapula (posterior aspect)

sternocleido mastoid muscle

C3

C4

clavicle

lateral supraclavicular n.'s

D

B

C

medial supraclavicular n.'s

intermediate supraclavicular n.'s

medial branches of supraorbital n.

lateral branches of supraorbital n.

E **supraorbital n.**

supraorbital n.

E

supratrochlear n.

G

infratrochlear n.

superior oblique muscle

frontal n.

opthalmic n.

maxillary n.

trigeminal ganglion

trigeminal n.

branches of infraorbital n.

infraorbital n.

mandibular n.

I **deep temporal n.'s**

chorda tympani n.

masseteric n.

buccal n.

lingual n.

sciatic n.

tibial n.

common peroneal n.

lateral sural cutaneous n.

medial sural cutaneous n.

sural communicating br. of common peroneal n.

sural n.

H

lateral malleolus

lateral cutaneous br.

lateral dorsal cutaneous n. of foot

© MELLONI

	NERVE	ORIGIN	BRANCHES	DISTRIBUTION
A	**n. tensoris tympani** *n. to tensor tympani*	medial pterygoid n.	filaments	tensor tympani muscle
B	**n. tensoris veli palatini** *n. to tensor veli palatini*	medial pterygoid n.	filaments	tensor veli palatini muscle
C	**n. tentorii** *tentorial n.* *recurrent tentorial n.*	ophthalmic n.	filaments	tentorium cerebelli
D	**nn. terminales** *terminal n.'s*	cerebral hemisphere close to anterior perforated substance	filaments	through cribriform plate to mucous membrane of nasal septum
E	**nn. thoracici** (12 pairs) *thoracic n.'s*	thoracic segments of spinal cord	dorsal, ventral	thoracic and upper abdominal walls
F	**n. thoracicus longus** *thoracic n., long* *n. of serratus anterior*	fifth, sixth, and seventh cervical n.'s	filaments	serratus anterior muscle
G	**n. thoracodorsalis** *thoracodorsal n.* *long subscapular n.* *n. of latissimus dorsi*	posterior cord of brachial plexus	filaments	latissimus dorsi muscle
H	**n. thyrohyoideus** *n. of thyrohyoid*	hypoglossal n.	filaments	thyrohyoid muscle
I	**nn. thyroideus** *thyroid n.'s*	middle cervical ganglion	none	thyroid and parathyroid glands

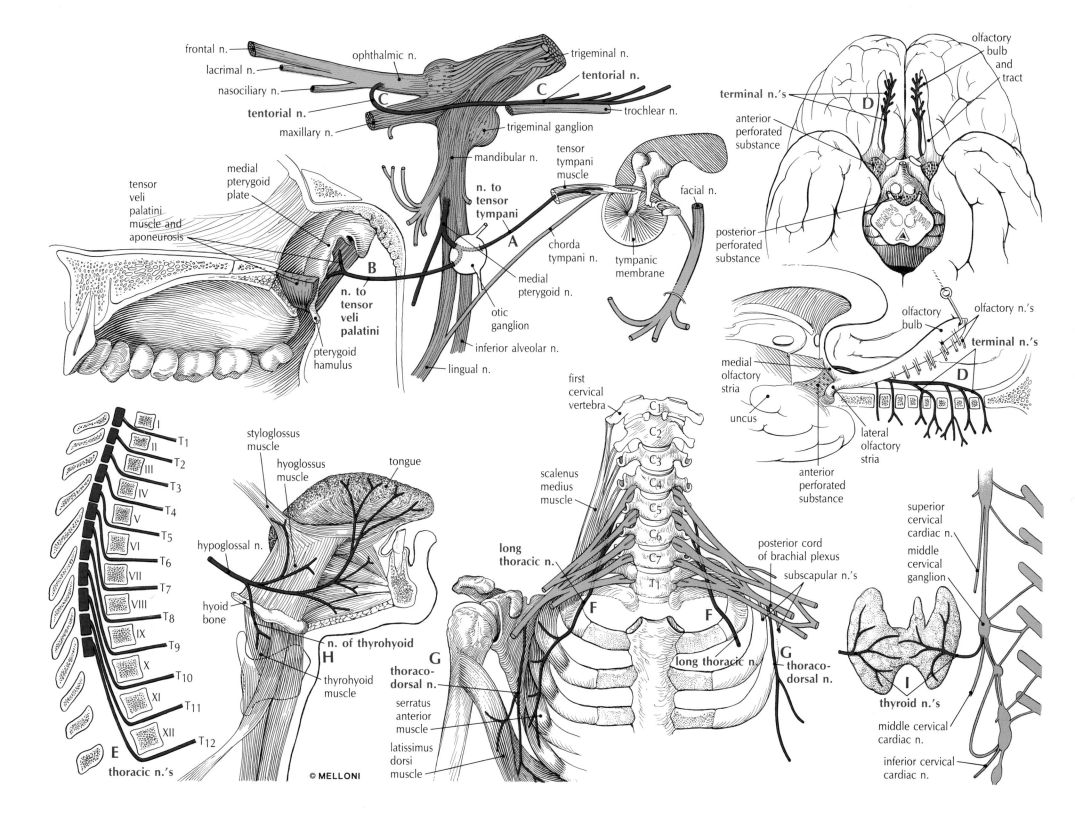

frontal n.

lacrimal n.

nasociliary n.

tentorial n.

maxillary n.

ophthalmic n.

C

C

tensor
veli
palatini
muscle and
aponeurosis

medial
pterygoid
plate

B

**n. to
tensor
veli
palatini**

pterygoid
hamulus

trigeminal n.

tentorial n.

trochlear n.

trigeminal ganglion

mandibular n.

tensor
tympani
muscle

facial n.

**n. to
tensor
tympani**

A

chorda
tympani n.

tympanic
membrane

medial
pterygoid n.

otic
ganglion

inferior alveolar n.

lingual n.

olfactory
bulb
and
tract

terminal n.'s

anterior
perforated
substance

D

posterior
perforated
substance

olfactory
bulb

terminal n.'s

medial
olfactory
stria

uncus

D

olfactory n.'s

anterior
perforated
substance

lateral
olfactory
stria

I
II
III
IV
V
VI
VII
VIII
IX
X
XI
XII

T1
T2
T3
T4
T5
T6
T7
T8
T9
T10
T11
T12

E

thoracic n.'s

styloglossus
muscle

hyoglossus
muscle

tongue

hypoglossal n.

hyoid
bone

n. of thyrohyoid

H

thyrohyoid
muscle

first
cervical
vertebra

C1
C2
C3
C4
C5
C6
C7
T1

scalenus
medius
muscle

**long
thoracic n.**

F

F

posterior cord
of brachial plexus

subscapular n.'s

long thoracic n.

G

**thoraco-
dorsal n.**

serratus
anterior
muscle

latissimus
dorsi
muscle

G

**thoraco-
dorsal n.**

superior
cervical
cardiac n.

middle
cervical
ganglion

I

thyroid n.'s

middle cervical
cardiac n.

inferior cervical
cardiac n.

© MELLONI

	NERVE	ORIGIN	BRANCHES	DISTRIBUTION
A	**n. tibialis** *tibial n.* *internal popliteal n.* *medial popliteal n.*	sciatic n.	medial cutaneous n. of calf, interosseous n. of leg, sural, medial plantar, lateral plantar, medial calcaneal, muscular	knee, ankle, and tibiofibular joints; muscles and skin on back of leg; plantar surface of foot; toes
B	**n. trigeminus** *trigeminal n.* *fifth cranial n.* *trifacial n.*	ventral surface of pons	motor root, intermediate fibers, sensory root (expands to form trigeminal ganglion that gives rise to ophthalmic, maxillary, and mandibular n.'s)	scalp, teeth, nasal cavity, mouth, muscles of mastication
C	**n. trochlearis** *trochlear n.* *fourth cranial n.*	midbrain below the inferior colliculus	filaments	superior oblique muscle of eyeball
D	**n. tympanicus** *tympanic n.* *n. of Jacobson*	glossopharyngeal n.	contributes to formation of tympanic plexus	mucous membrane of tympanic cavity, mastoid air cells, auditory tube, parotid gland
E	**n. ulnaris** *ulnar n.* *cubital n.*	medial cord of branchial plexus	dorsal, palmar, superficial, deep, muscular, articular	intrinsic muscles of hand; skin on medial part of hand; muscles of anterior part of forearm; elbow, wrist, and hand joints
F	**n. utricularis** *utricular n.*	vestibular n.	filaments	macula of the utricle of internal ear
G	**n. utriculoampullaris** *utriculoampullar n.*	A division of the vestibular part of the vestibulocochlear n. (8th cranial n.) that distributes to the macula of the utricle and the ampullae of the semicircular ducts.		
H	**nn. vaginales** *vaginal n.'s*	uterovaginal plexus	filaments	vagina

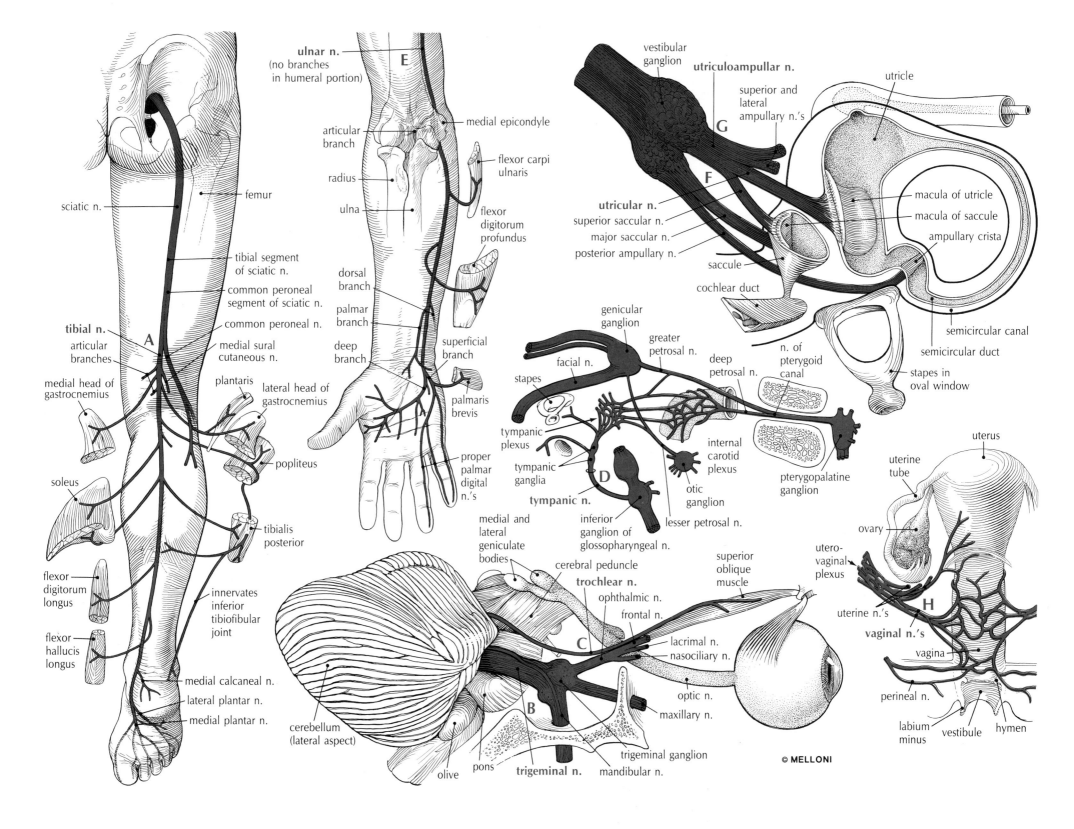

sciatic n.

femur

tibial segment of sciatic n.

common peroneal segment of sciatic n.

common peroneal n.

medial sural cutaneous n.

tibial n.

articular branches

A

medial head of gastrocnemius

plantaris

lateral head of gastrocnemius

popliteus

soleus

flexor digitorum longus

tibialis posterior

flexor hallucis longus

innervates inferior tibiofibular joint

medial calcaneal n.

lateral plantar n.

medial plantar n.

ulnar n.
(no branches in humeral portion)

E

articular branch

medial epicondyle

radius

flexor carpi ulnaris

ulna

flexor digitorum profundus

dorsal branch

palmar branch

deep branch

superficial branch

palmaris brevis

proper palmar digital n.'s

vestibular ganglion

utriculoampullar n.

superior and lateral ampullary n.'s

utricle

G

F

utricular n.

superior saccular n.

major saccular n.

posterior ampullary n.

saccule

cochlear duct

macula of utricle

macula of saccule

ampullary crista

semicircular canal

semicircular duct

stapes in oval window

n. of pterygoid canal

genicular ganglion

greater petrosal n.

deep petrosal n.

facial n.

stapes

tympanic plexus

tympanic ganglia

D

tympanic n.

inferior ganglion of glossopharyngeal n.

lesser petrosal n.

otic ganglion

internal carotid plexus

pterygopalatine ganglion

medial and lateral geniculate bodies

cerebral peduncle

trochlear n.

ophthalmic n.

frontal n.

superior oblique muscle

C

lacrimal n.

nasociliary n.

optic n.

maxillary n.

B

cerebellum (lateral aspect)

olive

pons

trigeminal n.

trigeminal ganglion

mandibular n.

uterus

uterine tube

ovary

utero-vaginal plexus

uterine n.'s

H

vaginal n.'s

vagina

perineal n.

labium minus

vestibule

hymen

© MELLONI

	NERVE	ORIGIN	BRANCHES	DISTRIBUTION
A	**n. vagus** *vagus n.* *tenth cranial n.*	medulla oblongata between the olive and the inferior cerebellar peduncle	auricular, meningeal, superior laryngeal, recurrent laryngeal, cardiac, pharyngeal, bronchial, hepatic, gastric, celiac, pulmonary, renal, esophageal, anterior trunk, posterior trunk	dura mater, skin over posterior region of external ear, pharynx and larynx, heart, esophagus and the back of the pericardium, stomach, trachea, bronchi, liver, and kidney
B	**n. vertebralis** *vertebral n.*	cervicothoracic (stellate) ganglion	filaments	meninges, vertebral artery
C	**n. vestibularis** *vestibular n.* *n. of equilibrium*	cells of the vestibular ganglion situated in the internal acoustic meatus	saccular, utricular	ampullae of semicircular ducts, utricle, and saccule
D	**n. vestibulocochlearis** *vestibulocochlear n.* *eighth cranial n.* *auditory n.* *acoustic n.* *otic n.*	connected to brainstem between pons and medulla oblongata by fibers from radix vestibularis and radix cochlearis	vestibular, cochlear	receptor organs of membranous labyrinth of internal ear
E	**n. zygomaticofacialis** *zygomaticofacial n.*	zygomatic n.	filaments	skin over zygomatic arch
F	**n. zygomaticotemporalis** *zygomaticotemporal n.*	zygomatic n.	filaments, lacrimal	skin of temple
G	**n. zygomaticus** *zygomatic n.* *orbital n.* *temporomalar n.*	maxillary n.	zygomaticofacial, zygomatico-temporal	skin of temple and over zygomatic arch

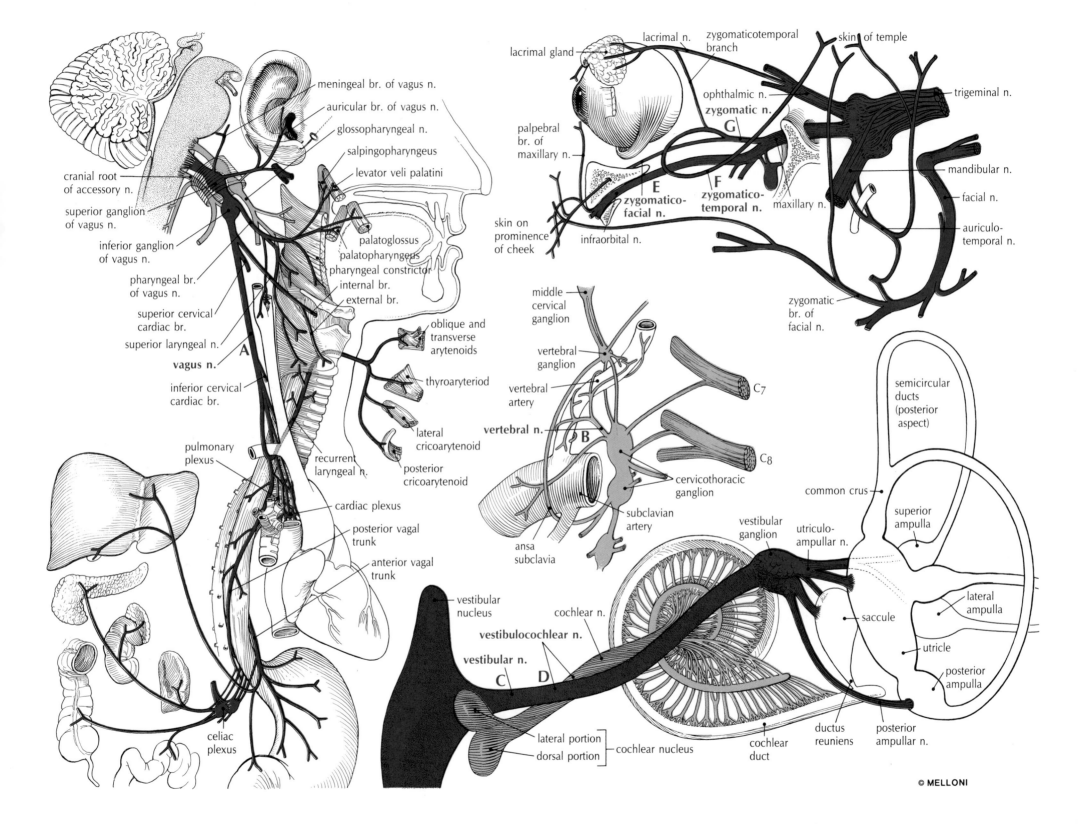

meningeal br. of vagus n.
auricular br. of vagus n.
glossopharyngeal n.
salpingopharyngeus
levator veli palatini
cranial root of accessory n.
superior ganglion of vagus n.
inferior ganglion of vagus n.
palatoglossus
palatopharyngeus
pharyngeal br. of vagus n.
pharyngeal constrictor
internal br.
external br.
superior cervical cardiac br.
superior laryngeal n.
vagus n.
A
inferior cervical cardiac br.
oblique and transverse arytenoids
thyroaryteriod
lateral cricoarytenoid
posterior cricoarytenoid
pulmonary plexus
recurrent laryngeal n.
cardiac plexus
posterior vagal trunk
anterior vagal trunk
celiac plexus

lacrimal n.
zygomaticotemporal branch
skin of temple
lacrimal gland
ophthalmic n.
zygomatic n.
G
trigeminal n.
palpebral br. of maxillary n.
E
F
mandibular n.
facial n.
zygomatico-facial n.
zygomatico-temporal n.
maxillary n.
auriculo-temporal n.
skin on prominence of cheek
infraorbital n.
zygomatic br. of facial n.

middle cervical ganglion
vertebral ganglion
vertebral artery
vertebral n.
B
C7
C8
cervicothoracic ganglion
subclavian artery
ansa subclavia

semicircular ducts (posterior aspect)
common crus
superior ampulla
vestibular ganglion
utriculo-ampullar n.
vestibular nucleus
cochlear n.
vestibulocochlear n.
vestibular n.
C
D
lateral ampulla
saccule
utricle
posterior ampulla
lateral portion
dorsal portion
cochlear nucleus
cochlear duct
ductus reuniens
posterior ampullar n.

© MELLONI

VEINS

	VEIN	LOCATION	DRAINS	TRIBUTARIES	EMPTIES INTO
A	**sinus cavernosus** (the internal carotid artery passes through it) *cavernous sinus*	on each side of the body of the sphenoid bone extending from the superior orbital fissure to the apex of the petrous portion of the temporal bone	base of brain, face, orbits	superior ophthalmic v., inferior ophthalmic v., superficial middle cerebral v., inferior cerebral v., sphenoparietal sinus, central v. of retina (occasionally), emissary v.'s, intercavernous sinus, basilar venous plexus	superior petrosal sinus, inferior petrosal sinus, plexus of v.'s on internal carotid artery, emissary v.'s
B	**sinus coronarius** *coronary sinus*	coronary sulcus on posterior heart wall	heart muscles	cardiac v.'s	right atrium
C	**sinus intercavernosi** *intercavernous sinus*	around the stalk of the hypophysis (pituitary gland)	connects the cavernous sinuses	venous sinuses under the hypophysis	cavernous sinuses
D	**sinus occipitalis** (smallest of cranial venous sinuses) *occipital sinus*	from vicinity of foramen magnum it courses backward and upward to confluence of the sinuses	venous plexus of foramen magnum	internal vertebral plexus, marginal sinuses	confluence of sinuses
E	**sinus petrosus inferior** *petrosal sinus, inferior*	courses along lower edge of petrosal bone from cavernous sinus to jugular foramen	base of brain, brain stem, internal ear	cavernous sinus, labyrinthine v's, and veins from the medulla oblongata, pons, and inferior part of cerebellum	internal jugular v.
F	**sinus petrosus superior** *petrosal sinus, superior*	courses along upper edge of petrosal bone (in margins of tentorium cerebelli) from cavernous sinus to sigmoid sinus	tympanic cavity, cerebellum, inferior part of cerebrum	cavernous sinus, and veins from tympanic cavity, cerebellum, and inferior surface of cerebrum	transverse sinus
G	**sinus rectus** *straight sinus*	dural fold at the junction of the falx cerebri and tentorium cerebelli toward the occipital protuberance	falx cerebri, upper part of cerebellum, midbrain, pons, choroid plexus	inferior sagittal sinus, great cerebral v., superior cerebellar v.'s	confluence of sinuses
H	**sinus sagittalis inferior** *sagittal sinus, inferior*	courses along the lower free margin of the falx cerebri	falx cerebri, medial surfaces of the cerebrum	veins from falx cerebri and medial surfaces of the cerebrum	straight sinus

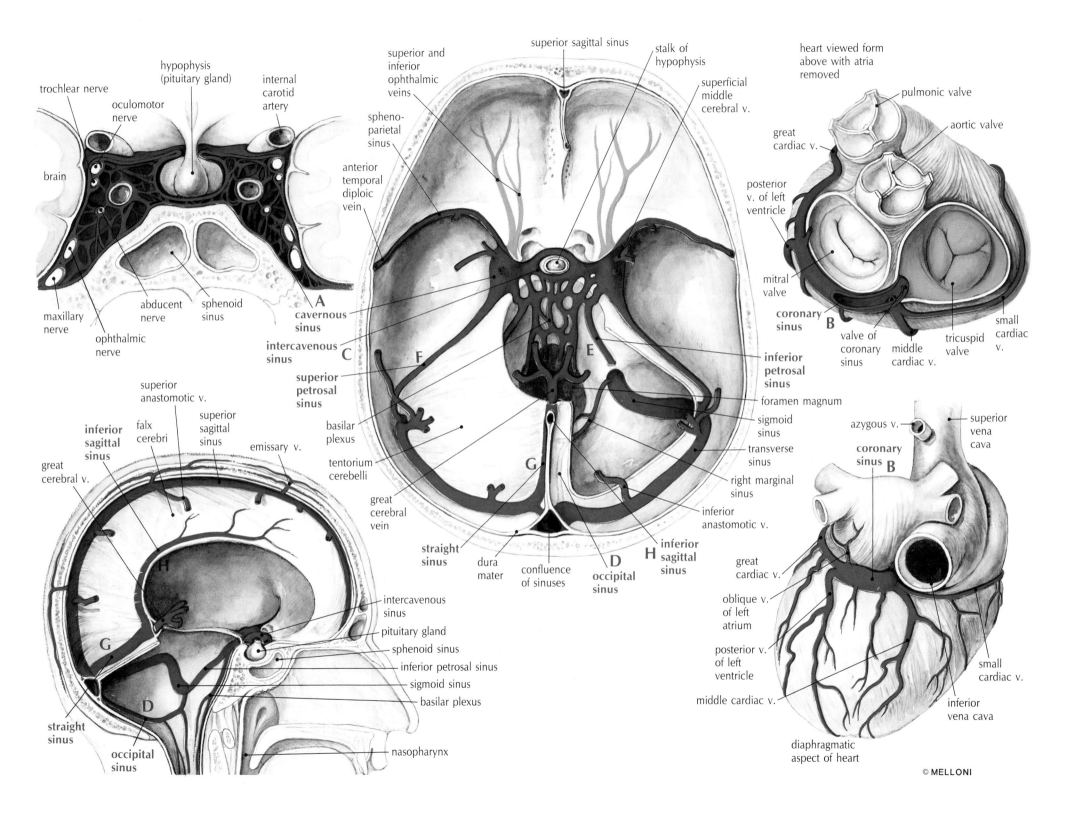

trochlear nerve

oculomotor nerve

hypophysis (pituitary gland)

internal carotid artery

brain

maxillary nerve

ophthalmic nerve

abducent nerve

sphenoid sinus

A

superior and inferior ophthalmic veins

spheno-parietal sinus

anterior temporal diploic vein

cavernous sinus

intercavenous sinus

C

superior sagittal sinus

stalk of hypophysis

superficial middle cerebral v.

F

superior petrosal sinus

basilar plexus

tentorium cerebelli

great cerebral vein

straight sinus

dura mater

confluence of sinuses

E

G

inferior petrosal sinus

foramen magnum

sigmoid sinus

transverse sinus

right marginal sinus

inferior anastomotic v.

D

occipital sinus

H

inferior sagittal sinus

heart viewed form above with atria removed

pulmonic valve

great cardiac v.

aortic valve

posterior v. of left ventricle

mitral valve

coronary sinus

B

valve of coronary sinus

middle cardiac v.

tricuspid valve

small cardiac v.

superior anastomotic v.

inferior sagittal sinus

falx cerebri

superior sagittal sinus

emissary v.

great cerebral v.

H

G

straight sinus

D

occipital sinus

intercavenous sinus

pituitary gland

sphenoid sinus

inferior petrosal sinus

sigmoid sinus

basilar plexus

nasopharynx

azygous v.

superior vena cava

coronary sinus

B

great cardiac v.

oblique v. of left atrium

posterior v. of left ventricle

middle cardiac v.

small cardiac v.

inferior vena cava

diaphragmatic aspect of heart

© MELLONI

	VEIN	LOCATION	DRAINS	TRIBUTARIES	EMPTIES INTO
A	**sinus sagittalis superior** *sagittal sinus, superior*	from foramen cecum, courses posteriorly to confluence of sinuses	superolateral and medial surfaces of cerebrum, meninges, cranium, pericranium, nasal cavity (occasionally)	superior cerebral v.'s, lateral venous lacunae (drain the diploic and meningeal veins), veins from pericranium, branch from nasal cavity	transverse sinus
B	**sinus sigmoideus** *sigmoid sinus*	in a groove on the mastoid part of temporal bone where it curves downward and medially toward the jugular foramen	transverse sinus	mastoid emissary v.'s, condylar emissary v.'s	internal jugular v.
C	**sinus sphenoparietalis** *sphenoparietal sinus*	from posterior edge of lesser wing of sphenoid bone, it courses backward and medially to front part of cavernous sinus	lower part of brain and supporting structures	middle meningeal v. (frontal branch), anterior temporal diploic v., veins of the dura mater	cavernous sinus
D	**sinus transversus** (two in number; the right one is usually larger) *transverse sinus*	from the confluence of sinuses near the internal occipital protuberance, coursing laterally and forward in the attached margin of the tentorium cerebelli to the sigmoid sinus	cerebrum and cerebellum	superior sagittal sinus, straight sinus, inferior cerebral v., inferior cerebellar v., diploic v.'s, inferior anastomotic v., superior petrosal sinus, mastoid and condylar emissary v.'s	sigmoid sinus
E	**v. alveolaris inferior** *alveolar v., inferior;* *dental v., inferior*	from lower teeth and interdental septa, some course to mental foramen and others to mandibular foramen	alveolar bone, lower teeth, body of mandible, lower lip	dental v., peridental v., mental v., mylohyoid v.	facial v. (via mental foramen) pterygoid plexus (via mandibular foramen) retromandibular v.
F	**v. alveolaris superior anterior** *alveolar v., anterior superior;* *dental v., anterior*	from nasal septum, cuspid and incisor teeth, and adjacent structures, courses upward to infraorbital v.	cuspid and incisor teeth of upper jaw, mucous membrane of maxillary sinus, gums, nasal cavity, and septum	dental v.'s, peridental v.'s, nasal v.	pterygoid plexus (via the infraorbital v.)
G	**v. alveolaris superior posterior** *alveolar v., posterior superior;* *dental v., posterior*	courses tortuously from upper molars and maxillary sinus to pterygoid plexus	molars and bicuspid teeth of upper jaw, maxillary sinus, gums, adjacent buccal mucosa	dental v.'s, peridental v.'s, maxillary sinus, penetrating branch of facial v.	pterygoid plexus

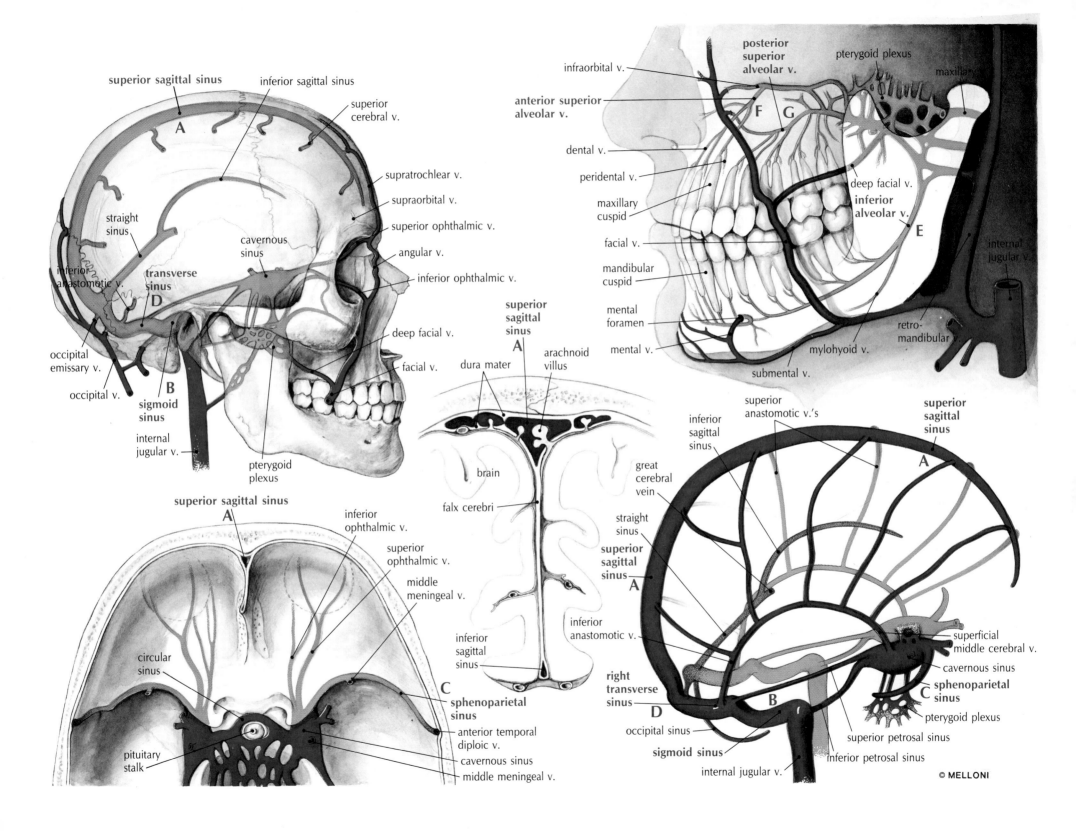

superior sagittal sinus

inferior sagittal sinus

superior cerebral v.

A

supratrochlear v.

supraorbital v.

superior ophthalmic v.

straight sinus

cavernous sinus

angular v.

inferior ophthalmic v.

inferior anastomotic v.

transverse sinus

D

deep facial v.

occipital emissary v.

facial v.

occipital v.

B

sigmoid sinus

internal jugular v.

pterygoid plexus

infraorbital v.

posterior superior alveolar v.

pterygoid plexus

maxillary

anterior superior alveolar v.

F G

dental v.

peridental v.

deep facial v.

inferior alveolar v.

maxillary cuspid

facial v.

E

mandibular cuspid

internal jugular v.

mental foramen

mental v.

retro-mandibular v.

mylohyoid v.

submental v.

superior sagittal sinus

A

arachnoid villus

dura mater

brain

falx cerebri

superior sagittal sinus

inferior ophthalmic v.

superior ophthalmic v.

middle meningeal v.

circular sinus

great cerebral vein

straight sinus

superior sagittal sinus

A

inferior sagittal sinus

superior anastomotic v.'s

superior sagittal sinus

A

pituitary stalk

sphenoparietal sinus

anterior temporal diploic v.

cavernous sinus

middle meningeal v.

C

inferior sagittal sinus

inferior anastomotic v.

right transverse sinus

D

occipital sinus

sigmoid sinus

internal jugular v.

B

superficial middle cerebral v.

cavernous sinus

sphenoparietal sinus

C

pterygoid plexus

superior petrosal sinus

inferior petrosal sinus

© MELLONI

	VEIN	LOCATION	DRAINS	TRIBUTARIES	EMPTIES INTO
A	**v. anastomotica inferior** *anastomotic v., inferior*	courses over posterior part of temporal lobe	temporal lobe	middle cerebral v.	transverse sinus
B	**v. anastomotica superior** *anastomotic v., superior*	from lateral sulcus of brain, courses across parietal lobe	parietal lobe	middle cerebral v.	superior sagittal sinus
C	**v. angularis** *angular v.*	between the eye and root of nose	lacrimal sac, eyelids, forehead, dorsum of nose, orbicularis oculi muscle	supratrochlear v.'s, supraorbital v., superior palpebral v.'s, inferior palpebral v.'s, external nasal v.'s	facial v. at junction with superior labial v.'s
D	**v. appendicularis** *appendicular v.*	courses along mesentery of vermiform appendix	vermiform appendix	none	ileocolic v.
E	**v. aqueductus cochleae** *v. of cochlear aqueduct*	along perilymphatic duct of internal ear from basal turn of cochlea through cochlear canaliculus	cochlea, saccule, utricle	spiral v. of modiolus, vestibular v.'s	internal jugular v.
F	**v. aqueductus vestibuli** *v. of aqueduct of vestibule*	in vestibular aqueduct (accompanies endolymphatic duct)	semicircular ducts of internal ear, utricle, saccule	vestibular v.'s of semicircular ducts	inferior petrosal sinus or superior petrosal sinus
G	**vv. arcuatae renis** *arcuate v.'s of the kidney*	corticomedullary border of kidney	corticomedullary area of kidney	interlobular v.'s, venulae rectae (straight venules)	interlobar v.
H	**vv. articulares** *articular v.'s*	temporomandibular joint	temporomandibular joint	none	retromandibular v.
I	**v. auricularis posterior** *posterior auricular v.*	from posterior part of parietal bone, courses down behind ear (auricle)	auricle, middle ear, mastoid air cells, parotid gland, adjacent neck muscles	stylomastoid v., auricular v., occipital v., superficial temporal v.'s	external jugular vein in union with retromandibular v.

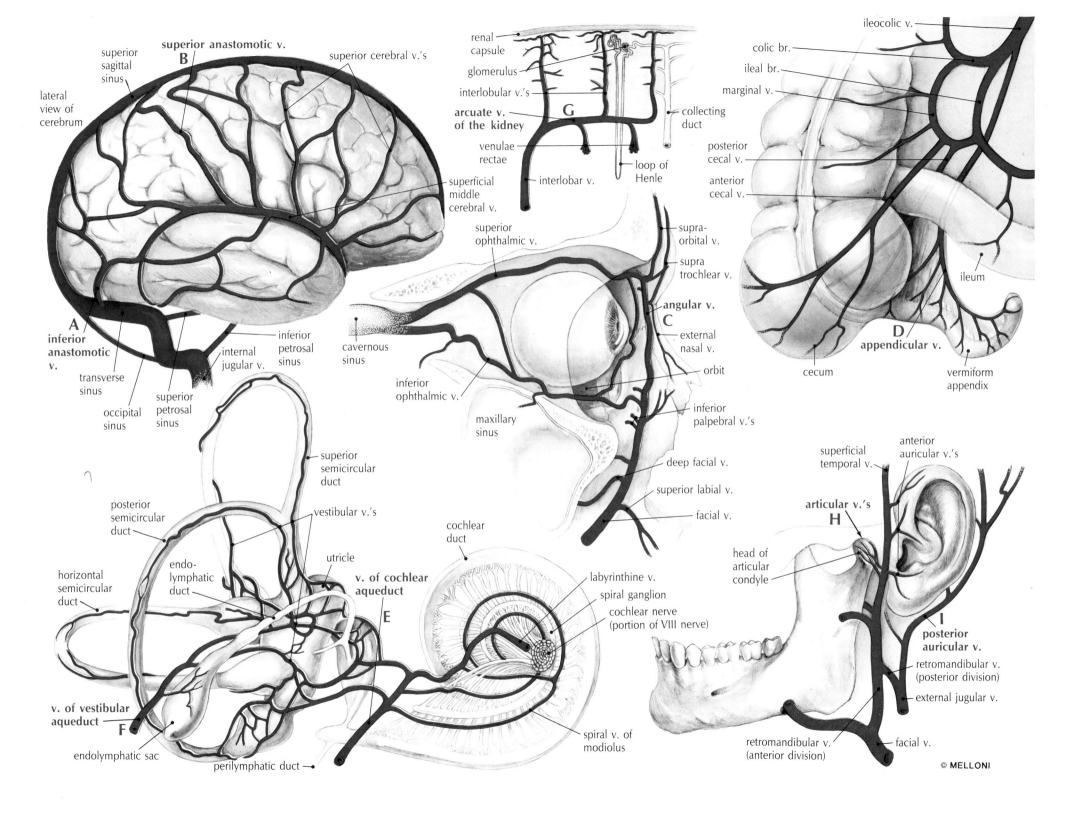

lateral view of cerebrum

superior sagittal sinus

superior anastomotic v.

B

superior cerebral v.'s

superficial middle cerebral v.

A

inferior anastomotic v.

transverse sinus

occipital sinus

superior petrosal sinus

internal jugular v.

inferior petrosal sinus

cavernous sinus

renal capsule

glomerulus

interlobular v.'s

arcuate v. of the kidney

G

venulae rectae

interlobar v.

collecting duct

loop of Henle

ileocolic v.

colic br.

ileal br.

marginal v.

posterior cecal v.

anterior cecal v.

ileum

D

appendicular v.

cecum

vermiform appendix

superior ophthalmic v.

supra-orbital v.

supra trochlear v.

angular v.

C

external nasal v.

orbit

inferior palpebral v.'s

inferior ophthalmic v.

maxillary sinus

deep facial v.

superior labial v.

facial v.

superior semicircular duct

posterior semicircular duct

vestibular v.'s

endolymphatic duct

utricle

horizontal semicircular duct

v. of cochlear aqueduct

E

v. of vestibular aqueduct

F

endolymphatic sac

perilymphatic duct

cochlear duct

labyrinthine v.

spiral ganglion

cochlear nerve (portion of VIII nerve)

spiral v. of modiolus

superficial temporal v.

anterior auricular v.'s

articular v.'s

H

head of articular condyle

I

posterior auricular v.

retromandibular v. (posterior division)

external jugular v.

retromandibular v. (anterior division)

facial v.

© MELLONI

	VEIN	LOCATION	DRAINS	TRIBUTARIES	EMPTIES INTO
A	**v. axillaris** *axillary v.*	from lower border of teres major muscle to lateral border of first rib	arm, axilla, superolateral chest wall	basilic v., brachial v.'s, cephalic v., subscapular v., highest thoracic v., thoracoacromial v., lateral thoracic v., posterior humeral circumflex v., anterior humeral circumflex v.	subclavian v.
B	**v. azygos** *azygos v.*	from right side of abdominal vertebral column, courses through diaphragm up to level T4 where it curves forward over roots of right lung	posterior wall of abdomen and thorax	right side: posterior intercostal v.'s (except 1st), superior intercostal v., subcostal v., hemiazygos v., accessory hemiazygos v., esophageal v.'s, mediastinal v.'s, pericardiac v.'s, bronchial v.'s, superior phrenic v.'s	superior vena cava, near its entrance into pericardium
C	**v. basalis** *basal v.*	from the anterior perforated substances it passes backward alongside the interpeduncular fossa and the midbrain	anterior perforated substances, superomedial surface of the cerebrum, insula, optic tract, optic chiasm, hypothalamus, medial aspect of cerebral peduncles, hippocampus, dentate gyrus, choroid plexus	deep middle cerebral v., anterior cerebral v., inferior thalamostriate v.'s, lateral atrial v., hippocampal and inferior ventricular v.'s, temporal v.'s, lateral mesencephalic v., anterior pontomesencephalic v.	great cerebral v., in union with internal cerebral v.'s (just under the splenium of the corpus callosum)
D	**v. basilica** *basilic v.*	from dorsum of hand, courses up arm (medial to biceps) to lower border of teres major muscle	upper limb	dorsal venous arch of hand, intermediate cubital v., intermediate antebrachial v.	axillary v. in union with brachial v.
E	**vv. basivertebrales** *basivertebral v.'s*	in vertebral bodies	vertebral bodies	none	anterior internal and external vertebral venous plexuses
F	**vv. brachiales** *brachial v.'s*	from neck of radius, courses upward to lower border of teres major muscle	forearm, elbow joint, arm, humerus	deep brachial v., nutrient v. of humerus, superior ulnar collateral v., inferior ulnar collateral v., radial v.'s, ulnar v.'s	axillary v., in union with basilic v.
G	**v. brachiocephalica dextra** *brachiocephalic v., right*	from behind medial end of right clavicle, it courses downward to first right costal cartilage	head and right arm	internal jugular v., right subclavian v.	superior vena cava in union with left brachiocephalic v.

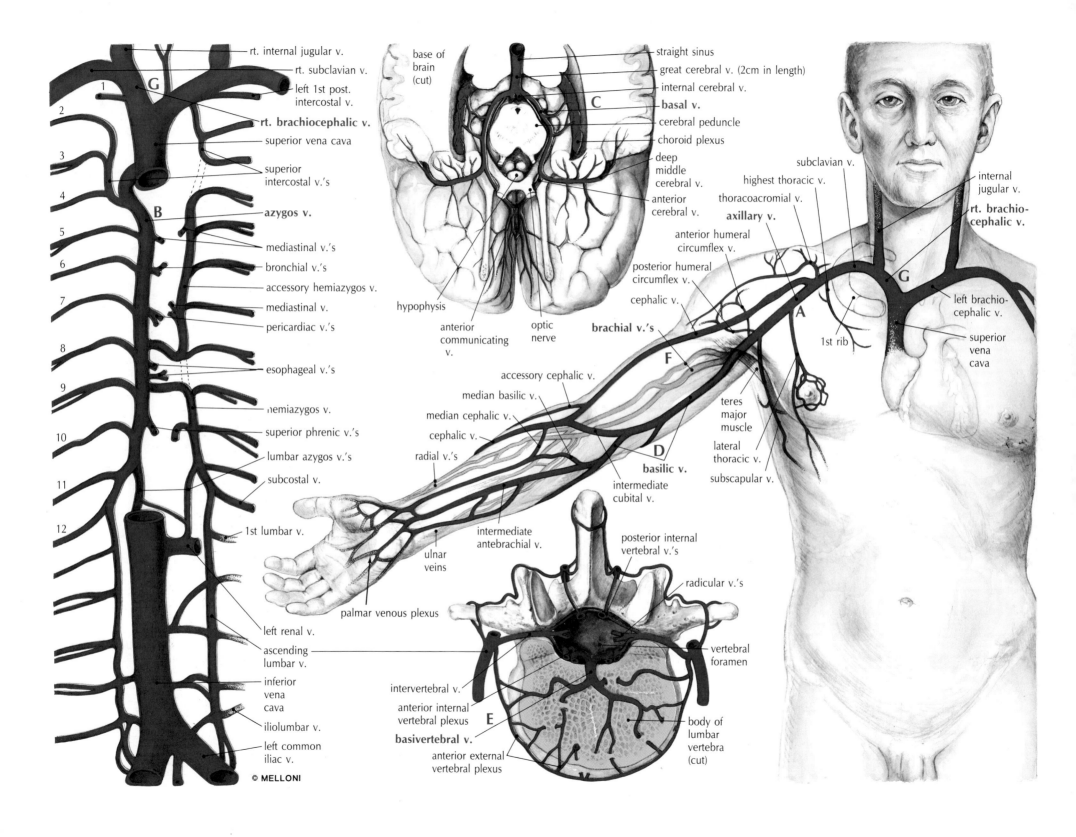

rt. internal jugular v.
rt. subclavian v.
left 1st post. intercostal v.
rt. brachiocephalic v.
superior vena cava
superior intercostal v.'s

1
2
3
4
B
5
6
7
8
9
10
11
12
G

azygos v.
mediastinal v.'s
bronchial v.'s
accessory hemiazygos v.
mediastinal v.
pericardiac v.'s
esophageal v.'s
hemiazygos v.
superior phrenic v.'s
lumbar azygos v.'s
subcostal v.
1st lumbar v.
left renal v.
ascending lumbar v.
inferior vena cava
iliolumbar v.
left common iliac v.

© MELLONI

base of brain (cut)
straight sinus
great cerebral v. (2cm in length)
internal cerebral v.
basal v.
cerebral peduncle
choroid plexus
deep middle cerebral v.
anterior cerebral v.
C
hypophysis
anterior communicating v.
optic nerve

subclavian v.
highest thoracic v.
thoracoacromial v.
axillary v.
anterior humeral circumflex v.
posterior humeral circumflex v.
cephalic v.
brachial v.'s
F
A
1st rib
internal jugular v.
rt. brachio-cephalic v.
G
left brachio-cephalic v.
superior vena cava
teres major muscle
lateral thoracic v.
subscapular v.

accessory cephalic v.
median basilic v.
median cephalic v.
cephalic v.
radial v.'s
D
basilic v.
intermediate cubital v.
intermediate antebrachial v.
ulnar veins
palmar venous plexus

posterior internal vertebral v.'s
radicular v.'s
vertebral foramen
intervertebral v.
anterior internal vertebral plexus
basivertebral v.
E
body of lumbar vertebra (cut)
anterior external vertebral plexus

	VEIN	LOCATION	DRAINS	TRIBUTARIES	EMPTIES INTO
A	**v. brachiocephalica sinistra** *brachiocephalic v., left*	from behind medial end of left clavicle, it courses downward obliquely to first right costal cartilage	head and left arm	internal jugular v., left subclavian v., thymic v.'s, left vertebral v.	superior vena cava in union with right brachiocephalic v.
B	**vv. bronchiales** *bronchial v.'s*	bronchi	bronchi and roots of lung	none	right side: azygos v. left side: left superior intercostal v. or accessory hemiazygos v.
C	**v. cardiaca magna** *cardiac v., great* *coronary v., left*	from apex of heart, courses up anterior interventricular sulcus	interventricular septum, anterior surface of ventricles and left atrium	anterior interventricular and circumflex branches	coronary sinus
D	**v. cardiaca media** *cardiac v., middle*	from apex of heart, courses up posterior interventricular sulcus	diaphragmatic surface of ventricular walls	none	coronary sinus, near its termination
E	**v. cardiaca parva** *cardiac v., small*	in coronary sulcus between right atrium and ventricles	walls of right atrium and ventricle	anterior cardiac v.'s	coronary sinus (near its termination) or middle cardiac v.
F	**vena cava inferior** *vena cava, inferior*	in front of vertebral column at 5th lumbar vertebra, ascends along right side of aorta, pierces diaphragm at level of 8th thoracic vertebra, and ends behind 6th right costal cartilage	lower half of the body (abdomen, pelvis, lower extremities)	both common iliac v.'s, median sacral v., lumbar v.'s, right gonadal v. (left drains into left renal v.), right suprarenal v. (left drains into left renal v.), hepatic v.'s, renal v.'s, inferior phrenic v.'s	lower part of right atrium of heart
G	**vena cava superior** (about 7 cm in length) *vena cava, superior*	courses vertically from the posterior surface of the 1st to 3rd costal cartilages close to margin of sternum	upper half of the body (head, neck, chest, upper extremities)	both brachiocephalic v.'s	upper part of right atrium of heart
H	**vv. centrales hepatis** *central v.'s of liver*	liver	liver lobules	peripheral and radial sinusoids	sublobular v. (interlobular v.)
I	**v. centralis retinae** *central v. of retina*	from optic disk it passes out of eyeball through optic nerve	retina	superior temporal venule, inferior temporal venule, superior nasal venule, inferior nasal venule, superior macular venule, inferior macular venule, medial venule	superior ophthalmic v. or cavernous sinus

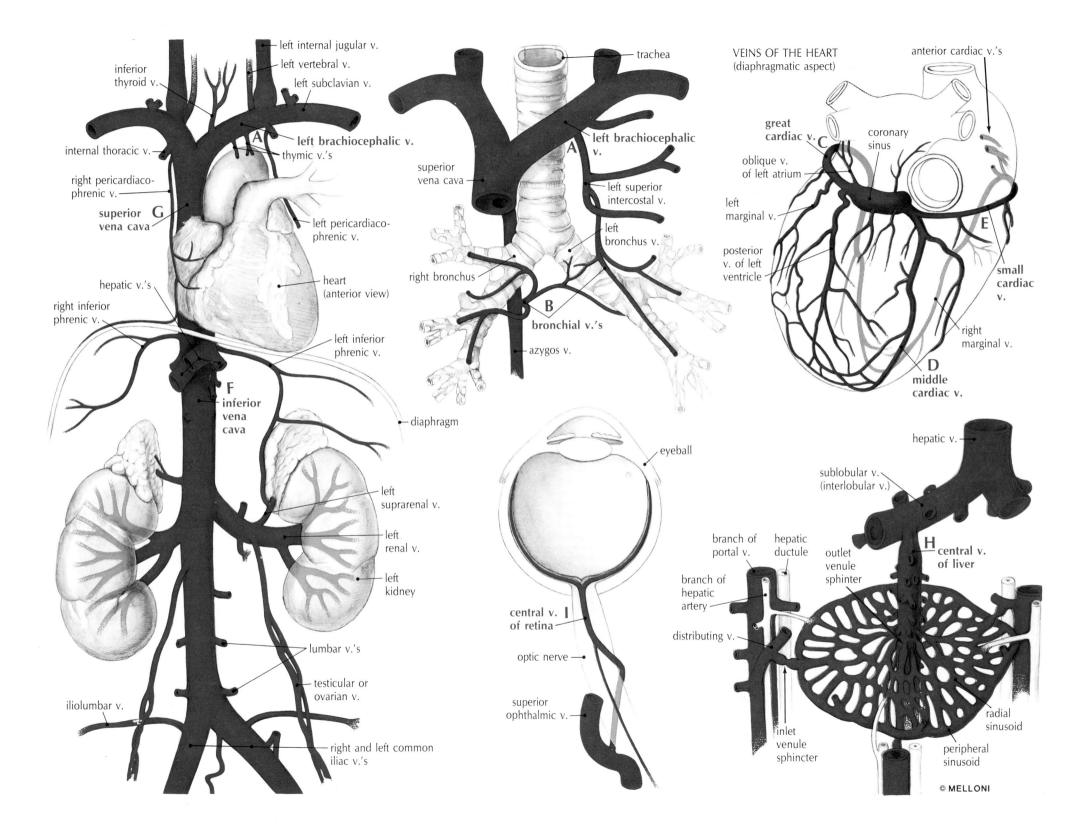

left internal jugular v.

left vertebral v.

left subclavian v.

inferior thyroid v.

left brachiocephalic v.

A

thymic v.'s

internal thoracic v.

right pericardiaco-phrenic v.

superior vena cava G

left pericardiaco-phrenic v.

heart (anterior view)

hepatic v.'s

right inferior phrenic v.

left inferior phrenic v.

F inferior vena cava

diaphragm

left suprarenal v.

left renal v.

left kidney

lumbar v.'s

testicular or ovarian v.

iliolumbar v.

right and left common iliac v.'s

trachea

left brachiocephalic v.

A

superior vena cava

left superior intercostal v.

left bronchus v.

right bronchus

B

bronchial v.'s

azygos v.

VEINS OF THE HEART
(diaphragmatic aspect)

anterior cardiac v.'s

great cardiac v. C

coronary sinus

oblique v. of left atrium

left marginal v.

posterior v. of left ventricle

E

small cardiac v.

right marginal v.

D

middle cardiac v.

eyeball

central v. of retina I

optic nerve

superior ophthalmic v.

hepatic v.

sublobular v. (interlobular v.)

branch of portal v.

hepatic ductule

outlet venule sphincter

H central v. of liver

branch of hepatic artery

distributing v.

inlet venule sphincter

radial sinusoid

peripheral sinusoid

© MELLONI

	VEIN	LOCATION	DRAINS	TRIBUTARIES	EMPTIES INTO
A	**v. cephalica** *cephalic v.*	from near base of thumb, courses up arm to just below the level of the clavicle	upper limb	dorsal venous arch of hand, accessory cephalic v.	axillary v.
B	**vv. cerebelli inferiores** *cerebellar v.'s, inferior*	from the lower surface of cerebellum they all course laterally except one, which runs backward on the inferior vermis	lower surface of cerebellum	neighboring v.'s	lateral v.'s: inferior petrosal sinus, transverse and sigmoid sinuses median v.: straight sinus or sigmoid sinus
C	**vv. cerebelli superiores** *cerebellar v.'s, superior*	from upper surface of cerebellum they course forward and medially across the superior vermis	upper region of cerebellum	neighboring v.'s	lateral v.'s: transverse sinus, superior petrosal sinus median v.'s: great cerebral v. or straight sinus
D	**v. cerebri anterior** *cerebral v. anterior*	from the upper surface of the posterior extremity of the corpus callosum, it runs forward in the longitudinal cerebral fissure, courses around the genu, and passes backward and laterally across the anterior perforated substance to the medial and of the lateral cerebral sulcus	diencaphalon, corpus striatum, internal capsule, choroid plexus of lateral ventricle, anterior third of corpus callosum, anterior part of medial surface of frontal lobe, medial orbital frontal gyri	central and cortical branches from neighboring v.'s (communicates with the contralateral anterior cerebral v. via the anterior communicating v.)	basal v., in union with the deep middle cerebral v.
E	**vv. cerebri inferiores** *cerebral v.'s, inferior*	lower part of brain	inferolateral surface of cerebral hemisphere	small v.'s from temporal lobe and orbital surface of frontal lobe, vein of the uncus	frontal: superior cerebral v.'s, superior sagittal sinus temporal: basal and deep cerebral v.'s., cavernous, superior petrosal and transverse sinuses occipital: straight sinus
F	**vv. cerebri internae** *cerebral v.'s, internal*	from near the interventricular foramen they pass backward through the tela choroidea (pia mater) of the 3rd ventricle	choroid plexus of 3rd and lateral ventricles, midbrain, pons, corpus callosum	superior choroidal v. anterior septal v., posterior septal v., direct lateral v., thalamostriate v.'s, v. of midbrain, veins of pons, medial atrial v.,	great cerebral v., in union with basal v.'s

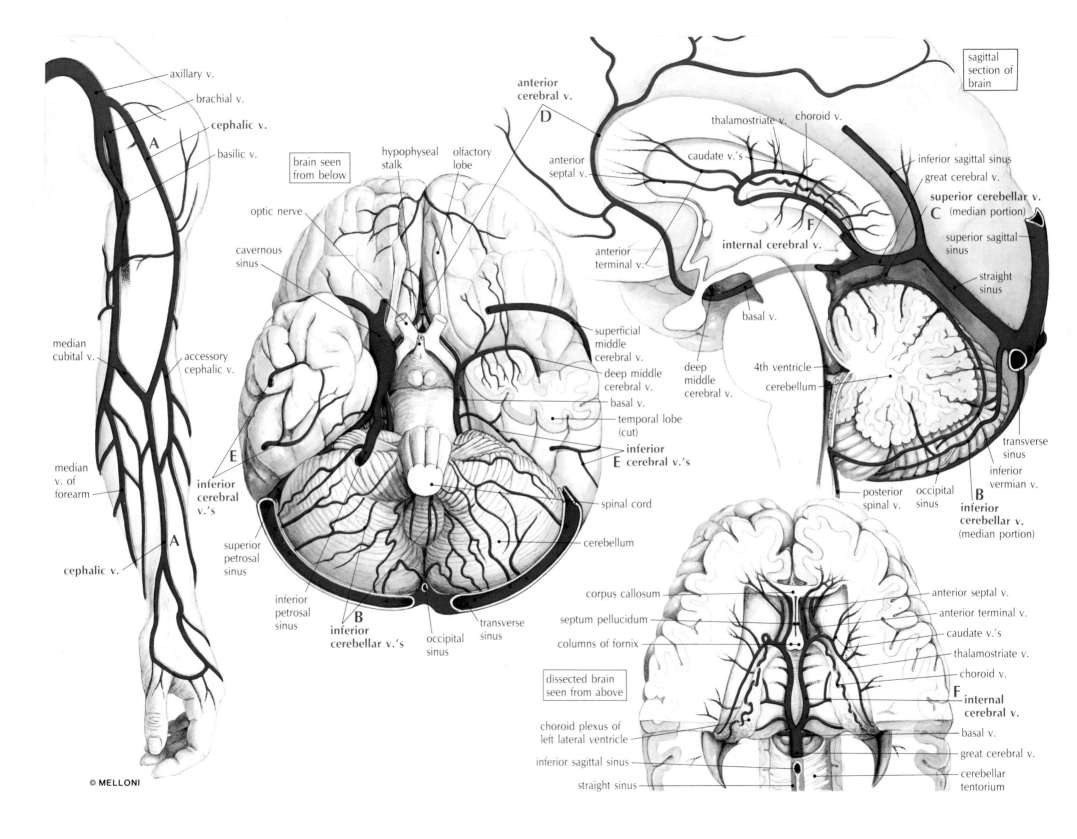

axillary v.

brachial v.

cephalic v.

basilic v.

A

median cubital v.

accessory cephalic v.

median v. of forearm

A

cephalic v.

© MELLONI

anterior cerebral v.

D

anterior septal v.

brain seen from below

hypophyseal stalk

olfactory lobe

optic nerve

cavernous sinus

superficial middle cerebral v.

deep middle cerebral v.

basal v.

temporal lobe (cut)

inferior
E cerebral v.'s

inferior cerebral v.'s

E

superior petrosal sinus

spinal cord

cerebellum

inferior petrosal sinus

inferior cerebellar v.'s

B

occipital sinus

transverse sinus

sagittal section of brain

thalamostriate v.

choroid v.

caudate v.'s

inferior sagittal sinus

great cerebral v.

superior cerebellar v.
C (median portion)

superior sagittal sinus

straight sinus

internal cerebral v.

F

anterior terminal v.

deep middle cerebral v.

basal v.

deep middle cerebral v.

4th ventricle

cerebellum

transverse sinus

inferior vermian v.

posterior spinal v.

occipital sinus

B
inferior cerebellar v. (median portion)

corpus callosum

anterior septal v.

septum pellucidum

anterior terminal v.

columns of fornix

caudate v.'s

thalamostriate v.

choroid v.

dissected brain seen from above

F internal cerebral v.

choroid plexus of left lateral ventricle

basal v.

inferior sagittal sinus

great cerebral v.

straight sinus

cerebellar tentorium

	VEIN	LOCATION	DRAINS	TRIBUTARIES	EMPTIES INTO
A	**v. cerebri magna** (2 cm in length) *cerebral v., great; great v. of Galen*	between junction of the two internal cerebral veins and straight sinus, curving sharply upward around the splenium of the corpus callosum	midbrain, pons, choroid plexus of 3rd and lateral ventricles, superomedial surface of the cerebrum, insula	basal v.'s, internal cerebral v.'s, posterior pericallosal v., internal occipital v., posterior mesencephalic v., precentral cerebellar v., superior vermian v., medial atrial v., lateral atrial v., superior cerebellar v. (occasionally)	straight sinus, in union with the inferior sagittal sinus
B	**v. cerebri media profunda** *cerebral v., deep middle*	on the insula, floor of lateral sulcus of the cerebrum	cortex of insula, lateral surface of the cerebrum, inferior part of corpus callosum	veins of lateral surface of the cerebrum, insula v.	basal v. in union with anterior cerebral v.
C	**v. cerebri media superficialis** *cerebral v., superficial middle*	from the lateral surface of cerebral hemisphere it passes along the lateral sulcus (between frontal and parietal lobes above and temporal lobe below)	most of the orbital, frontal, parietal, and temporal cortex, corpus striatum, internal capsule	inferior anastomotic v., superior anastomotic v.	cavernous sinus or sphenoparietal sinus
D	**vv. cerebri superiores** (9 to 12 in number on each cerebral hemisphere) *cerebral v.'s, superior*	the sulci between the gyri	superolateral and medial surfaces of the cerebrum	prefrontal v.'s, frontal v.'s, parietal v.'s, occipital v.'s	superior sagittal sinus
E	**v. cervicalis profunda** *cervical v., deep*	from suboccipital region, courses down neck to level of first rib	back of head and neck	occipital v., cervical spine plexus, veins of back of neck	vertebral v. or brachiocephalic v.
F	**vv. ciliares anteriores** *ciliary v.'s, anterior*	from ciliary body they pierce the sclera near the cornea	scleral venous sinus (canal of Schlemm), conjunctiva	episcleral v.'s, anterior conjunctival v.'s, scleral v.'s	superior ophthalmic v.
G	**vv. ciliares posteriores** (usually four in number) *ciliary v.'s, posterior*	from vascular tunic of eyeball (choroid layer) they pierce the sclera obliquely	uveal tract (choroid, ciliary body and iris)	veins from ciliary body, iris, and network of choroidal veins, bulbus venae vorticosae, episcleral v.'s	upper v.'s: superior ophthalmic v. lower v.'s: inferior ophthalmic v.
H	**vv. circumflexae femoris laterales** *circumflex femoral v.'s, lateral*	posterolateral thigh	head and neck of femur, thigh muscles	ascending, descending, transverse branches	femoral v. or deep femoral v.
I	**vv. circumflexae femoris mediales** *circumflex femoral v.'s, medial*	posteromedial thigh	hip joint, adductor muscles of thigh	deep, ascending transverse acetabular branches	femoral v. or deep femoral v.

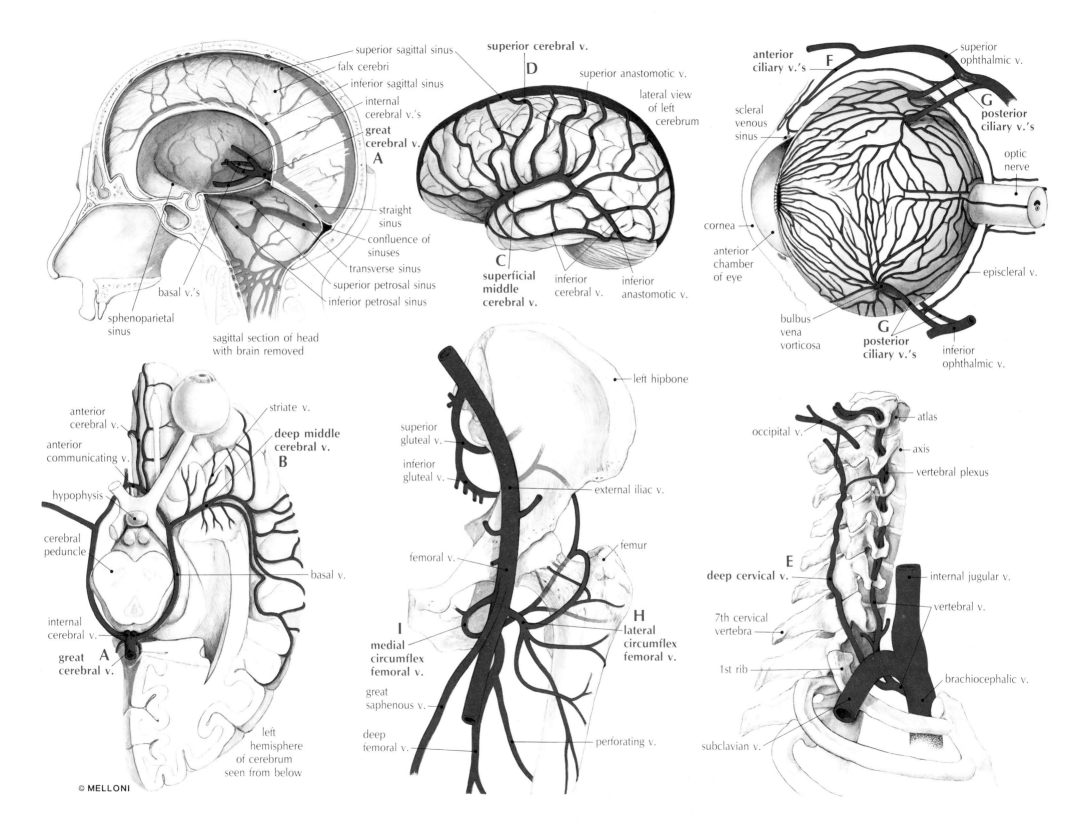

superior sagittal sinus

falx cerebri

inferior sagittal sinus

internal cerebral v.'s

great cerebral v.

A

straight sinus

confluence of sinuses

transverse sinus

superior petrosal sinus

inferior petrosal sinus

basal v.'s

sphenoparietal sinus

sagittal section of head with brain removed

superior cerebral v.

D

superior anastomotic v.

lateral view of left cerebrum

C

superficial middle cerebral v.

inferior cerebral v.

inferior anastomotic v.

anterior ciliary v.'s

F

superior ophthalmic v.

G

posterior ciliary v.'s

scleral venous sinus

optic nerve

cornea

anterior chamber of eye

bulbus vena vorticosa

G

posterior ciliary v.'s

episcleral v.

inferior ophthalmic v.

anterior cerebral v.

anterior communicating v.

hypophysis

cerebral peduncle

internal cerebral v.

great cerebral v.

A

striate v.

deep middle cerebral v.

B

basal v.

left hemisphere of cerebrum seen from below

© MELLONI

left hipbone

superior gluteal v.

inferior gluteal v.

external iliac v.

femur

femoral v.

H

lateral circumflex femoral v.

I

medial circumflex femoral v.

great saphenous v.

deep femoral v.

perforating v.

occipital v.

atlas

axis

vertebral plexus

E

deep cervical v.

internal jugular v.

7th cervical vertebra

vertebral v.

1st rib

brachiocephalic v.

subclavian v.

	VEIN	LOCATION	DRAINS	TRIBUTARIES	EMPTIES INTO
A	**v. circumflexa ilium profunda** *circumflex iliac v., deep*	lower abdomen	internal oblique, transversus abdominis, iliacus, psoas, and sartorius muscles	ascending branch	external iliac v. (about 2 cm above level of inguinal ligament)
B	**v. circumflexa ilium superficialis** *circumflex iliac v., superficial*	from ilium, courses downward obliquely to level of inguinal ligament	superficial inguinal lymph nodes, skin of groin	none	great saphenous v. or femoral v.
C	**v. colica dextra** *colic v., right*	along medial side of ascending colon and right colic (hepatic) flexure	ascending colon and right flexure	colic and ileal branches, marginal v.'s	superior mesenteric v.
D	**v. coloca media** *colic v., middle*	just behind transverse colon	transverse colon	right and left branches, marginal v.'s	superior mesenteric v.
E	**v. colica sinistra** (may be divided into superior and inferior left colic veins) *colic v., left*	along the medial side of descending colon and left colic (splenic) flexure	descending colon and left flexure	ascending and descending branches, marginal v.'s	inferior mesenteric v.
F	**v. comitans n. hypoglossi** *v. accompanying hypoglossal nerve* *ranine v.*	near hypoglossal nerve in tongue	tip and inferior part of tongue, sublingual salivary gland	deep lingual v., sublingual v.	lingual v. or facial v. or internal jugular v.
G	**v. cystica** *cystic v.*	from fundus of gallbladder, courses dorsocephalically into substance of liver	gallbladder, areolar tissue between liver and gallbladder	superficial and deep branches	right branch of portal v. (intrahepatic)
H	**vv. digitales dorsales manus** *digital v.'s of hand, dorsal*	along side of fingers	fingers	oblique communicating branches	dorsal metacarpal v.'s, after uniting with each other
I	**vv. digitales dorsales pedis** *digital v.'s of foot, dorsal*	dorsum of toes and clefts between toes	dorsum of foot, toes	perforating v.'s, plantar digital v.'s	dorsal metatarsal v.'s, after uniting with each other

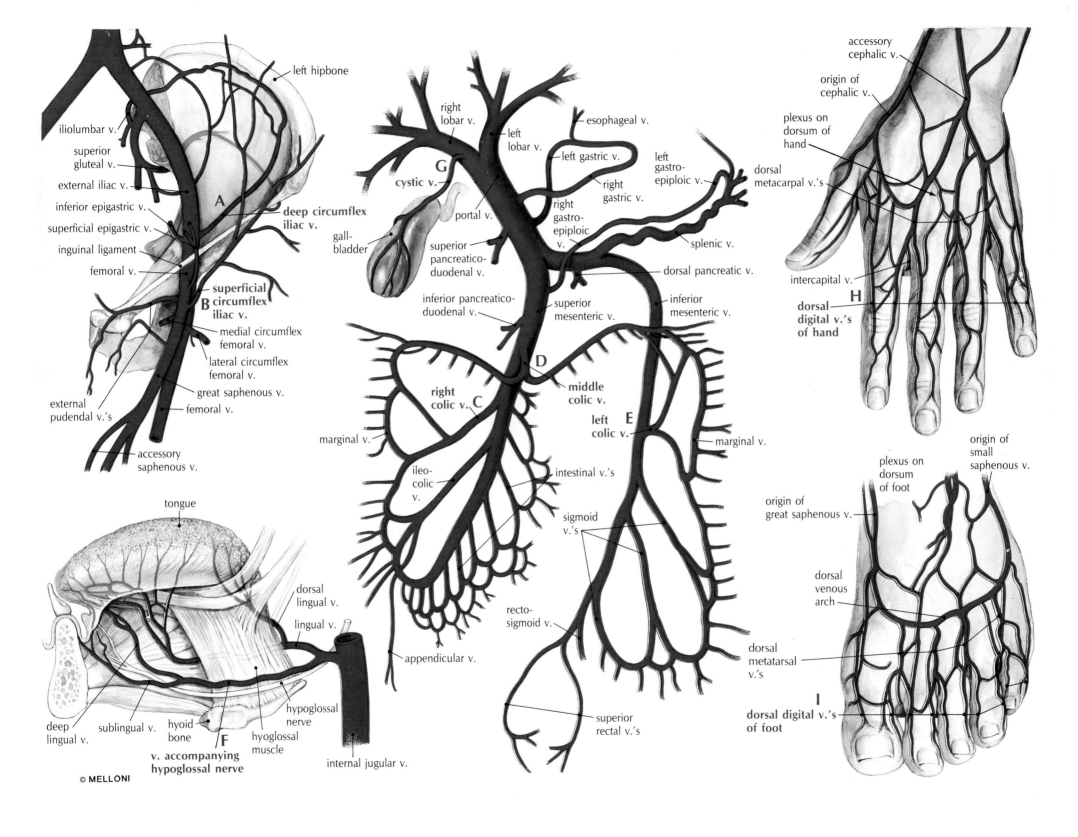

left hipbone

iliolumbar v.

superior gluteal v.

external iliac v.

inferior epigastric v.

superficial epigastric v.

inguinal ligament

femoral v.

A

deep circumflex iliac v.

B **superficial circumflex iliac v.**

medial circumflex femoral v.

lateral circumflex femoral v.

great saphenous v.

femoral v.

external pudendal v.'s

accessory saphenous v.

right lobar v.

G

cystic v.

gallbladder

portal v.

superior pancreatico-duodenal v.

inferior pancreatico-duodenal v.

left lobar v.

esophageal v.

left gastric v.

right gastric v.

left gastro-epiploic v.

right gastro-epiploic v.

splenic v.

dorsal pancreatic v.

superior mesenteric v.

inferior mesenteric v.

D

right colic v. **C**

middle colic v.

left colic v. **E**

marginal v.

marginal v.

ileo-colic v.

intestinal v.'s

sigmoid v.'s

recto-sigmoid v.

appendicular v.

superior rectal v.'s

accessory cephalic v.

origin of cephalic v.

plexus on dorsum of hand

dorsal metacarpal v.'s

intercapital v.

H

dorsal digital v.'s of hand

origin of small saphenous v.

plexus on dorsum of foot

origin of great saphenous v.

dorsal venous arch

dorsal metatarsal v.'s

I

dorsal digital v.'s of foot

tongue

dorsal lingual v.

lingual v.

hypoglossal nerve

deep lingual v.

sublingual v.

hyoid bone

F

hyoglossal muscle

v. accompanying hypoglossal nerve

internal jugular v.

© MELLONI

	VEIN	LOCATION	DRAINS	TRIBUTARIES	EMPTIES INTO
A	**vv. diploicae** *diploic v.'s*	A series of endothelium-lined channels located in cancellous tissue (diploe) between the inner and outer tables of cranial bones (calvaria) that communicate with the sinuses of the dura mater and pericranial v.'s; the major channels include frontal diploic v., anterior temporal diploic v., posterior temporal diploic v., and occipital diploic v.; the channels generally start to appear at the age of about 2 years.			
B	**vv. dorsales clitoridis superficiales** *dorsal v.'s of clitoris, superficial*	on dorsum of clitoris	prepuce and mucosa of clitoris and surrounding area	small branches from mucosa of clitoris and surrounding area	external pudendal v.'s or femoral v.
C	**v. dorsalis clitoridis profunda** *dorsal v. of clitoris, deep*	on dorsum of midline of clitoris, deep to the fascia; passes under the pubic symphysis	glans clitoris, corpus cavernosum (right and left)	small branches from clitoris	vesical venous plexus, internal pudendal v.
D	**vv. dorsales linguae** *dorsal lingual v.'s* *dorsal v. of tongue*	dorsum of tongue	dorsum and sides of tongue	none	lingual v.
E	**vv. dorsales penis superficiales** *dorsal v.'s of penis, superficial*	on dorsum of penis	skin of penis including prepuce	small branches from skin and mucosa of penis	external pudendal veins, superficial epigastric v.
F	**v. dorsalis penis profunda** *dorsal v. of penis, deep*	from dorsum of midline of penis (between deep fascia and tunica albuginea) it courses under the pubic symphysis	glans penis, corpus cavernosum of penis	branches from glans penis and upper surface of corpus cavernosum	prostatic venous plexus, internal pudendal v.
G	**vv. emissarias** *emissary v.'s*	Veins that pass through foramina in the skull to link the venous sinuses and diploic veins with the veins on the surface of the skull; the more constant emissary veins include condylar emissary v., mastoid emissary v., occipital emissary v., and parietal emissary v.			
H	**v. epigastrica inferior** *epigastric v., inferior*	from substance of rectus muscle in abdominal wall, descends to a level just above the inguinal ligament	rectus abdominis muscle, cremaster muscle, skin	superior epigastric v.'s, pubic v., v. of round ligament, muscular and cutaneous branches	external iliac v.
I	**v. epigastrica superficialis** *epigastric v., superficial*	lower anterior abdominal wall	lower anterior abdominal wall	thoracoepigastric v.	great saphenous v. or femoral v.

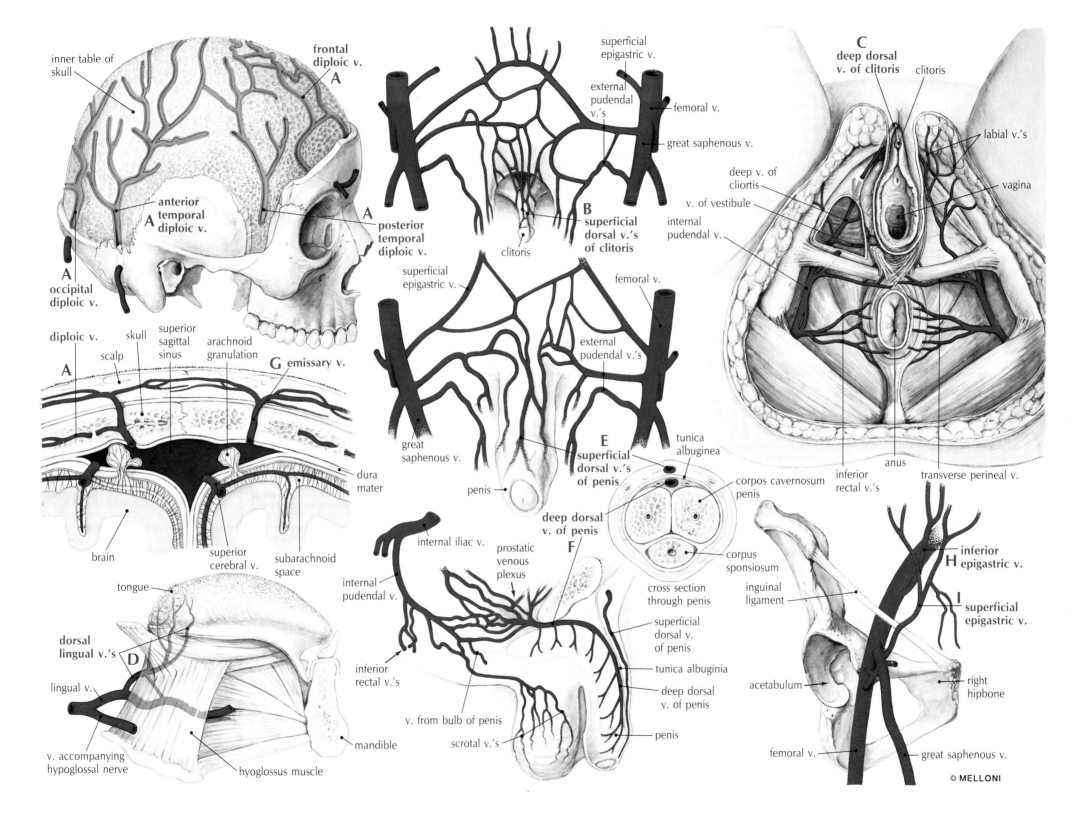

inner table of skull

frontal diploic v.

A

anterior temporal diploic v.

A

A

A posterior temporal diploic v.

A occipital diploic v.

diploic v.

scalp

skull

superior sagittal sinus

arachnoid granulation

A

G emissary v.

brain

superior cerebral v.

subarachnoid space

dura mater

tongue

dorsal lingual v.'s

D

lingual v.

v. accompanying hypoglossal nerve

hyoglossus muscle

mandible

superficial epigastric v.

external pudendal v.'s

femoral v.

great saphenous v.

B superficial dorsal v.'s of clitoris

clitoris

superficial epigastric v.

femoral v.

external pudendal v.'s

great saphenous v.

E superficial dorsal v.'s of penis

penis

deep dorsal v. of penis

F

internal iliac v.

prostatic venous plexus

internal pudendal v.

inferior rectal v.'s

v. from bulb of penis

scrotal v.'s

superficial dorsal v. of penis

tunica albuginia

deep dorsal v. of penis

penis

tunica albuginea

corpos cavernosum penis

corpus sponsiosum

cross section through penis

C deep dorsal v. of cliortis

clitoris

labial v.'s

deep v. of cliortis

vagina

v. of vestibule

internal pudendal v.

inferior rectal v.'s

anus

transverse perineal v.

inguinal ligament

H inferior epigastric v.

I superficial epigastric v.

acetabulum

right hipbone

femoral v.

great saphenous v.

© MELLONI

	VEIN	LOCATION	DRAINS	TRIBUTARIES	EMPTIES INTO
A	**vv. epigastricae superiores** *epigastric v.'s, superior*	upper anterior abdominal wall to costal cartilages	upper anterior abdominal wall	subcutaneous abdominal v.'s	internal thoracic v.'s
B	**vv. esophageales** *esophageal v.'s*	esophagus	esophagus	none	azygos v., left gastric v., left brachiocephalic v.
C	**v. facialis** *facial v.*	from side of face, it courses obliquely downward, crossing lower margin of body of mandible	face, tonsil, soft palate, submandibular gland, pterygoid venous plexus (through deep facial v.), cavernous sinus (through superior ophthalmic v.)	superior ophthalmic v., deep facial v., angular v., retromandibular v. (anterior division), superior labial v., inferior labial v.'s, inferior palpebral v.'s, superior palpebral v.'s, parotid v.'s, masseteric v.'s, submental v., external palatine v., pharyngeal v.'s, superior thyroid v.	internal jugular v.
D	**v. faciei profunda** *facial v., deep*	from infratemporal fossa, courses downward on maxilla just below the zygomatic bone	pterygoid plexus	none	facial v.
E	**v. femoralis** *femoral v.*	from adductor canal of thigh, courses upward to level of inguinal ligament	lower abdominal wall, external genitalia, muscles of thigh, superficial lymph nodes	popliteal v., deep femoral v., great saphenous v., lateral circumflex femoral v.'s, medial circumflex femoral v.'s	external iliac v., at level of inguinal ligament
F	**vv. gastricae breves** *gastric v.'s, short*	courses within gastrolienal ligament between fundus of stomach and spleen	fundus and left side of greater curvature of stomach	none	splenic v.
G	**v. gastrica dextra** *gastric v., right;* *short pyloric v.*	along lesser curvature of stomach	both surfaces of upper stomach, pyloris	prepyloric v.	portal v.
H	**v. gastrica sinistra** *gastric v., left;* *coronary v.*	from lower esophagus and upper stomach, courses downward and to the right	both surfaces of cardia of stomach	esophageal v.'s	portal v.

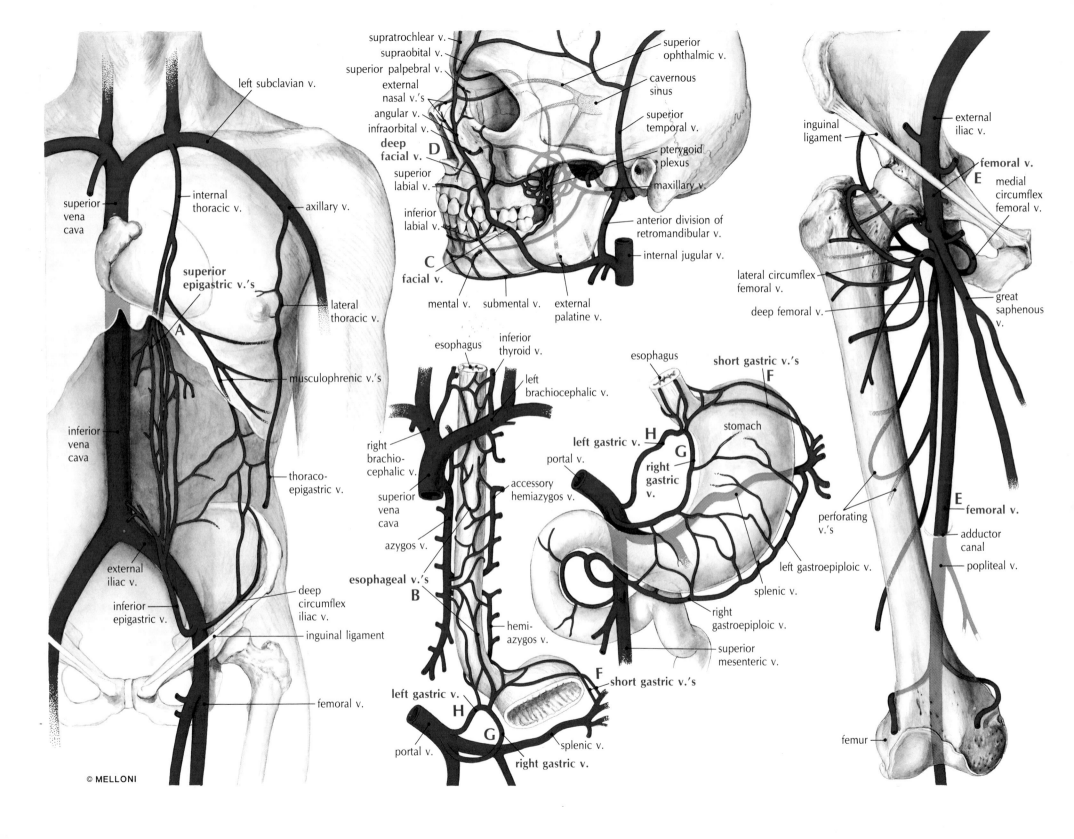

left subclavian v.

internal thoracic v.

axillary v.

superior vena cava

superior epigastric v.'s

A

lateral thoracic v.

musculophrenic v.'s

inferior vena cava

thoraco-epigastric v.

external iliac v.

deep circumflex iliac v.

inferior epigastric v.

inguinal ligament

femoral v.

© MELLONI

supratrochlear v.

supraobital v.

superior palpebral v.

external nasal v.'s

angular v.

infraorbital v.

deep facial v.

D

superior labial v.

inferior labial v.

C

facial v.

mental v.   submental v.   external palatine v.

superior ophthalmic v.

cavernous sinus

superior temporal v.

pterygoid plexus

maxillary v.

anterior division of retromandibular v.

internal jugular v.

esophagus   inferior thyroid v.

left brachiocephalic v.

right brachio-cephalic v.

superior vena cava

azygos v.

accessory hemiazygos v.

esophageal v.'s

B

hemi-azygos v.

left gastric v.

H

G

portal v.

right gastric v.

splenic v.

esophagus   **short gastric v.'s**

F

left gastric v. **H**

G

portal v.

right gastric v.

stomach

left gastroepiploic v.

splenic v.

right gastroepiploic v.

superior mesenteric v.

F   **short gastric v.'s**

inguinal ligament

external iliac v.

medial circumflex femoral v.

femoral v.

E

lateral circumflex femoral v.

deep femoral v.

great saphenous v.

perforating v.'s

E **femoral v.**

adductor canal

popliteal v.

femur

	VEIN	LOCATION	DRAINS	TRIBUTARIES	EMPTIES INTO
A	**v. gastroepiploica dextra** *gastroepiploic v., right; gastro-omental v., right*	from left to right along lower part of greater curvature of stomach	both surfaces of lower stomach and adjacent greater omentum	branches from both surfaces of lower part of stomach and greater omentum	superior mesenteric v., below level of neck of pancreas
B	**v. gastroepiploica sinistra** *gastroepiploic v., left; gastro-omental v., left*	from right to left along upper part of greater curvature of stomach	both surfaces of upper stomach and adjacent greater omentum	branches from both surfaces of upper part of stomach and greater omentum	splenic v.
C	**vv. geniculares** *genicular v.'s*	knee	structures around knee	none	popliteal v.
D	**vv. gluteae inferiores** *gluteal v.'s, inferior*	from upper part of posterior surface of thigh, they course into pelvis through lower part of greater sciatic foramen	muscles of buttock and back of thigh	medial circumflex femoral v.'s, first perforating v.,	internal iliac v.
E	**vv. gluteae superiores** *gluteal v.'s, superior*	short v.'s under gluteus maximus muscle, coursing forward into pelvis through greater sciatic foramen (above piriformis muscle)	muscles of buttock, ilium, skin over sacrum	nutrient v. of hipbone, muscular (deep and superficial) and cutaneous branches, inferior gluteal v.'s	internal iliac v.
F	**v. hemiazygos** *hemiazygos v.*	from left side of vertebral column at level of 2nd lumbar vertebra, it courses upward through diaphragm to eighth thoracic vertebra, where it turns obliquely to the right and crosses the vertebral column behind the aorta and esophagus	intercostal spaces, muscles of back, vertebral bodies, mediastinum, esophagus	posterior intercostal v's, IX–XI, accessory hemiazygos v., left esophageal v.'s left mediastinal v.'s, union of left ascending lumbar and subcostal v.'s, superior phrenic v.'s	azygos v. at level of 9th thoracic vertebra
G	**v. hemiazygos accessoria** *hemiazygos v., accessory*	vertically situated in posterior mediastinum on left side of thoracic vertebrae 5 to 8	intercostal space, mediastinum, bronchus	intercostal v.'s 4 to 8, left posterior bronchial v.'s	hemiazygos v. or azygos v.
H	**vv. hepaticae** *hepatic v.'s*	posterior surface of right, left, and caudate lobes of liver	liver	right hepatic v.: sublobular v.'s from right lobe of liver intermediate hepatic v.: sublobular v.'s from caudate lobe of liver left hepatic v.: sublobular v.'s from left lobe of liver	inferior vena cava

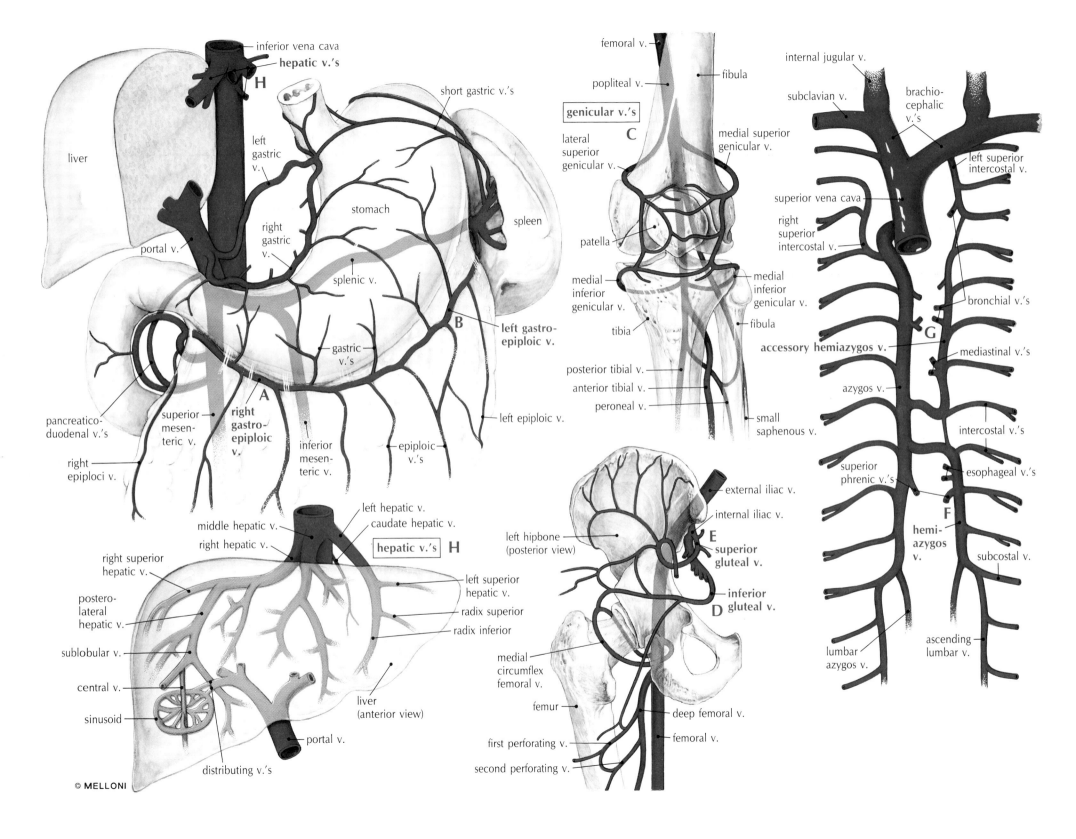

inferior vena cava
hepatic v.'s
H
liver
portal v.
left gastric v.
right gastric v.
short gastric v.'s
stomach
spleen
splenic v.
left gastro-epiploic v.
B
pancreatico-duodenal v.'s
superior mesenteric v.
right gastro-epiploic v.
gastric v.'s
A
inferior mesenteric v.
left epiploic v.
epiploic v.'s
right epiploci v.

femoral v.
popliteal v.
fibula
genicular v.'s
C
lateral superior genicular v.
medial superior genicular v.
patella
medial inferior genicular v.
medial inferior genicular v.
tibia
fibula
posterior tibial v.
anterior tibial v.
peroneal v.
small saphenous v.

internal jugular v.
subclavian v.
brachio-cephalic v.'s
left superior intercostal v.
superior vena cava
right superior intercostal v.
G
bronchial v.'s
accessory hemiazygos v.
mediastinal v.'s
azygos v.
intercostal v.'s
superior phrenic v.'s
esophageal v.'s
F
hemi-azygos v.
subcostal v.
lumbar azygos v.
ascending lumbar v.

middle hepatic v.
left hepatic v.
caudate hepatic v.
right hepatic v.
hepatic v.'s **H**
right superior hepatic v.
left superior hepatic v.
postero-lateral hepatic v.
radix superior
radix inferior
sublobular v.
central v.
sinusoid
liver (anterior view)
portal v.
distributing v.'s

external iliac v.
internal iliac v.
left hipbone (posterior view)
E
superior gluteal v.
inferior gluteal v. **D**
medial circumflex femoral v.
femur
deep femoral v.
first perforating v.
femoral v.
second perforating v.

© MELLONI

	VEIN	LOCATION	DRAINS	TRIBUTARIES	EMPTIES INTO

A	**vv. intercostales posterior**
	intercostal v.'s, posterior
		intercostal spaces	intercostal spaces, muscles and skin of back	dorsal and spinal branches, intervertebral v.'s	right side:
					  1st—right brachiocephalic v.
					  2nd, 3rd, 4th—right superior intercostal v.
					  5th, 6th, 7th—azygos v.
					  8th, 9th, 10th, 11th, 12th—azygos v.
					
					left side:
					  1st—left brachiocephalic v.
					  2nd, 3rd, 4th—left superior intercostal v.
					  5th, 6th, 7th, 8th—accessory hemiazygos v.
					  9th, 10th, 11th, 12th—hemiazygos v.

B	**v. intercostalis superior dextra** *intercostal v., right superior*	from the upper right intercostal spaces, it courses to the area of the back side of the superior vena cava	intercostal spaces	2nd, 3rd, and occasionally 4th posterior intercostal v.'s	azygos v.
C	**v. intercostalis superior sinistra** *intercostal v., left superior*	from upper left intercostal spaces, course obliquely to area of left side of aortic arch	left 2nd, 3rd, and occasionally 4th intercostal spaces	left 2nd, 3rd, and occasionally 4th left posterior intercostal v.'s, left bronchial v.'s, left pericardiacophrenic v. (occasionally)	left brachiocephalic v.
D	**v. intercostalis suprema** *intercostal v., highest*	1st intercostal space	1st intercostal space	none	brachiocephalic v. or vertebral v.
E	**vv. interlobares renis** *interlobar v.'s of kidney*	from corticomedullary junction of kidney, course down between pyramids (renal lobes)	venous arcades of kidney	arcuate v.'s	renal v.
F	**vv. interlobulares renis** *interlobular v.'s of kidney*	from superficial part of renal cortex, they course toward the corticomedullary junction	peritubular capillary network of the corticomedullary area of kidney	cortical capillary plexus, stellate venules, perforating v.'s, capsular venous plexus	arcuate v.'s

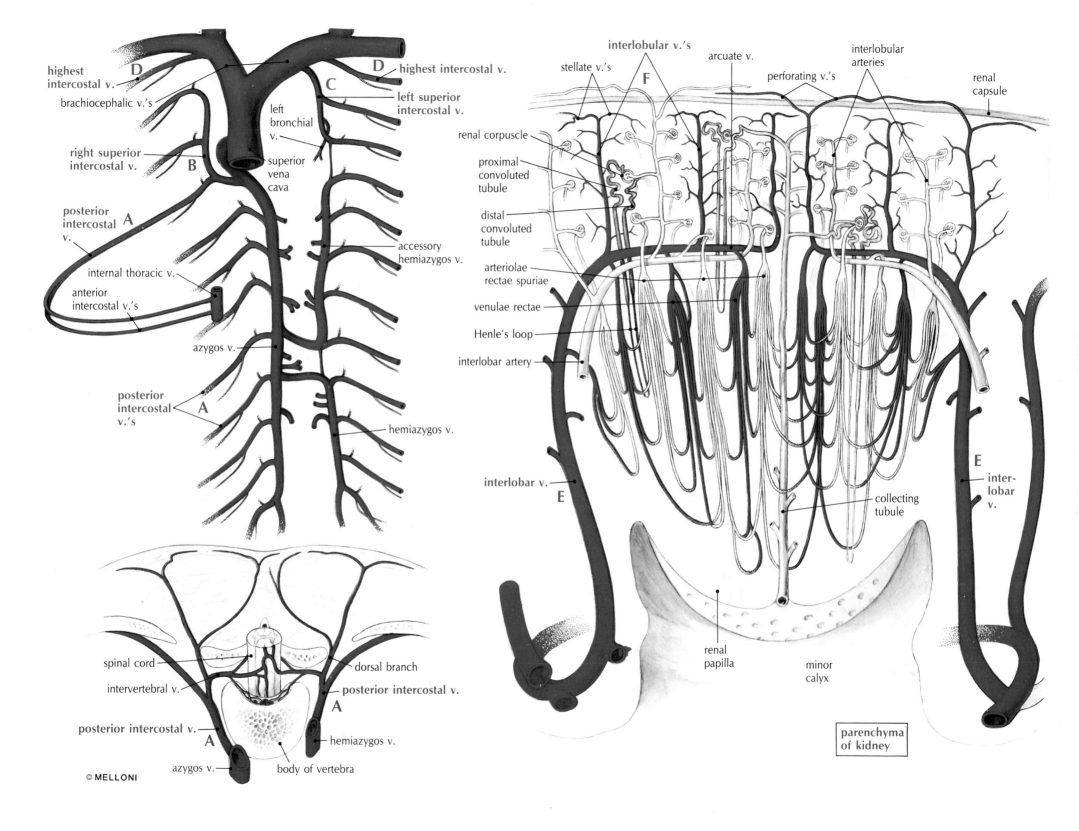

highest intercostal v.

D

brachiocephalic v.'s

right superior intercostal v.

B

posterior intercostal v.

A

internal thoracic v.

anterior intercostal v.'s

azygos v.

posterior intercostal v.'s

A

left bronchial v.

superior vena cava

D highest intercostal v.

C

left superior intercostal v.

accessory hemiazygos v.

hemiazygos v.

spinal cord

intervertebral v.

posterior intercostal v.

A

azygos v.

dorsal branch

posterior intercostal v.

A

hemiazygos v.

body of vertebra

© MELLONI

stellate v.'s

interlobular v.'s

F

arcuate v.

interlobular arteries

perforating v.'s

renal capsule

renal corpuscle

proximal convoluted tubule

distal convoluted tubule

arteriolae rectae spuriae

venulae rectae

Henle's loop

interlobar artery

interlobar v.

E

E

inter- lobar v.

collecting tubule

renal papilla

minor calyx

parenchyma of kidney

	VEIN	LOCATION	DRAINS	TRIBUTARIES	EMPTIES INTO
A	**v. intermedia antebrachii** *intermediate antebrachial v; median antebrachial v. median v. of forearm*	front of forearm	forearm, palm of hand	superficial palmar venous plexus, subcutaneous venous network of forearm	basilic v. or intermediate (median) cubital v.
B	**v. intermedia cubiti** *intermediate cubital v; median cubital v.*	passes across the bend of the elbow from lateral below obliquely to medial above	forearm	cephalic v., communicating branches from deep v.'s of forearm	basilic v.
C	**v. intervertebralis** *intervertebral v.*	intervertebral foramen	vertebral column	veins from spinal cord, internal and external vertebral venous plexuses	neck: vertebral v. thorax: posterior intercostal v. abdomen: lumbar v.'s pelvis: lateral sacral v.'s
D	**vv. jejunales** *jejunal v.'s*	adjacent to jejunum	jejunum	marginal v.'s	superior mesenteric v.
E	**v. jugularis anterior** *jugular v., anterior*	from just above hyoid bone, courses downward along medial border of sternocleidomastoid muscle to lower neck, where it turns laterally to area behind middle of clavicle	anterior neck region	superficial veins just below the chin, facial v., jugular arch, laryngeal v.'s	external jugular v.
F	**v. jugularis externa** *jugular v., external*	from level of mandibular angle, it courses downward to middle of clavicle just under the platysma	superficial and deep parts of the scalp and face	posterior auricular v., retromandibular v. (posterior division), posterior external jugular v., transverse cervical v.'s, supraclavicular v., anterior jugular v.	subclavian v. or internal jugular v.
G	**v. jugularis externa posterior** *jugular v., posterior external*	from occipital region, courses downward somewhat parallel to the posterior border of the sternocleidomastoid muscle	skin and superficial muscles of back of neck	muscular v.'s, occasionally the occipital v.	about the middle of the external jugular vein

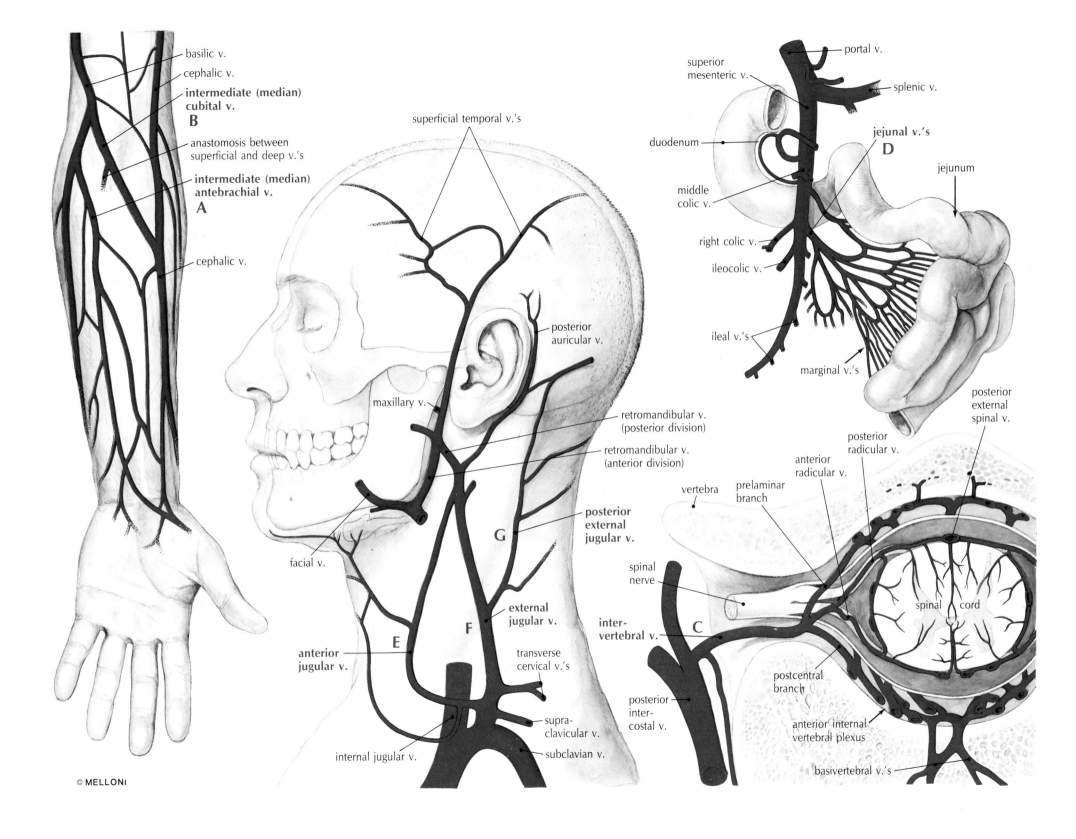

basilic v.

cephalic v.

intermediate (median) cubital v.

B

anastomosis between superficial and deep v.'s

intermediate (median) antebrachial v.

A

cephalic v.

superficial temporal v.'s

posterior auricular v.

maxillary v.

retromandibular v. (posterior division)

retromandibular v. (anterior division)

posterior external jugular v.

facial v.

G

external jugular v.

E

F

anterior jugular v.

transverse cervical v.'s

supra-clavicular v.

internal jugular v.

subclavian v.

portal v.

superior mesenteric v.

splenic v.

jejunal v.'s

D

jejunum

duodenum

middle colic v.

right colic v.

ileocolic v.

ileal v.'s

marginal v.'s

posterior external spinal v.

posterior radicular v.

anterior radicular v.

vertebra

prelaminar branch

spinal nerve

inter-vertebral v.

C

posterior inter-costal v.

spinal cord

postcentral branch

anterior internal vertebral plexus

basivertebral v.'s

© MELLONI

	VEIN	LOCATION	DRAINS	TRIBUTARIES	EMPTIES INTO
A	**v. jugularis interna** *jugular v., internal*	from jugular foramen at base of skull, it courses downward behind the medial end of clavicle	brain, face, and neck	sigmoid sinus, inferior petrosal sinus, facial v., lingual v., pharyngeal v.'s, superior thyroid v., middle thyroid v., occipital v. (occasionally)	brachiocephalic v., after union with subclavian v.
B	**vv. labiales** *labial v.'s*	labia majora	labia majora	none	anterior v.: external pudendal v.'s posterior v.: internal pudendal v.
C	**vv. labiales inferiores** *labial v.'s, inferior*	lower lip	lower lip and chin	none	facial v. or submental v.
D	**v. labialis superior** *labial v., superior*	upper lip	upper lip and philtrum	none	facial v.
E	**vv. labyrinthi** *labyrinthine v.'s;* *auditory v.'s, internal*	pass through internal acoustic meatus from the vestibule, semicircular canals, and cochlea of the internal ear	utricle, saccule, semicircular canals, lamina spiralis, basilar membrane	cochlear and vestibular v.'s	inferior petrosal sinus or sigmoid sinus
F	**v. laryngea inferior** *laryngeal v., inferior*	dorsal part of larynx	muscles and mucous membrane of larynx	none	inferior thyroid v.
G	**v. laryngea superior** *laryngeal v., superior*	larynx	glands, muscles, and mucous membrane of larynx	none	superior thyroid v.
H	**v. lienalis** *splenic v.*	from hilum of spleen to posterior neck of pancreas	spleen, pancreas, greater curvature of stomach	short gastric v.'s, left gastroepiploic v., pancreatic v.'s, inferior mesenteric v.	portal v., in union with superior mesenteric v.
I	**v. lingualis** *lingual v.*	from underside of tongue, descends tortuously to level of hyoid bone	tongue, sublingual gland, tonsil, gums, epiglottis	dorsal lingual v.'s, deep lingual v. (occasionally), submental c. (occasionally), v. comitans nervi hypoglossi	internal jugular v. (near the greater cornu of hyoid bone) or facial v.
J	**vv. lumbales** (usually four in number on each side) *lumbar v.'s*	lumbar walls	muscles and skin of the loins and walls of the abdomen	vertebral plexuses, dorsal and abdomenal branches	1st and 2nd: ascending lumbar v. 3rd and 4th: inferior vena cava

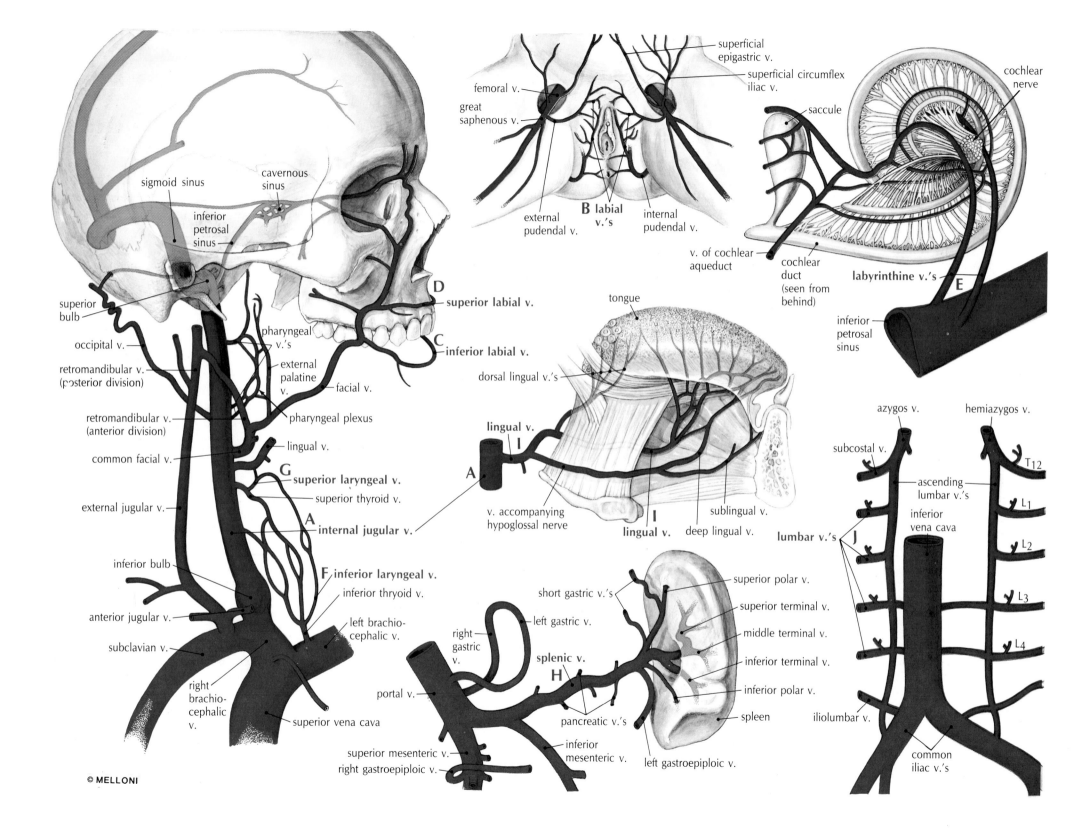

sigmoid sinus

cavernous sinus

inferior petrosal sinus

superior bulb

occipital v.

retromandibular v. (posterior division)

retromandibular v. (anterior division)

common facial v.

external jugular v.

inferior bulb

anterior jugular v.

subclavian v.

right brachio-cephalic v.

pharyngeal v.'s

external palatine v.

facial v.

pharyngeal plexus

lingual v.

G superior laryngeal v.

superior thyroid v.

A internal jugular v.

F inferior laryngeal v.

inferior thyroid v.

left brachio-cephalic v.

superior vena cava

© MELLONI

superficial epigastric v.

superficial circumflex iliac v.

femoral v.

great saphenous v.

external pudendal v.

B labial v.'s

internal pudendal v.

D superior labial v.

C inferior labial v.

cochlear nerve

saccule

v. of cochlear aqueduct

cochlear duct (seen from behind)

labyrinthine v.'s E

inferior petrosal sinus

tongue

dorsal lingual v.'s

lingual v.

I

A

v. accompanying hypoglossal nerve

I

sublingual v.

lingual v.

deep lingual v.

azygos v.

hemiazygos v.

subcostal v.

ascending lumbar v.'s

inferior vena cava

lumbar v.'s J

T_{12}

L_1

L_2

L_3

L_4

iliolumbar v.

common iliac v.'s

short gastric v.'s

left gastric v.

right gastric v.

splenic v.

H

portal v.

pancreatic v.'s

superior mesenteric v.

right gastroepiploic v.

inferior mesenteric v.

left gastroepiploic v.

superior polar v.

superior terminal v.

middle terminal v.

inferior terminal v.

inferior polar v.

spleen

	VEIN	LOCATION	DRAINS	TRIBUTARIES	EMPTIES INTO
A	**v. lumbalis ascendens** *lumbar v., ascending*	ventral to transverse process of lumbar vertebrae	lumbar plexus, back muscles, spinal cord	lateral sacral v.'s, lumbar v.'s	right side: azygos v., in union with subcostal v. left side: hemiazygos v., in union with subcostal v.
B	**vv. massetericae** *masseteric v.'s*	cheek over masseter muscle	masseter muscle and overlying skin	none	facial v., retromandibular v., pterygoid plexus, or transverse facial v.
C	**v. maxillaris** *maxillary v.*	short trunk from posterior end of pterygoid plexus, courses laterally between sphenomandibular ligament and neck of mandible	temporomandibilar joint, pterygoid and temporalis muscles, auditory tube, sinuses, teeth, ear	pterygoid plexus	retromandibular vein in union with superficial temporal v.
D	**vv. meningeae** *meningeal v.'s*	in endosteal layer of dura mater	dura mater covering the convexity of the cerebrum, falx cerebri, tentorium cerebelli, falx cerebelli, cranium	venous sinuses, diploic v.'s	regional sinuses and efferent v.'s outside the cranial cavity
E	**vv. meningeae mediae** *meningeal v's, middle*	in endosteal layer of dura mater	cranium, dura mater, tensor tympani muscle	meningeal tributaries (frontal, parietal, petrosal, superior tympanic), inferior cerebral v.'s, diploic v.'s, superficial middle cerebral v.	pterygoid venous plexus, via the foramina spinosum, ovale, or lacerum
F	**v. mesenterica inferior** *mesenteric v., inferior*	from area of upper rectum, it ascends to level of body of pancreas	upper rectum, sigmoid, and descending colon	superior rectal (hemorrhoi-dal) v., sigmoid v.'s, left colic v., rectosigmoid v.	splenic v. or junction of splenic v. and superior mesenteric v.
G	**v. mesenterica superior** *mesenteric v., superior*	from right iliac fossa, it ascends between the two layers of the mesentary to the level of the neck of the pancreas	small intestine (except proximal half of duodenum), cecum, vermiform appendix, ascending colon, transverse colon	right colic v., middle colic v., ileocolic v., jejunal v.'s, right gastroepiploic v., inferior pancreatico-duodenal v., ileal v.'s	portal v., in union with splenic v.
H	**vv. metacarpales dorsales** *metacarpal v.'s, dorsal*	on dorsum of hand over distal $\frac{2}{3}$ of metacarpus	fingers	dorsal digital v.'s of adjacent fingers	venous network on dorsum of hand

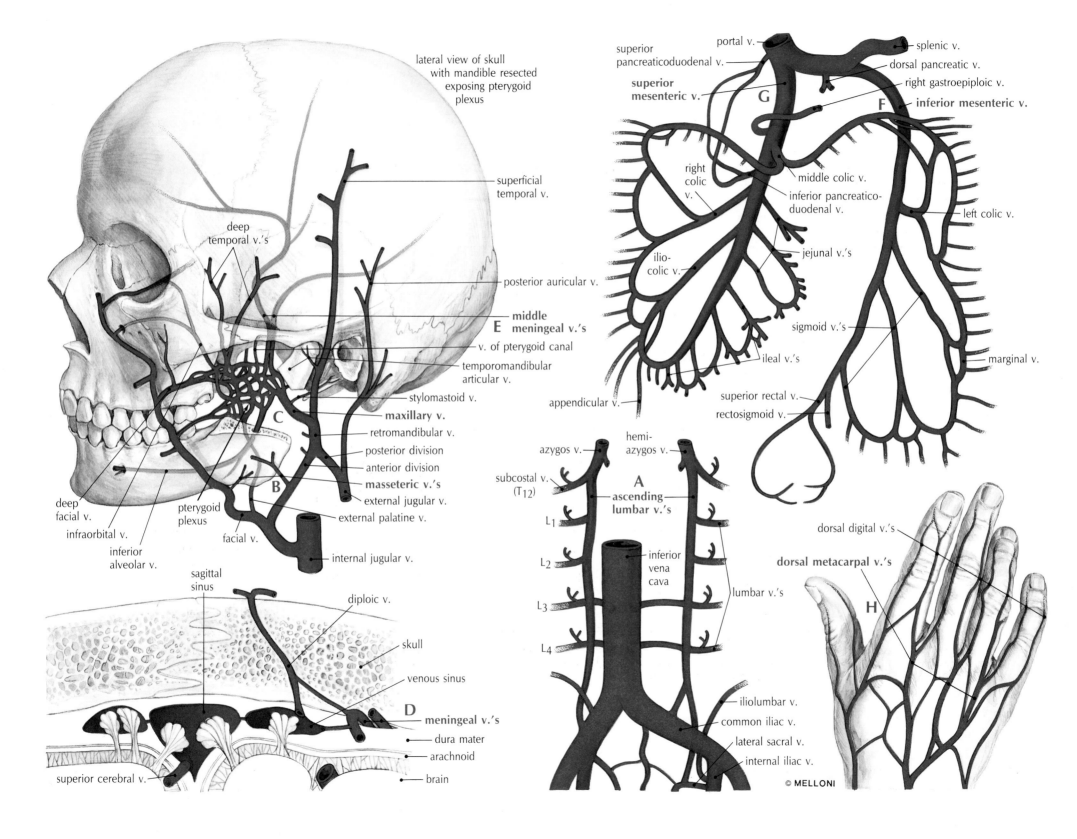

lateral view of skull
with mandible resected
exposing pterygoid
plexus

superficial temporal v.

deep temporal v.'s

posterior auricular v.

E **middle meningeal v.'s**

v. of pterygoid canal

temporomandibular articular v.

stylomastoid v.

maxillary v.

retromandibular v.

posterior division

anterior division

masseteric v.'s

external jugular v.

external palatine v.

internal jugular v.

deep facial v.

infraorbital v.

inferior alveolar v.

pterygoid plexus

facial v.

C

B

sagittal sinus

diploic v.

skull

venous sinus

D **meningeal v.'s**

dura mater

arachnoid

brain

superior cerebral v.

portal v.

splenic v.

superior pancreaticoduodenal v.

dorsal pancreatic v.

right gastroepiploic v.

superior mesenteric v.

G

F **inferior mesenteric v.**

right colic v.

middle colic v.

inferior pancreatico-duodenal v.

left colic v.

ilio-colic v.

jejunal v.'s

sigmoid v.'s

marginal v.

ileal v.'s

appendicular v.

superior rectal v.

rectosigmoid v.

azygos v.

hemi-azygos v.

subcostal v. (T$_{12}$)

A

ascending lumbar v.'s

L$_1$

L$_2$

inferior vena cava

lumbar v.'s

L$_3$

L$_4$

iliolumbar v.

common iliac v.

lateral sacral v.

internal iliac v.

dorsal digital v.'s

dorsal metacarpal v.'s

H

© MELLONI

	VEIN	LOCATION	DRAINS	TRIBUTARIES	EMPTIES INTO
A	**vv. metacarpales palmares** *metacarpal v.'s, palmar*	palmar side of metacarpus	fingers, metacarpus	perforating v.'s	deep palmar venous arch
B	**vv. metatarsales dorsales pedis** *metatarsal v.'s of foot, dorsal*	dorsal surface of foot	toes and dorsal part of foot	dorsal digital v.'s of toes	dorsal venous arch
C	**vv. metatarsales plantares** *metatarsal v.'s, plantar*	plantar side of metatarsus	toes	plantar digital v.'s, perforating v.'s	deep plantar venous arch
D	**vv. musculophrenicae** *musculophrenic v.'s*	just under costal cartilages of lower ribs	diaphragm, abdominal wall, lower intercostal spaces	anterior intercostal, deep circumflex iliac v.	internal thoracic v.'s
E	**vv. nasales externae** *external nasal v.'s*	external surface of nose	ala and dorsum of nose	none	angular v.
F	**vv. obturatoriae** *obturator v.'s*	from high in thigh, enters pelvis through obturator canal	adductor region of thigh, hip joint, ilium, pelvic muscles	anterior branch, posterior branch, pubic v.'s, vesical v.'s, acetabular branch, medial circumflex femoral v., iliac v.'s, iliolumbar v.	internal iliac v., sometimes the inferior epigastric or common iliac v.
G	**v. occipitalis** *occipital v.*	from back of scalp, courses downward over the occipital bone to the suboccipital triangle	scalp, dura mater, mastoid air cells, adjacent muscles of neck	posterior auricular v., superficial temporal v.'s, superior sagittal sinus, transverse sinus, occipital diploic v., meningeal v.'s, mastoid v.	deep cervical v. and vertebral v., internal jugular v. (occasionally)
H	**v. ophthalmica inferior** *ophthalmic v., inferior*	from floor and medial wall of orbit, it courses through the superior orbital fissure (sometimes indirectly by joining the superior ophthalmic v.)	lower eyelid, lacrimal sac, rectus inferior muscle, oblique inferior muscle, eyeball	angular v., venous plexus on floor of orbit, muscular and ciliary branches	cavernous sinus or superior ophthalmic v.
I	**v. ophthalmica superior** *ophthalmic v., superior*	from upper medial part of orbit, it courses through the superior orbital fissure	orbit, upper eyelid, lacrimal gland, eyeball	supraorbital v., angular v., supratrochlear v., lacrimal v., ethmoidal v.'s, dorsal nasal v., vorticose v.'s	cavernous sinus

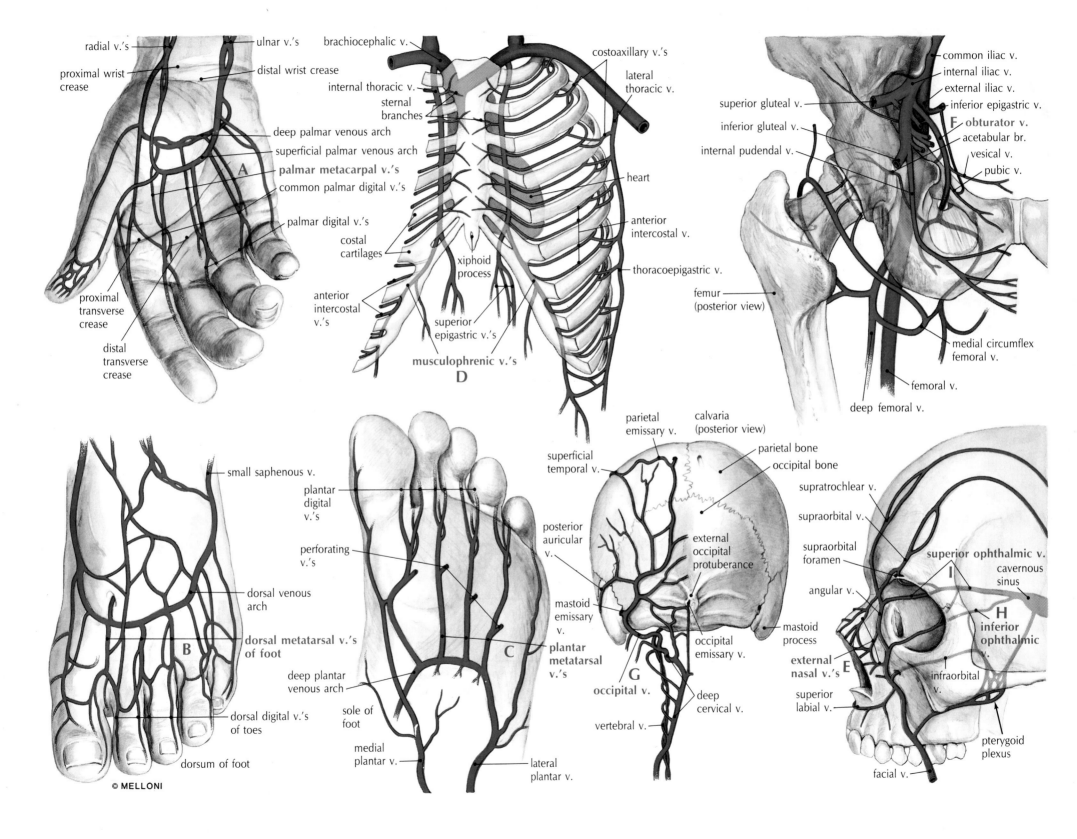

A

radial v.'s
ulnar v.'s
proximal wrist crease
distal wrist crease
deep palmar venous arch
superficial palmar venous arch
palmar metacarpal v.'s
common palmar digital v.'s
palmar digital v.'s
proximal transverse crease
distal transverse crease

B

small saphenous v.
dorsal venous arch
dorsal metatarsal v.'s of foot
dorsal digital v.'s of toes
dorsum of foot

© MELLONI

C

plantar digital v.'s
perforating v.'s
deep plantar venous arch
sole of foot
medial plantar v.
plantar metatarsal v.'s
lateral plantar v.

D

brachiocephalic v.
costoaxillary v.'s
lateral thoracic v.
internal thoracic v.
sternal branches
heart
anterior intercostal v.
thoracoepigastric v.
costal cartilages
xiphoid process
superior epigastric v.'s
musculophrenic v.'s
anterior intercostal v.'s

F

common iliac v.
internal iliac v.
external iliac v.
inferior epigastric v.
superior gluteal v.
F obturator v.
inferior gluteal v.
acetabular br.
internal pudendal v.
vesical v.
pubic v.
medial circumflex femoral v.
femur (posterior view)
femoral v.
deep femoral v.

G

parietal emissary v.
calvaria (posterior view)
superficial temporal v.
parietal bone
occipital bone
posterior auricular v.
external occipital protuberance
mastoid emissary v.
mastoid process
occipital emissary v.
occipital v.
deep cervical v.
vertebral v.

E / H / I

supratrochlear v.
supraorbital v.
supraorbital foramen
angular v.
superior ophthalmic v.
cavernous sinus
H inferior ophthalmic
external nasal v.'s E
infraorbital v.
superior labial v.
pterygoid plexus
facial v.

	VEIN	LOCATION	DRAINS	TRIBUTARIES	EMPTIES INTO
A	**v. ovarica** *ovarian v.*	from ovary and uterine tube, it courses through deep inguinal ring to abdomen up to level of about L2	ovary, uterine tube, uterus, ureter	uterine plexus, pampiniform plexus, ureteric v.	right: inferior vena cava left: left renal v.
B	**v. palatina externa** *palatine v., external* *paratonsillar v.*	from pharyngeal tonsil, it courses downward to angle of mandible	tonsil, soft palate, pharyngeal wall, auditory tube	none	facial v.
C	**vv. palpebrales inferiores** *palpebral v.'s, inferior*	from lower eyelid, courses downward over cheek	lower eyelid, conjunctiva, nasolacrimal duct	infraorbital v., tributaries of cheek	angular v.
D	**vv. palpebrales superiores** *palpebral v.'s, superior*	upper eyelid	upper eyelid, conjunctiva	middle temporal v.	angular v. or supraorbital v.
E	**vv. pancreaticae** *pancreatic v.'s*	from superior part of body and tail of pancreas, it courses upward a short distance	body and tail of pancreas	none	splenic v., superior mesenteric v. (occasionally)
F	**vv. pancreaticoduodenales** *pancreaticoduodenal v.'s*	between pancreas and duodenum	pancreas, duodenum	small branches from duodenum and head of pancreas	superior v. (anterior branch): portal v. or right gastroepiploic v. superior v. (posterior branch): portal v. inferior v.: upper part of superior mesenteric v.
G	**vv. paraumbilicales** *paraumbilical v.'s*	from umbilicus, they course along the round ligament (ligamentum teres) of the liver and the median umbilical ligament of the bladder	drain umbilicus (part of collateral circulation between v.'s of anterior abdominal wall and portal v.)	superior epigastric v.'s, inferior epigastric v., superior vesical v.'s, lateral thoracic v., superficial epigastric v.	portal v.
H	**vv. parotideae** *parotid v.'s*	cheek over parotid gland	parotid gland and overlying skin	none	anterior v.'s: facial v. posterior v.'s: retromandibular v. or superficial temporal v.
I	**vv. pectorales** *pectoral v.'s*	pectoral muscles	pectoral region	none	subclavian v.

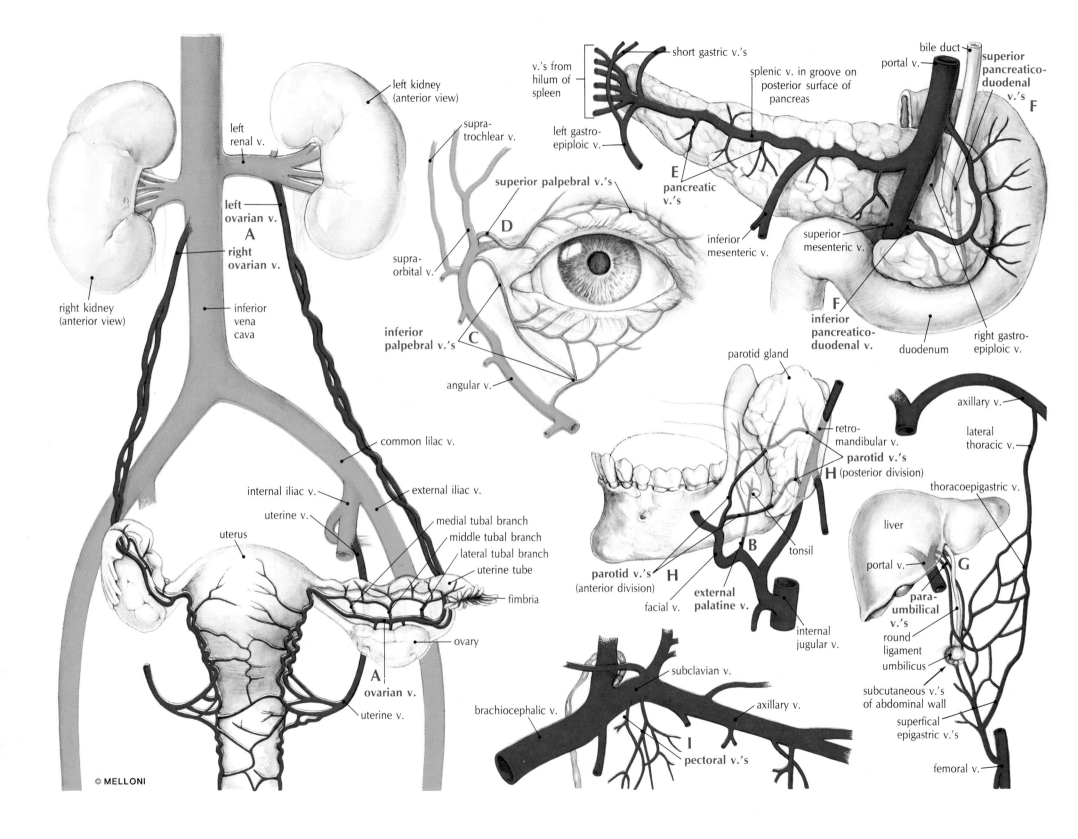

left kidney (anterior view)

left renal v.

left ovarian v.

A

right ovarian v.

right kidney (anterior view)

inferior vena cava

common lilac v.

internal iliac v.

external iliac v.

uterine v.

uterus

medial tubal branch
middle tubal branch
lateral tubal branch
uterine tube
fimbria

ovary

A
ovarian v.

uterine v.

© MELLONI

supra-trochlear v.

supra-orbital v.

superior palpebral v.'s

D

inferior palpebral v.'s

C

angular v.

short gastric v.'s

v.'s from hilum of spleen

left gastro-epiploic v.

E

pancreatic v.'s

splenic v. in groove on posterior surface of pancreas

inferior mesenteric v.

superior mesenteric v.

bile duct

portal v.

superior pancreatico-duodenal v.'s

F

F

inferior pancreatico-duodenal v.

duodenum

right gastro-epiploic v.

parotid gland

retro-mandibular v.

parotid v.'s (posterior division)

H

B

tonsil

parotid v.'s (anterior division)

H

facial v.

external palatine v.

internal jugular v.

axillary v.

lateral thoracic v.

thoracoepigastric v.

liver

portal v.

G

para-umbilical v.'s

round ligament

umbilicus

subcutaneous v.'s of abdominal wall

superfical epigastric v.'s

femoral v.

brachiocephalic v.

subclavian v.

axillary v.

I

pectoral v.'s

	VEIN	LOCATION	DRAINS	TRIBUTARIES	EMPTIES INTO
A	**vv. perforantes** *perforating v.'s*	back of thigh	vastus lateralis and hamstring muscles, femur	inferior gluteal v., popliteal v.	deep femoral v.
B	**vv. pericardiales** *pericardial v.'s*	over pericardium	pericardium	none	brachiocephalic v., azygos v., or superior vena cava
C	**vv. pericardiacophrenicae** *pericardiacophrenic v.'s*	from diaphragm and pericardium, they course upward to level just below first rib	diaphragm, pleura, pericardium	none	brachiocephalic v. or superior vena cava or internal thoracic v.
D	**vv. peroneae** *peroneal v.'s* *fibular v.'s*	from lateral side of heel, courses up back of leg to just below knee	back of leg, especially calf muscles	superficial v.'s of leg	popliteal v., after uniting with posterior tibial v.
E	**vv. pharyngeales** *pharyngeal v.'s*	pharynx	pharyngeal musculature	pharyngeal plexus, meningeal v.'s, v. of pterygoid canal	internal jugular v., facial v. (occasionally)
F	**vv. phrenicae inferiores** *phrenic v.'s, inferior*	undersurface of diaphragm	diaphragm	none	right side: inferior vena cava left side: left suprarenal v. and inferior vena cava
G	**vv. phrenicae superiores** *phrenic v.'s, superior*	upper surface of diaphragm	diaphragm	none	azygos v., hemiazygos v.
H	**v. poplitea** *popliteal v.*	from distal border of popliteus muscle, it courses upward to tendinous hiatus of adductor canal	skin and muscles of thigh and calf around region of knee	anterior tibial v., posterior tibial v., small saphenous v., medial inferior genicular v., lateral inferior genicular v., middle genicular v., medial superior genicular v., lateral superior genicular v.	femoral v., at the adductor canal
I	**v. portae** (about 7 cm in length) *portal v.*	from behind the neck of the pancreas at level of 2nd lumbar vertebra, it inclines obliquely to transverse fissure of liver	gastrointestinal tract from lower part of esophagus to upper part of anal canal, pancreas, gallbladder, bile ducts, spleen	superior mesenteric v., splenic v., cystic v., right gastric v., left gastric v., paraumbilical v.'s, prepyloric v., superior pancreaticoduodenal v.	right and left terminal branches in liver

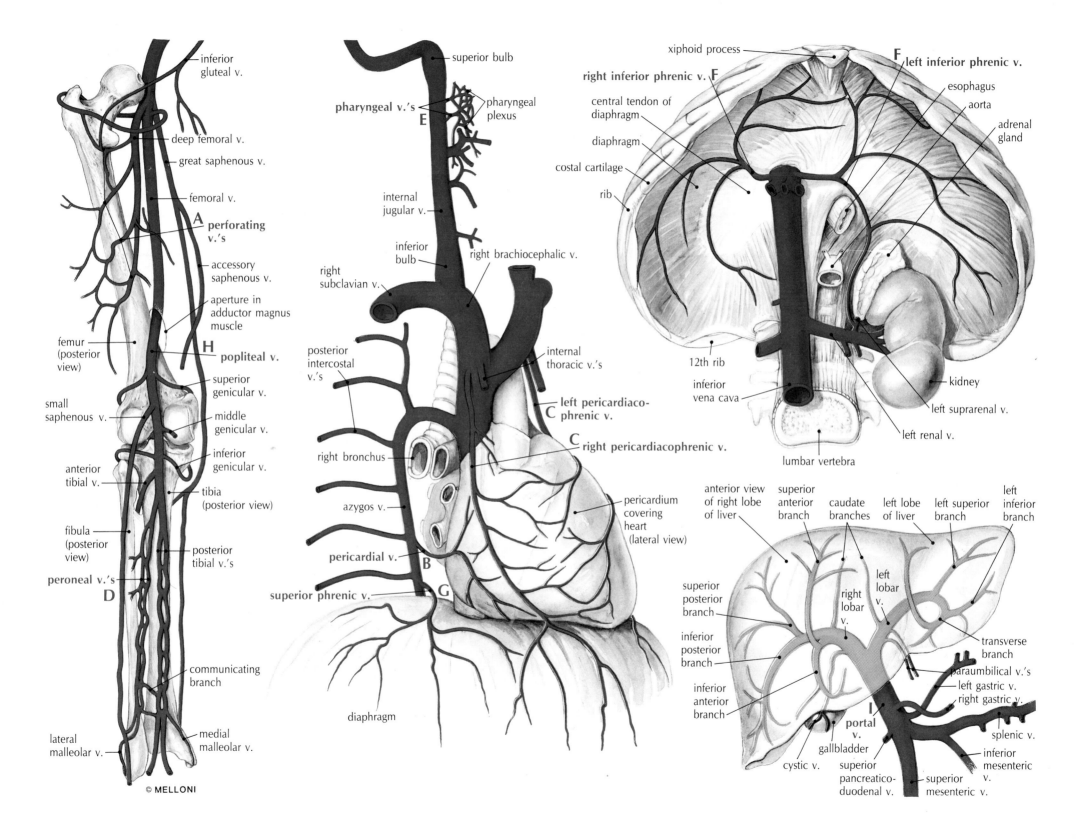

inferior gluteal v.

deep femoral v.

great saphenous v.

femoral v.

A **perforating v.'s**

accessory saphenous v.

aperture in adductor magnus muscle

femur (posterior view)

H **popliteal v.**

superior genicular v.

small saphenous v.

middle genicular v.

inferior genicular v.

anterior tibial v.

tibia (posterior view)

fibula (posterior view)

posterior tibial v.'s

peroneal v.'s

D

communicating branch

lateral malleolar v.

medial malleolar v.

© MELLONI

superior bulb

pharyngeal plexus

pharyngeal v.'s

E

internal jugular v.

inferior bulb

right brachiocephalic v.

right subclavian v.

posterior intercostal v.'s

internal thoracic v.'s

left pericardiaco-phrenic v.

C

right bronchus

C **right pericardiacophrenic v.**

azygos v.

pericardium covering heart (lateral view)

pericardial v.

B

superior phrenic v.

G

diaphragm

xiphoid process

right inferior phrenic v. **F**

F

left inferior phrenic v.

esophagus

aorta

central tendon of diaphragm

adrenal gland

diaphragm

costal cartilage

rib

12th rib

inferior vena cava

kidney

left suprarenal v.

left renal v.

lumbar vertebra

anterior view of right lobe of liver

superior anterior branch

caudate branches

left lobe of liver

left superior branch

left inferior branch

superior posterior branch

left lobar v.

right lobar v.

inferior posterior branch

transverse branch

inferior anterior branch

paraumbilical v.'s

left gastric v.

right gastric v.

I

portal v.

cystic v.

gallbladder

superior pancreatico-duodenal v.

superior mesenteric v.

splenic v.

inferior mesenteric v.

VEIN	LOCATION	DRAINS	TRIBUTARIES	EMPTIES INTO
v. portae hypophysialis *portal vein, hypophyseal*	stalk of pituitary gland (hypophysis)	Hypothalamus, stalk of pituitary gland, median eminence	superior hypophyseal arteries	sinusoids of anterior lobe of pituitary gland
v. posterior ventriculi sinistri *posterior v. of left ventricle*	from left margin of heart, courses upward to coronary sulcus	posterior wall of left ventricle	none	coronary sinus of great cardiac v.
v. prepylorica *prepyloric v.*	anterior to pylorus	pylorus	none	right gastric v.
v. profunda linguae *deep lingual v.* *deep v. of tongue*	from tip of tongue, courses backward on its inferior surface near frenulum	deep aspect and sides of front of tongue	none	vena comitans of the hypoglossal nerve, in union with sublingual v.
vv. pudendae externae *pudendal v.'s, external*	external genitalia, lower and medial part of abdomen	skin of lower part of abdomen, external genitalia	male: superficial dorsal v. of penis, anterior scrotal v.'s female: superficial dorsal v. of clitoris. anterior labial v.'s	great saphenous vein or femoral vein
v. pudenda interna *pudendal v., internal*	from the region of the ischial tuberosity it passes to pelvis through the greater sciatic foramen	perineum and genitalia	male: deep dorsal v. of penis, prostatic venous plexus, scrotal v.'s, inferior rectal v.'s, v.'s from bulb of penis female: deep dorsal v. of clitoris, vesical venous plexus, labial v.'s, inferior rectal v.'s, v.'s from bulb of vestibule	internal iliac v. (distal part)
vv. pulmonales (four in number) *pulmonary v.'s*	from lungs to heart	lungs	v.'s from inferior and superior lobes of left lung and from superior, middle, and inferior lobes of right lung	left atrium of heart
vv. radiales *radial v.'s*	from lateral side of wrist, they course up arm to front of elbow	muscles of forearm, wrist, and hand, radius, ulnar, elbow joint, skin of thumb, intercarpal articulations	deep palmar venous arch, dorsal metacarpal v.'s, palmar metacarpal v.'s, deep v.'s of dorsum of hand, muscular v.'s	brachial v.'s, after uniting with ulnar v.'s

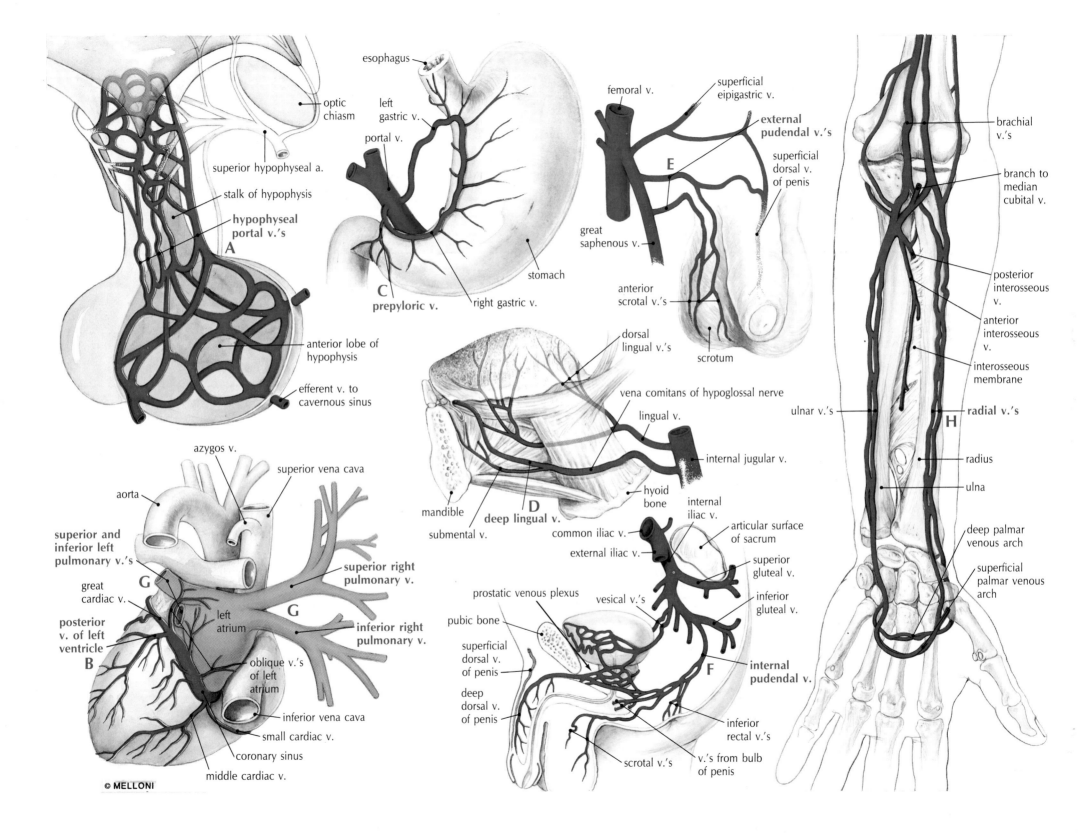

optic chiasm

superior hypophyseal a.

stalk of hypophysis

hypophyseal portal v.'s

A

anterior lobe of hypophysis

efferent v. to cavernous sinus

esophagus

left gastric v.

portal v.

C

prepyloric v.

right gastric v.

stomach

femoral v.

superficial eipigastric v.

external pudendal v.'s

superficial dorsal v. of penis

E

great saphenous v.

anterior scrotal v.'s

scrotum

dorsal lingual v.'s

vena comitans of hypoglossal nerve

lingual v.

internal jugular v.

hyoid bone

D

mandible

deep lingual v.

submental v.

azygos v.

superior vena cava

aorta

superior and inferior left pulmonary v.'s

great cardiac v.

G

left atrium

posterior v. of left ventricle

B

oblique v.'s of left atrium

superior right pulmonary v.

G

inferior right pulmonary v.

inferior vena cava

small cardiac v.

coronary sinus

middle cardiac v.

© MELLONI

common iliac v.

internal iliac v.

external iliac v.

articular surface of sacrum

superior gluteal v.

inferior gluteal v.

prostatic venous plexus

vesical v.'s

pubic bone

superficial dorsal v. of penis

deep dorsal v. of penis

internal pudendal v.

F

inferior rectal v.'s

scrotal v.'s

v.'s from bulb of penis

brachial v.'s

branch to median cubital v.

posterior interosseous v.

anterior interosseous v.

interosseous membrane

ulnar v.'s

radial v.'s

H

radius

ulna

deep palmar venous arch

superficial palmar venous arch

	VEIN	LOCATION	DRAINS	TRIBUTARIES	EMPTIES INTO
A	**vv. rectales inferiores** *rectal v.'s, inferior* *hemorrhoidal v.'s, inferior*	anal region	lower part of anal canal (anastomoses with middle and superior rectal v.'s)	external rectal plexus	internal pudendal v.
B	**vv. rectales mediae** *rectal v.'s, middle;* *hemorrhoidal v.'s, middle*	middle of rectum in lesser pelvis	muscular wall of middle of rectum and surrounding organs (anastomoses with superior and inferior rectal v.'s)	lower part of perimuscular rectal plexus, middle part of external rectal plexus, v.'s from the bladder, prostate, and seminal vesicle	internal iliac v. or inferior gluteal v.
C	**v. rectalis superior** (unpaired commencement of inferior mesenteric v.) *rectal v., superior* *hemorrhoidal v., superior*	upper rectum to brim of pelvis	upper rectum	upper part of perimuscular rectal plexus, about six branches encircling upper rectum, internal and external rectal plexuses	inferior mesenteric v.
D	**v. renalis dextra** (2.5 cm in length) *renal v., right*	from hilus of right kidney, courses medially	right kidney	segmental v.'s of right kidney, right ureteric v.	inferior vena cava, at level of 2nd lumbar vertebra
E	**v. renalis sinistra** (7 cm in length) *renal v., left*	from hilus of left kidney, courses medially	left kidney, left suprarenal gland, left gonad, diaphragm, body wall	segmental v.'s of left kidney, left gonadal v., left suprarenal v., left ureteric v., left inferior phrenic v.	inferior vena cava, at level of 2nd lumbar vertebra
F	**v. retromandibularis** *retromandibular v.;* *facial v., posterior*	from upper parotid gland, it courses downward, alongside of ramus to angle of mandible	parotid gland, temporomandibular joint, muscles of mastication, auricle, external acoustic canal, auditory tube, sinuses, mandible, scalp on side of head	maxillary v., superficial temporal v.'s, transverse facial v. (occasionally)	anterior branch: facial v. posterior branch: external jugular v., in union with posterior auricular v.
G	**vv. sacrales laterales** *sacral v.'s, lateral*	from dorsum of sacrum and coccyx, they course through sacral foramina to upper part of pelvis	sacrum, skin and muscles on dorsum of sacrum and coccyx	spinal v.'s, sacral venous plexus	superior gluteal v.'s or internal iliac v.
H	**v. sacralis media** (unpaired) *sacral v., middle;* *sacral v., median*	front of sarcum	sacrum, rectum	rectal (hemorrhoidal) v.'s, small lumbar v.'s	left common iliac v. or junction of two common iliac v.'s

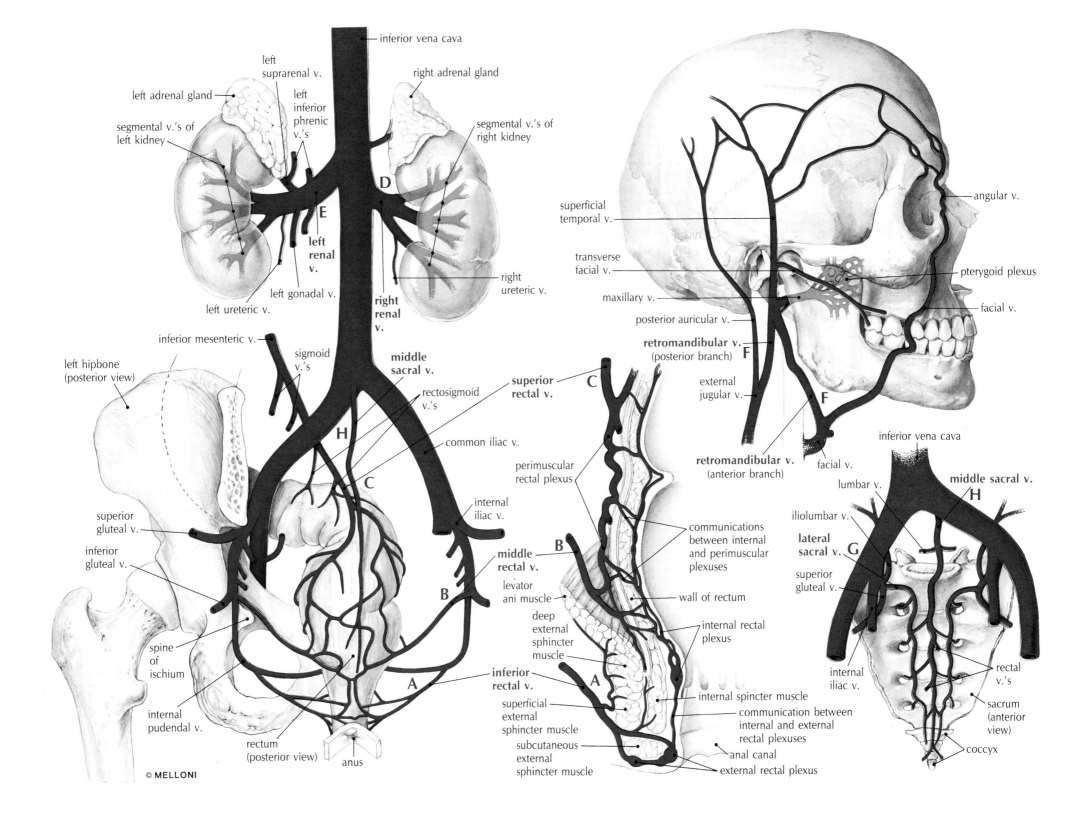

inferior vena cava

left suprarenal v.

left adrenal gland

left inferior phrenic v.'s

right adrenal gland

segmental v.'s of left kidney

segmental v.'s of right kidney

D

E

left renal v.

right renal v.

left gonadal v.

left ureteric v.

right ureteric v.

inferior mesenteric v.

sigmoid v.'s

middle sacral v.

superior rectal v.

C

left hipbone (posterior view)

rectosigmoid v.'s

common iliac v.

H

C

internal iliac v.

superior gluteal v.

inferior gluteal v.

B

spine of ischium

internal pudendal v.

rectum (posterior view)

anus

A

© MELLONI

superficial temporal v.

transverse facial v.

maxillary v.

posterior auricular v.

angular v.

pterygoid plexus

facial v.

retromandibular v. (posterior branch)

F

external jugular v.

F

retromandibular v. (anterior branch)

facial v.

inferior vena cava

middle sacral v.

H

lumbar v.

iliolumbar v.

lateral sacral v.

G

superior gluteal v.

internal iliac v.

rectal v.'s

sacrum (anterior view)

coccyx

C

perimuscular rectal plexus

communications between internal and perimuscular plexuses

B

middle rectal v.

levator ani muscle

deep external sphincter muscle

wall of rectum

internal rectal plexus

inferior rectal v.

A

superficial external sphincter muscle

subcutaneous external sphincter muscle

internal spincter muscle

communication between internal and external rectal plexuses

anal canal

external rectal plexus

	VEIN	LOCATION	DRAINS	TRIBUTARIES	EMPTIES INTO
A	**v. saphena accessoria** *saphenous v., accessory*	posteromedial part of thigh	posteromedial part of thigh	small saphenous v., numerous small v.'s from posterior and medial thigh	great saphenous v.
B	**v. saphena magna** (longest vein in body) *saphenous v., great;* *saphenous v., long*	medial marginal v. of foot, courses medially up left to about 4 cm below the pubic tubercle	thigh, sole of foot, leg, lower part of abdominal wall, scrotum	medial marginal v. of foot, accessory saphenous v., medial superficial v.'s, anterior femoral cutaneous v., superficial epigastric v., superficial circumflex iliac v., external pudendal v.'s, small saphenous v., deep and perforating v.'s	femoral v.
C	**v. saphena parva** *saphenous v., small;* *saphenous v., short*	from lateral margin of foot, courses along posterior side of leg to 5 cm above knee joint	foot, back of leg	dorsal venous arch of foot, lateral marginal v. of foot, small v.'s from back of leg, communicating v.'s from deep v.'s of foot	popliteal v. or great saphenous v. or deep posterior v. of thigh
D	**v. scapularis dorsalis** *scapular v., dorsal*	scapula	muscles of back	muscular branches	subclavian v., external jugular v., or tranverse cervical v.
E	**vv. scrotales** *scrotal v.'s*	scrotum	scrotum	none	anterior v.: external pudendal v.'s posterior v.: internal pudendal v.'s
F	**vv. sigmoideae** *sigmoid v.'s*	adjacent to sigmoid colon	sigmoid colon	marginal v.'s	inferior mesenteric v.
G	**v. spiralis modioli** *spiral v. of modiolus*	modiolus of cochlea	cochlea	none	labyrinthine v.'s, v. of cochlear aqueduct
H	**v. subclavia** *subclavian v.*	from lateral border of 1st rib to medial end of clavicle	arm, neck, thoracic wall	axillary v., external jugular v., dorsal scapular v., pectoral v.'s, anterior jugular v. (occasionally), vertebral v. (occasionally)	brachiocephalic v., in union with internal jugular v.
I	**v. subcostalis** *subcostal v.*	beneath the 12th rib	upper abdominal wall below the 12th rib, spinal cord	dorsal and spinal branches, intervertebral v.	right side: azygos v., in union with ascending lumbar v. left side: hemiazygos v., in union with ascending limbar v.

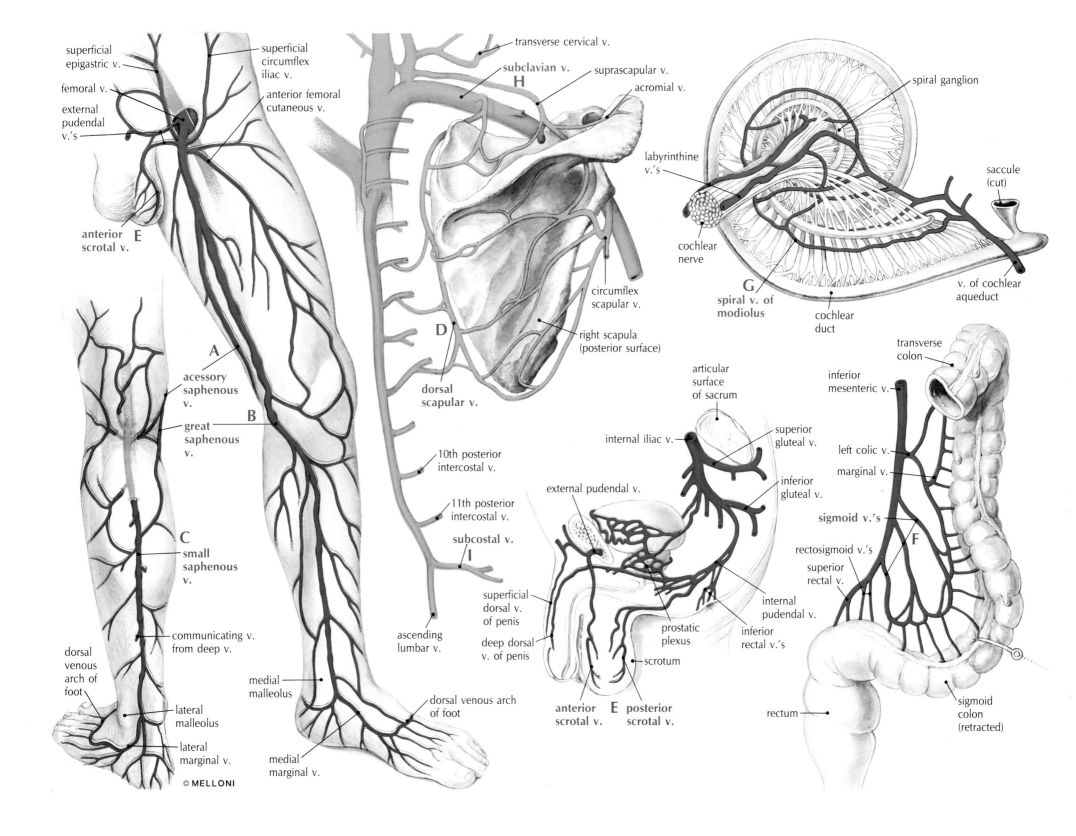

superficial
epigastric v.

superficial
circumflex
iliac v.

femoral v.

anterior femoral
cutaneous v.

external
pudendal
v.'s

**anterior
scrotal v.** **E**

A

**acessory
saphenous
v.**

B

**great
saphenous
v.**

C

**small
saphenous
v.**

communicating v.
from deep v.

dorsal
venous
arch of
foot

lateral
malleolus

lateral
marginal v.

© MELLONI

medial
malleolus

medial
marginal v.

medial
malleolus

dorsal venous arch
of foot

transverse cervical v.

subclavian v. suprascapular v.

acromial v.

H

circumflex
scapular v.

D

right scapula
(posterior surface)

**dorsal
scapular v.**

10th posterior
intercostal v.

11th posterior
intercostal v.

subcostal v.

I

ascending
lumbar v.

spiral ganglion

labyrinthine
v.'s

saccule
(cut)

cochlear
nerve

G

**spiral v. of
modiolus**

cochlear
duct

v. of cochlear
aqueduct

articular
surface
of sacrum

superior
gluteal v.

internal iliac v.

inferior
gluteal v.

external pudendal v.

prostatic
plexus

internal
pudendal v.

inferior
rectal v.'s

superficial
dorsal v.
of penis

deep dorsal
v. of penis

scrotum

**anterior
scrotal v.** **E** **posterior
scrotal v.**

transverse
colon

inferior
mesenteric v.

left colic v.

marginal v.

sigmoid v.'s

F

rectosigmoid v.'s

superior
rectal v.

rectum

sigmoid
colon
(retracted)

	VEIN	LOCATION	DRAINS	TRIBUTARIES	EMPTIES INTO
A	**v. sublingualis** *sublingual v.*	below the tongue	sublingual gland, mylohyoid and geniohyoid muscles, mucous membrane of mouth and gums	deep lingual v., submental v.	lingual v. or facial v. or internal jugular v.
B	**v. submentalis** *submental v.*	chin	muscles in region of chin and lower lip, submandibular gland	inferior labial v.'s, superficial and deep v.'s, (anastomoses with sublingual and anterior jugular v.'s)	facial v.
C	**v. supraorbitalis** *supraorbital v.*	over frontal eminence, it courses medially and downward to medial angle of eye	forehead, eyebrow, frontal sinus, superior rectus and levator palpebral muscles	middle temporal v., frontal diploic v., superior ophthalmic v., superficial temporal v.	angular v. (beginning of facial v.), in union with supratrochlear v.
D	**v. suprarenalis dextra** *suprarenal v., right*	from hilus of right suprarenal gland, it courses downward	right suprarenal gland	v.'s of renal capsule, intercostal v.'s	inferior vena cava, inferior phrenic v. (occasionally)
E	**v. suprarenalis sinistra** *suprarenal v., left*	from hilus of left suprarenal gland, it courses downward	left suprarenal gland	left inferior phrenic v., v.'s of renal capsule, intercostal v.'s	left renal v., inferior phrenic v. (occasionally)
F	**v. suprascapularis** *suprascapular v.* *scapular v., transverse*	from supraspinous and infraspinous fossae of scapula, it courses upward and medially across the anterior scalene muscle	clavicle, scapula, skin of chest, muscles of scapular region, acromioclavicular and shoulder joints	suprasternal, articular, and acromial branches, nutrient v.'s of clavicle and scapula	external jugular v.
G	**v. supratrochlearis** *supratrochlear v.;* *frontal v.*	from forehead near midline, it courses to medial angle of orbit	scalp of medial forehead, dorsum of nose	nasal venous arch, superficial temporal v.	angular v. (part of facial v.), in union with supraorbital v.
H	**vv. temporales profundae** *temporal v.'s, deep*	from side of head, course down just behind zygomatic arch	temporal muscle	temporal venous plexus	pterygoid venous plexus
I	**vv. temporales superficiales** (anterior and posterior branches) *temporal v.'s, superficial*	over lateral part of scalp, they course downward to area in front of ear	parotid gland, temporomandibular joint, masseter and temporal muscles, orbit, auricle, external acoustic canal	middle temporal v., transverse facial v., anterior auricular v., parotid v.'s, articular v.'s	retromandibular v., in union with maxillary v.

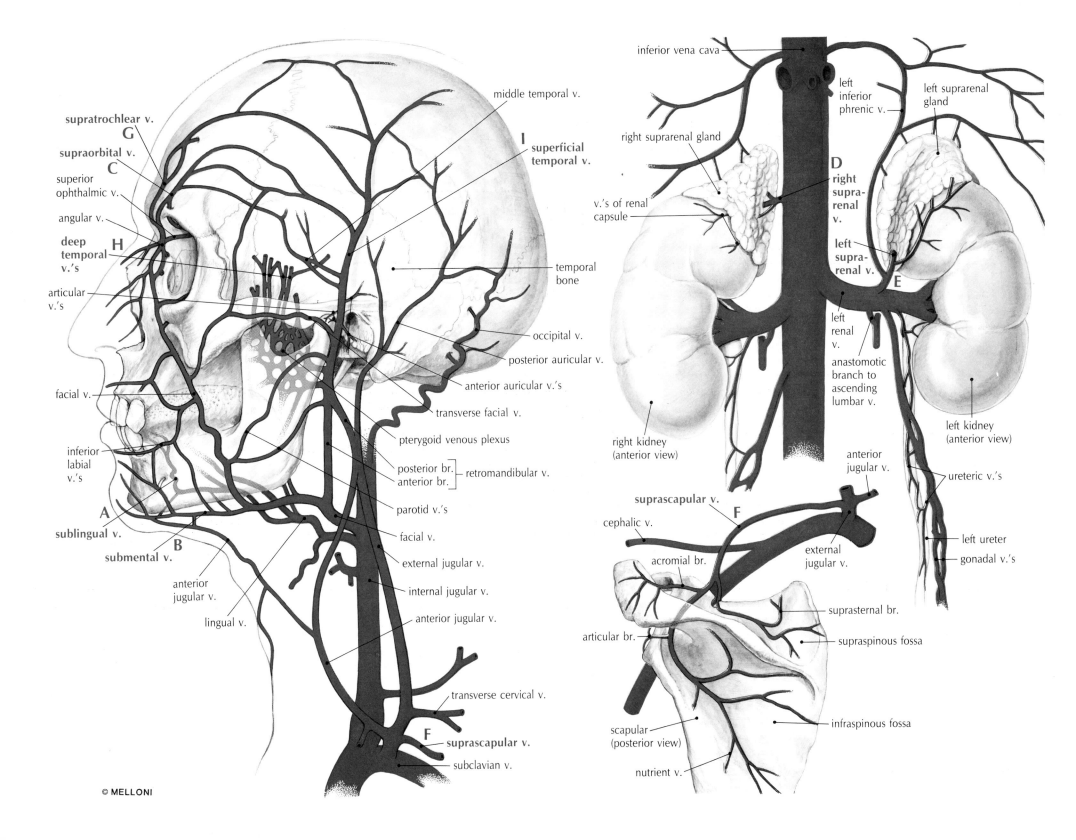

middle temporal v.

supratrochlear v.

G

supraorbital v.

C

superior ophthalmic v.

angular v.

deep temporal v.'s

H

articular v.'s

facial v.

inferior labial v.'s

A

sublingual v.

B

submental v.

anterior jugular v.

lingual v.

I **superficial temporal v.**

temporal bone

occipital v.

posterior auricular v.

anterior auricular v.'s

transverse facial v.

pterygoid venous plexus

posterior br.
anterior br. } retromandibular v.

parotid v.'s

facial v.

external jugular v.

internal jugular v.

anterior jugular v.

transverse cervical v.

F

suprascapular v.

subclavian v.

inferior vena cava

left inferior phrenic v.

left suprarenal gland

right suprarenal gland

D **right suprarenal v.**

v.'s of renal capsule

left suprarenal v.

E

left renal v.

anastomotic branch to ascending lumbar v.

right kidney (anterior view)

left kidney (anterior view)

anterior jugular v.

ureteric v.'s

left ureter

gonadal v.'s

suprascapular v.

cephalic v.

acromial br.

F

external jugular v.

suprasternal br.

supraspinous fossa

articular br.

scapular (posterior view)

nutrient v.

infraspinous fossa

© MELLONI

	VEIN	LOCATION	DRAINS	TRIBUTARIES	EMPTIES INTO
A	**v. temporalis media** *temporal v., middle*	from within temporal muscle, it courses posteriorly downward to just above the zygomatic arch	temporal muscle	deep temporal v.'s, supraorbital v. (occasionally)	superficial temporal v.'s
B	**vv. testiculares** *testicular v.'s;* *spermatic v.'s, internal*	from back of testis, they course through deep inguinal ring to abdomen up to level of about L2	testis, epididymis, ureter, cremaster muscle	epididymal v., ureteral v., pampiniform plexus	right: inferior vena cava left: left renal v.
C	**vv. thoracicae internae** *thoracic v.'s, internal;* *mammary v.'s, internal*	from chest, they course upward just beyond level of clavicle	anterior thoracic wall, mediastinal lymph nodes, diaphragm	pericardiacophrenic v.'s, mediastinal v.'s, anterior intercostal v.'s, musculophrenic v.'s, superior epigastric v.'s, thymic v.'s, abdominal subcutaneous v.'s	brachiocephalic v.
D	**v. thoracica lateralis** *thoracic v., lateral*	lateral thoracic wall	chest muscles, mammary gland (in female), axillary lymph nodes	lateral mammary v. (in female), thoracoepigastric v., intercostal v.'s	axillary v.
E	**v. thoracoacromialis** *thoracoacromial v.* *acromiothoracic v.*	top of shoulder	pectoralis major and minor, subclavius and deltoid muscles, sternoclavicular joint, acromion	pectoral, acromial, deltoid, and clavicular branches	axillary v. (sometimes in union with cephalic v.) subclavian v. (occasionally)
F	**v. thoracoepigastrica** *thoracoepigastric v.*	on anterolateral wall of trunk connecting the superficial epigastric vein with the lateral thoracic vein	skin and subcutaneous tissue of lower anterolateral wall of trunk	alveolar venous plexus, superficial v.'s of anterolateral trunk	superiorly: lateral thoracic v. inferiorly: superficial epigastric v. or femoral v.
G	**vv. thymicae** *thymic v.'s*	thymus gland	thymus gland	none	left brachiocephalic v.
H	**v. thyroidea inferior** *thyroid v., inferior*	the lower part of the thyroid gland, anterior to the 5th, 6th, and 7th tracheal rings	thyroid gland, esophagus, trachea, and lower part of larynx	thyroid venous plexus, inferior laryngeal v., tracheal v.'s, esophageal v.'s	brachiocephalic v. (sometimes just the left brachiocephalic v.)

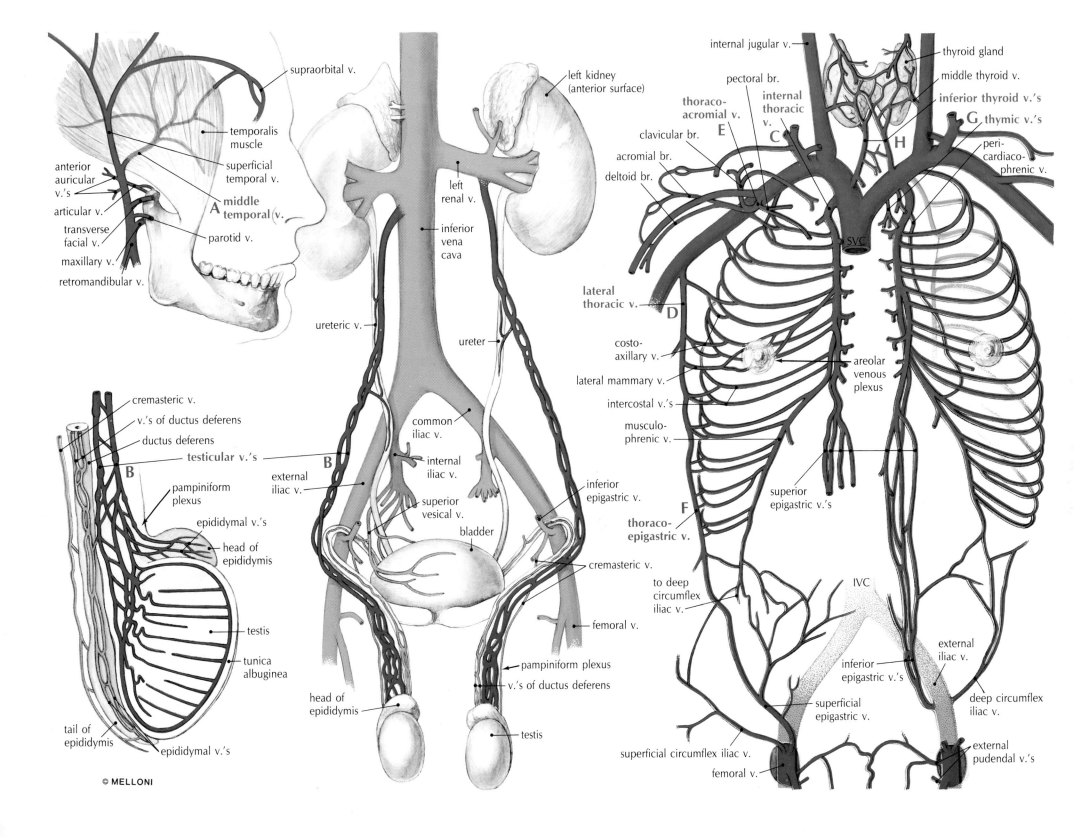

supraorbital v.

temporalis muscle

superficial temporal v.

anterior auricular v.'s

articular v.

transverse facial v.

maxillary v.

retromandibular v.

A middle temporal v.

parotid v.

cremasteric v.

v.'s of ductus deferens

ductus deferens

testicular v.'s

B

pampiniform plexus

epididymal v.'s

head of epididymis

testis

tunica albuginea

tail of epididymis

epididymal v.'s

© MELLONI

left kidney (anterior surface)

left renal v.

inferior vena cava

ureteric v.

ureter

common iliac v.

internal iliac v.

inferior epigastric v.

B

external iliac v.

superior vesical v.

bladder

cremasteric v.

femoral v.

pampiniform plexus

v.'s of ductus deferens

head of epididymis

testis

internal jugular v.

thyroid gland

middle thyroid v.

pectoral br.

inferior thyroid v.'s

thoraco-acromial v.

internal thoracic v.

E

C

G thymic v.'s

H

clavicular br.

peri-cardiaco-phrenic v.

acromial br.

deltoid br.

SVC

lateral thoracic v.

D

costo-axillary v.

areolar venous plexus

lateral mammary v.

intercostal v.'s

musculo-phrenic v.

superior epigastric v.'s

F

thoraco-epigastric v.

to deep circumflex iliac v.

IVC

inferior epigastric v.'s

external iliac v.

superficial epigastric v.

deep circumflex iliac v.

superficial circumflex iliac v.

external pudendal v.'s

femoral v.

	VEIN	LOCATION	DRAINS	TRIBUTARIES	EMPTIES INTO
A	**v. thyroidea media** *thyroid v., middle*	from lower part of thyroid gland, it courses downward and laterally	lower part of thyroid gland, larynx, trachea	thyroid plexus, v.'s from larynx and trachea	internal jugular v. just below level of the cricoid cartilage
B	**v. thyroidea superior** *thyroid v., superior*	from upper part of thyroid gland, it courses upward and laterally	upper part of thyroid gland, larynx, and neighboring muscles	thyroid venous plexus, superior laryngeal v., sternohyoid, sternothyroid, and thyrohyoid branches, cricothyroid v.	internal jugular v. or facial v.
C	**vv. tibiales anteriores** *tibial v.'s, anterior*	from top of foot, courses up front of leg about 5 cm below knee joint	foot, ankle, front of leg, knee joint	dorsal v. of foot, anterior lateral malleolar v., anterior medial malleolar v., anterior tibial recurrent v., posterior tibial recurrent v., dorsal venous arch	popliteal v., in union with posterior tibial v.
D	**vv. tibiales posteriores** *tibial v.'s, posterior*	from back of foot, courses upward on posterior leg to lower border of popliteus muscle	foot, muscles, bones, and articulations of leg	plantar venous arch, medial plantar v., lateral plantar v., fibular circumflex v., peroneal v.'s, medial malleolar v., calcaneal v., nutrient v. of tibia, venous plexus of soleus muscle	popliteal v., in union with anterior tibial v.
E	**vv. tracheales** *tracheal v.'s*	trachea	trachea	none	brachiocephalic v., thyroid v.'s
F	**vv. transversae colli** *transverse cervical v.'s*	posterior triangle of neck	levator scapulae, trapezius, and supraspinatus muscles	superficial cervical and dorsal scapular v.'s, intercostal v.'s	external jugular v. or subclavian v.
G	**v. transversa faciei** *transverse facial v.*	across masseter muscle about a finger's width below the zygomatic arch, it courses deeply into the parotid gland	parotid gland, masseter gland, skin of face	infraorbital v., masseteric v.'s, parotid v.'s, lateral palpebral v.'s, buccal v., facial v.	retromandibular v. or superficial temporal v.
H	**vv. ulnares** *ulnar v.'s*	from medial side of wrist, it courses up arm to front of elbow	muscles and skin of forearm, wrist, and hand	superficial palmar venous arch, superficial v.'s of wrist, anterior and posterior interosseous v.'s, deep palmar venous arch	brachial v.s, in union with radial v.'s

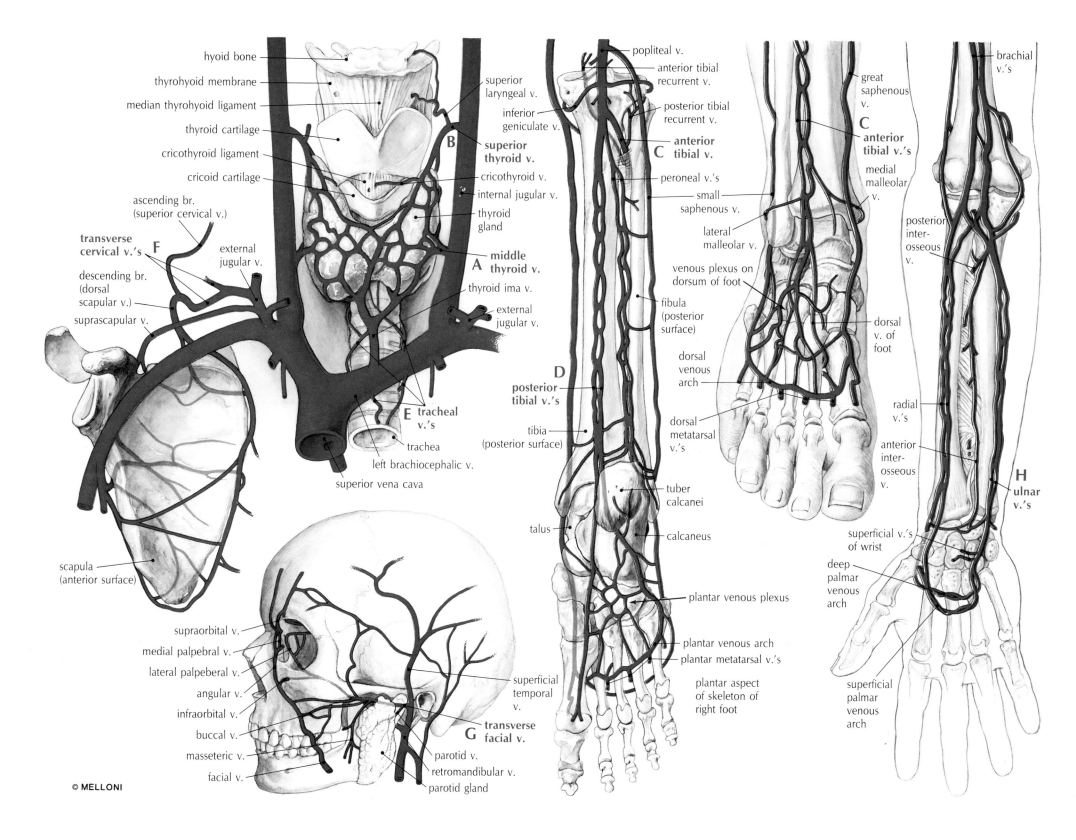

hyoid bone
thyrohyoid membrane
median thyrohyoid ligament
thyroid cartilage
cricothyroid ligament
cricoid cartilage

superior laryngeal v.
superior thyroid v.
cricothyroid v.
internal jugular v.
thyroid gland
middle thyroid v.
thyroid ima v.
external jugular v.
tracheal v.'s
trachea
left brachiocephalic v.
superior vena cava

ascending br. (superior cervical v.)
transverse cervical v.'s **F**
external jugular v.
descending br. (dorsal scapular v.)
suprascapular v.

scapula (anterior surface)

supraorbital v.
medial palpebral v.
lateral palpeberal v.
angular v.
infraorbital v.
buccal v.
masseteric v.
facial v.

superficial temporal v.
transverse facial v. **G**
parotid v.
retromandibular v.
parotid gland

B
A
E

© MELLONI

popliteal v.
anterior tibial recurrent v.
inferior geniculate v.
posterior tibial recurrent v.
anterior tibial v. **C**
peroneal v.'s
small saphenous v.
fibula (posterior surface)
posterior tibial v.'s **D**
tibia (posterior surface)
dorsal venous arch
dorsal metatarsal v.'s
tuber calcanei
talus
calcaneus
plantar venous plexus
plantar venous arch
plantar metatarsal v.'s
plantar aspect of skeleton of right foot

great saphenous v.
anterior tibial v.'s **C**
medial malleolar v.
lateral malleolar v.
venous plexus on dorsum of foot
dorsal v. of foot

brachial v.'s
posterior interosseous v.
radial v.'s
anterior interosseous v.
ulnar v.'s **H**
superficial v.'s of wrist
deep palmar venous arch
superficial palmar venous arch

	VEIN	LOCATION	DRAINS	TRIBUTARIES	EMPTIES INTO
A	**v. ureteric** *ureteric v.*	along entire length of ureter	ureter	none	renal v., inferior vena cava, common iliac v., testicular and ovarian v.'s, superior and inferior vesical v.'s
B	**vv. uterinae** *uterine v.'s*	lateral side of uterus	uterus, upper part of vagina, round ligament of uterus, cervix, uterine tube	uterine venous plexus, ovarian v., vaginal and tubal branches	internal iliac v.
C	**v. vaginalis** *vaginal v.*	lateral side of vagina	vagina, fundus of urinary bladder, rectum	none	internal iliac v., uterine v. (occasionally)
D	**v. vertebralis** *vertebral v.*	from suboccipital triangle, it descends through transverse foramina of upper cervical vertebrae as dense plexus around vertebral artery, emerging from transverse foramen of 6th cervical vertebra as single v.	deep muscles of back and neck, spinal cord, cerebellum, medulla oblongata	sigmoid sinus, occipital v., internal and external vertebral plexuses, anterior vertebral v., deep cervical v., first intercostal v. (occasionally)	brachiocephalic v.
E	**v. vertebralis accessoria** *vertebral v., accessory*	from posterior surface of transverse processes of upper cervical vertebrae, it descends through foramen of transverse process of C7	suboccipital venous plexus, venous plexus around vertebral artery	venous plexuses	brachiocephalic v.
F	**v. vertebralis anterior** *vertebral v., anterior*	from transverse processes of upper cervical vertebrae, it courses along ascending cervical artery	vertebral canal and bodies of cervical vertebrae, muscles of neck	spinal v.'s	vertebral v.
G	**vv. vesicales** *vesical v.'s*	urinary bladder	urinary bladder and adjacent structures	vesical venous plexus	internal iliac v.
H	**vv. vestibulares** *vestibular v.'s*	vestibule of internal ear	utricle, saccule, semicircular ducts	none	labyrinthine v.'s and v. of vestibular aqueduct, v. of cochlear aqueduct
I	**vv. vorticosae** (four in number) *vorticose v.'s*	eyeball, piercing sclera obliquely	choroid layer of eyeball	branches from iris, ciliary process and choroid, episcleral veins	superior branches: superior ophthalmic v. inferior branches: inferior ophthalmic v.

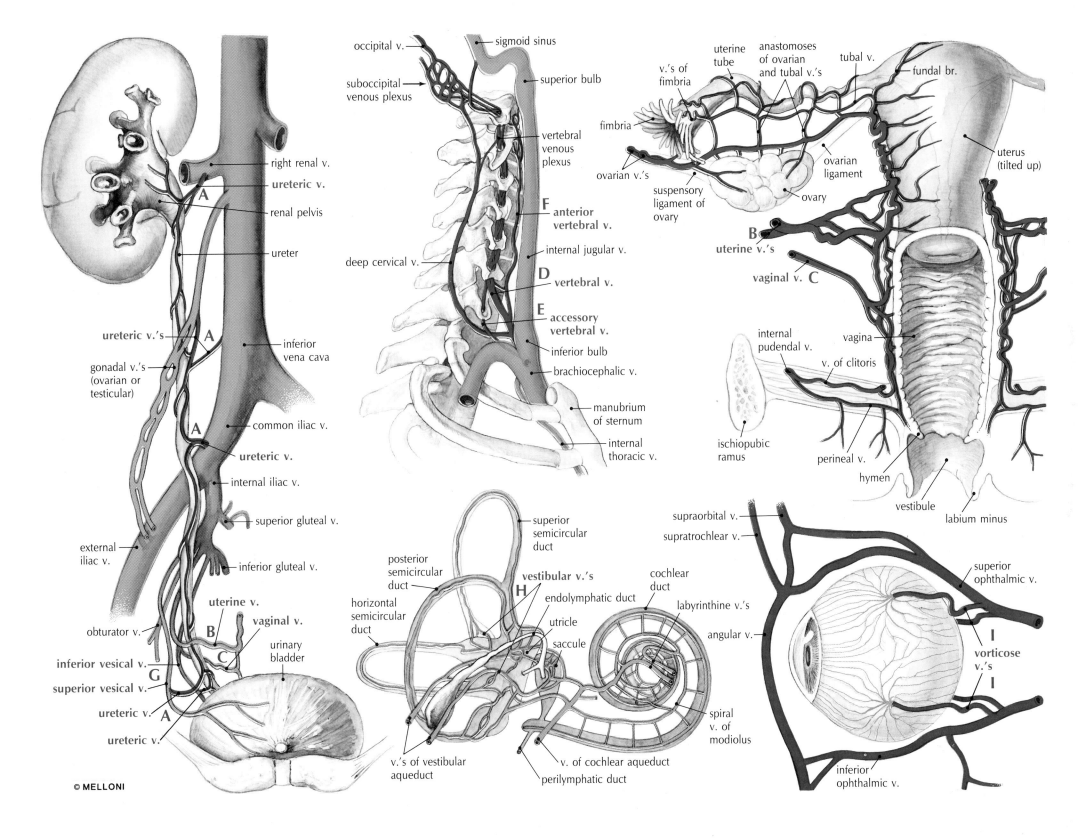

occipital v.

sigmoid sinus

suboccipital venous plexus

superior bulb

vertebral venous plexus

F **anterior vertebral v.**

deep cervical v.

internal jugular v.

D **vertebral v.**

E **accessory vertebral v.**

inferior bulb

brachiocephalic v.

manubrium of sternum

internal thoracic v.

right renal v.

ureteric v.

renal pelvis

ureter

A

A **ureteric v.'s**

gonadal v.'s (ovarian or testicular)

inferior vena cava

A **ureteric v.**

common iliac v.

internal iliac v.

superior gluteal v.

external iliac v.

inferior gluteal v.

uterine v.

vaginal v.

obturator v.

B

C

urinary bladder

inferior vesical v.

G

superior vesical v.

ureteric v. **A**

ureteric v.

uterine tube

anastomoses of ovarian and tubal v.'s

tubal v.

fundal br.

v.'s of fimbria

fimbria

ovarian v.'s

suspensory ligament of ovary

ovarian ligament

ovary

uterus (tilted up)

B

uterine v.'s

vaginal v. C

internal pudendal v.

vagina

v. of clitoris

ischiopubic ramus

perineal v.

hymen

vestibule

labium minus

superior semicircular duct

posterior semicircular duct

vestibular v.'s

H

cochlear duct

horizontal semicircular duct

endolymphatic duct

utricle

saccule

labyrinthine v.'s

spiral v. of modiolus

v.'s of vestibular aqueduct

v. of cochlear aqueduct

perilymphatic duct

supraorbital v.

supratrochlear v.

superior ophthalmic v.

angular v.

I

vorticose v.'s

I

inferior ophthalmic v.

© MELLONI

BONES

MUSCLES

biceps
  of arm, 98D
  of thigh, 98E
brachial, 98F
brachioradial, 98G
bronchoesophageal, 98H
buccinator, 98I
bulbocavernous, 100A
canine, 120E
ceratocricoid, 100B
chin, 126B
chondroglossus, 100C
ciliary, 100D
coccygeus, 100E
compressor
  of nose, 100F
constrictor
  of pharynx, inferior, 100G
  of pharynx, middle, 100H
  of pharynx, superior, 102A
coracobrachial, 102B
corrugator
  cutis ani, 102C
  superciliary, 102D
cremaster, 102E
cricoarytenoid
  lateral, 102F
  posterior, 102G
cricothyroid, 104A
deltoid, 104B
depressor
  of angle of mouth, 104C
  of lower lip, 104D
  of nasal septum, 104E
  superciliary, 104F
detrusor
  of urinary bladder, 104G
diaphragm, 104H
  pelvic, 106A
  urogenital, 106B
digastric, 106C
dilator
  of nose, 106D
  of pupil, 106E
diventer cervicis, 148G
epicranial, 106F
erector
  of clitoris, 120C
  of penis, 120C
  of spine, 106G
extensor
  of big toe, long, 108F
  of big toe, short, 108E
  of fingers, 108B
  of index finger, 108G
  of little finger, 108A
  of thumb, long, 108I
  of thumb, short, 108H
  of toes, long, 108D
  of toes, short, 108C
  of wrist, long radial, 106I
  of wrist, short radial, 106H
  of wrist, ulnar, 106J
fibular

long, 134E
short, 134D
third, 134F
flexor
  accessory, 138I
  of big toe, long, 110H
  of big toe, short, 110G
  of fingers, deep, 110E
  of fingers, superficial, 110F
  of little finger, short, 110A
  of little toe, short, 110B
  of thumb, long, 110J
  of thumb, short, 110I
  of toes, long, 110D
  of toes, short, 110C
  of wrist, radial, 108J
  of wrist, ulnar, 108K
of floor of mouth, 126D
gastrocnemius, 112A
gemellus
  inferior, 112B
  superior, 112C
genioglossus, 112D
geniohyoid, 112E
gluteal
  greatest, 112F
  least, 112H
  middle, 112G
gracilis, 112I
great
  intermediate, 158D
  lateral, 158E
  medial, 158F
helicis
  larger, 114A
  major, 114A
  minor, 114B
  smaller, 114B
hyoglossus, 114C
iliacus, 114D
iliococcygeal, 114E
iliocostal, 114F
  of back, 114I
  of loins, 114H
  of neck, 114G
  of thorax, 114I
iliopsoas, 114J
incisure
  of helix, 114K
  of lower lip, 114L
  of upper lip, 116A
infrahyoid, 116B
infraspinous, 116C
intercostal
  external, 116D
  innermost, 116F
  internal, 116E
interosseous
  of foot, dorsal, 116H
  of hand, dorsal, 116G
  palmar, 116I
  plantar, 116J
interspinal, 118A
  of loins, 118C

of neck, 118B
of thorax, 118D
intertransverse, 118E
  lumbar, lateral, 118G
  lumbar, medial, 118H
  of neck, anterior, 118F
  of neck, posterior, 120A
  of thorax, 120B
ischiocavernous, 120C
latissimus dorsi, 120D
levator
  of anus, 120F
  of eyelid, upper, 122D
  of lip, upper, 122B
  of lip, upper and nose, ala, 122C
  of mouth, angle, 120E
  of palate, soft, 122H
  of prostate, 122E
  of ribs, 120G
  of ribs, long, 120I
  of ribs, short, 120H
  of scapula, 122F
  of soft palate, 122H
  of thyroid gland, 122A
  of vagina, 122G
long
  of head, 124E
  of neck, 124F
longissimus, 122I
  of back, 124B
  of head, 122J
  of neck, 124A
  of thorax, 124B
longitudinal
  of tongue, inferior, 124C
  of tongue, superior, 124D
lumbrical
  of foot, 124H
  of hand, 124G
masseter, 126A
mental, 126B
multifidus, 126C
mylohyoid, 126D
nasal, 126E
oblique
  of abdomen, external, 128C
  of abdomen, internal, 128E
  of auricle, 126F
  of eyeball, inferior, 128D
  of eyeball, superior, 128F
  of head, inferior, 128A
  of head, superior, 128B
obturator
  external, 128G
  internal, 128H
occipitofrontal, 128I
omohyoid, 130A
opposing
  of finger, little, 130B
  of thumb, 130C
orbicular
  of eye, 130D
  of mouth, 130E
orbital, 130F

palatoglossus, 132A
palatopharyngeal, 132B
palmar
  long, 132D
  short, 132C
papillary, 132E
  of left ventricle, anterior, 132G
  of left ventricle, posterior, 132I
  of right ventricle, anterior, 132F
  of right ventricle, posterior, 132H
  of right ventricle, septal, 132J
pectinate, 132K
pectineal, 134A
pectoral
  greater, 134B
  smaller, 134C
peroneal
  long, 134E
  short, 134D
  third, 134F
piriform, 134G
plantar, 134H
platysma, 134I
pleuroesophageal, 136A
popliteal, 136B
procerus, 136C
pronator
  quadrate, 136D
  round, 136E
psoas
  greater, 136F
  smaller, 136G
pterygoid
  external, 136H
  internal, 136I
  lateral, 136H
  medial, 136I
pubococcygeal, 136J
puboprostatic, 138A
puborectal, 138B
pubovaginal, 138C
pubovesical, 138D
pyramidal, 138E
  of auricle, 138F
quadrate
  of loins, 138H
  of lower lip, 104D
  of sole, 138I
  of thigh, 138G
quadriceps
  of thigh, 138J
rectococcygeal, 138K
rectourethral, 138L
rectouterine, 140A
rectovesical, 140B
rectus
  of abdomen, 140C
  of eyeball, inferior, 140I
  of eyeball, lateral, 140J
  of eyeball, medial, 142A
  of eyeball, superior, 142B
  of head, anterior, 140D
  of head, greater posterior, 140F
  of head, lateral, 140E

NERVES

VEINS

0825